Obstetric Hemorrhage
Evidence-based Management and Recent Advances

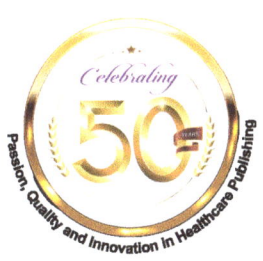

Obstetric Hemorrhage
Evidence-based Management and Recent Advances

Editors

Sheela V Mane MBBS MD FICOG FICMCH
Former Professor
Department of Obstetrics and Gynecology
DNB Faculty
KC General Hospital, Bengaluru
Organizing Secretary, AICOG, 2019
Past President, BSOG
Vice President, FOGSI, 2014
National PPH Workshop Convenor, FOGSI
Chairperson
Safe Motherhood Committee, FOGSI, 2008-11
Senior Consultant
Anugraha Nursing Home
Bengaluru, Karnataka, India

Shobha N Gudi MD DNB FICOG CIMP
Professor and Head
Department of Obstetrics and Gynecology
St Philomena's Hospital, Bengaluru
Consultant
Manipal Sagar and Excel Care Hospitals
Bengaluru, Karnataka, India
Chairperson, Family Welfare Committee, FPGSI
FOGSI, 2019-21
Past President, BSOG
Secretary, BMS, 2018-20
Board Member, FPAI
Distinguished NBE Teacher
Peer Reviewer, JOGI

Co-Editor

Priyanka Dilip Kumar MBBS DNB
Obstetrician and Gynecologist
Reproductive Medicine Specialist
Department of Obstetrics and Gynecology
Anugraha Nursing Home
Bengaluru, Karnataka, India

Forewords

CN Purandare   **Nandita Palshetkar**   **Sabaratnam Arulkumaran**

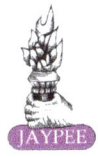

JAYPEE BROTHERS MEDICAL PUBLISHERS
The Health Sciences Publisher
New Delhi | London

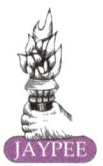
Jaypee Brothers Medical Publishers (P) Ltd

Headquarters
Jaypee Brothers Medical Publishers (P) Ltd
4838/24, Ansari Road, Daryaganj
New Delhi 110 002, India
Phone: +91-11-43574357
Fax: +91-11-43574314
E-mail: jaypee@jaypeebrothers.com

Overseas Office
JP Medical Ltd
83 Victoria Street, London
SW1H 0HW (UK)
Phone: +44 20 3170 8910
Fax: +44 (0)20 3008 6180
E-mail: info@jpmedpub.com

Website: www.jaypeebrothers.com
Website: www.jaypeedigital.com

© 2020, Jaypee Brothers Medical Publishers

The views and opinions expressed in this book are solely those of the original contributor(s)/author(s) and do not necessarily represent those of editor(s) of the book.

All rights reserved. No part of this publication may be reproduced, stored or transmitted in any form or by any means, electronic, mechanical, photocopying, recording or otherwise, without the prior permission in writing of the publishers.

All brand names and product names used in this book are trade names, service marks, trademarks or registered trademarks of their respective owners. The publisher is not associated with any product or vendor mentioned in this book.

Medical knowledge and practice change constantly. This book is designed to provide accurate, authoritative information about the subject matter in question. However, readers are advised to check the most current information available on procedures included and check information from the manufacturer of each product to be administered, to verify the recommended dose, formula, method and duration of administration, adverse effects and contraindications. It is the responsibility of the practitioner to take all appropriate safety precautions. Neither the publisher nor the author(s)/editor(s) assume any liability for any injury and/or damage to persons or property arising from or related to use of material in this book.

This book is sold on the understanding that the publisher is not engaged in providing professional medical services. If such advice or services are required, the services of a competent medical professional should be sought.

Every effort has been made where necessary to contact holders of copyright to obtain permission to reproduce copyright material. If any have been inadvertently overlooked, the publisher will be pleased to make the necessary arrangements at the first opportunity. The **CD/DVD-ROM** (if any) provided in the sealed envelope with this book is complimentary and free of cost. **Not meant for sale**.

Inquiries for bulk sales may be solicited at: jaypee@jaypeebrothers.com

Obstetric Hemorrhage: Evidence-based Management and Recent Advances

First Edition: **2020**
ISBN: 978-93-5270-898-7

Dedication

This work is dedicated to my beloved parents, late Dr VU Mane and Mrs Bharati Devi Mane, whose blessings have always guided me, my wonderful husband Dr V Dilip Kumar and my dear children Drs Priyanka and Anup, my son-in-law Dr Vijay Korvi and my little fairy grand-daughter Avani.

— Sheela V Mane

This work is dedicated to my beloved parents, late Prof S Ranganna and Mrs Ahalya Bai, their sacrifice and affection has made me what I am today, my dear husband Dr Narayan S Gudi who is a constant source of inspiration and my charming son Varun.

—Shobha N Gudi

We dedicate this manuscript to all those mothers who are true martyrs: they lost their precious lives in order to birth new lives.

Contributors

Alpesh Gandhi MBBS DGO FRCOG(Hon)
President, FOGSI, 2020
Secretary, Gestosis-India Chapter
Senior Consultant
Department of Obstetrics and Gynecology
High Risk and Critical Care in Obstetric Specialist
Arihant Women's Hospital
Ahmedabad, Gujarat, India

Amitha Indersen MD(Obs/Gyne)
Postdoctoral Fellowship in Fetal Medicine
Fellowship in Advanced Obstetric and Gynecologic Ultrasound
Fetal Medicine Consultant
Apollo Cradle Hospitals
Hyderabad, Telangana, India

Anahita Chauhan MD DGO DFP FICOG
Joint Secretary, FOGSI, 2019-20
Obstetrician and Gynecologist
Former Professor and Unit Head
Seth GS Medical College and
KEM Hospital, Mumbai
Honorary Consultant
Saifee and St Elizabeth Hospital
Mumbai, Maharashtra, India

Ashakiran T Rathod MBBS MS(Obs/Gyne) MRCOG
Assistant Professor
Department of Obstetrics and Gynecology
Bangalore Medical College and Research Institute
Bengaluru, Karnataka, India

Ashis Kumar Mukhopadhyay
MBBS(Cal) DGO (Cal) DNBOG (NBE) FICOG FICMCH
Vice-President, FOGSI, 2016-17
WHO Fellow, Maternal Health
Principal, Professor and Unit-Chief
Department of Obstetrics and Gynecology
CSS College of Obstetrics Gynecology and Child Health
Kolkata, West Bengal, India

Asmita Kaundal MS DNB
Scientist
Department of Obstetrics and Gynecology
All India Institute of Medical Sciences
New Delhi, India

Bhavana Girish MBBS MD DNB
Fellow of Minimally Invasive Gynecology
Radhakrishna Multispeciality Hospital and IVF Centre
Bengaluru, Karnataka, India

BS Susheela Rani
MD(Obs/Gyne) PGDMLE FICOG
Past President of BSOG
Co-ordinator, BSOG PG CME
Consultant Obstetrician and Gynecologist and Medical Director
Manjushree Speciality Hospital
Bengaluru, Karnataka, India

Garima Kachhawa MS FICOG FIMSA
Associate Professor
Department of Obstetrics and Gynecology
All India Institute of Medical Sciences
New Delhi, India

Girija Wagh
MD FICOG Dip Endoscopy FICS
Chairperson, Medical Disorders in Pregnancy Committee, FOGSI, 2012-16
Vice-President, Gestosis India Chapter
Professor
Department of Obstetrics and Gynecology
Bharati Vidyapeeth University Medical College, Pune
Consultant, Apollo Spectra Hospitals
Pune, Maharashtra, India

Gomathy Narayanan MD DGO FICS FICOG
Former Professor
Department of Obstetrics and Gynecology
Kempegowda Institute of Medical Sciences, Bengaluru
Senior Consultant
Cloud Nine Hospital
Bengaluru, Karnataka, India

Indusekhara S DMRD MD
Consultant Interventional Radiologist
HCG Hospital, Bengaluru
Visiting Consultant
Mahaveer Jain Hospital and Columbia Asia Hospital
Bengaluru, Karnataka, India

Isha Wadhawan MBBS MD(USA)
Diplomate to the American Board
Junior Consultant
Sant Parmanand Hospital
New Delhi, India

Jaideep Malhotra
MD FICMCH FICOG FICS FMAS FIAJAGO FRCOG FRCPI
Professor, Dubrovnik International University, Croatia
Past President, FOGSI
President Elect, SAFOMS, 2019-21
President Elect, ISPAT
Editor-in-Chief, SAFOMS & SAFOG Journal
Member FIGO–Reproductive Endocrinology and Infertility
ART Rainbow IVF
Agra, Uttar Pradesh, India

Jyothika A Desai MD DGO PGDMLE FICOG
Past President of BSOG
President, BMS
Senior Consultant
Department of Obstetrics and Gynecology
Dr PR Desai Hospital, Bengaluru
DNB Faculty
CSI Hospital
Bengaluru, Karnataka, India

Madhva Prasad MS DNB PGDMLS PGDCR
Assistant Professor
Vydehi Institute of Medical Sciences and Research Centre, Whitefield, Bengaluru
Seth GS Medical College and KEM Hospital
Mumbai, Maharashtra, India

Mala Arora FRCOG FICOG FICMCH DA(UK)
Past ICOG Chairperson
Senior Consultant
Department of Obstetrics and Gynecologist
Fortis La Femme and Noble IVF Centre
Faridabad, Haryana, India

Manisha Singhal MBBS MS FMAS
Senior Resident
American Institute of Medical Sciences Udaipur
Former Clinical Fellow in Reproductive Medicine and Gynaec Endoscopy at Nadkarni Test Tube Baby Center Killa Pardi
Gujarat, India

MB Bellad MD(Obs/Gyne) FICOG
Past President, KSOGA
Professor
Department of Obstetrics and Gynecology
KAHER's Jawaharlal Nehru Medical College, Belgaum
Chief Consultant
Department of Obstetrics and Gynecology
KLES'S Dr PK Hospital
Belgaum, Karnataka, India

Mousumi Das Ghosh MD FICOG
Consultant
Department of Obstetrics and Gynecology
Tata Steel Limited
Tata Main Hospital
Jamshedpur, Jharkhand, India

Muralidhar V Pai MBBS DGO MD FICOG MRCOG
Associate Professor and Head
Department of Obstetrics and Gynecology
Kasturba Medical College, Manipal
Manipal Academy of Higher Education
Manipal, Karnataka, India

Contributors

Narayanan R MBBS MD DGO
Past President of BSOG
Senior Gynecologist and Obstetrician
Former Professor and Head
Department of Obstetrics and Gynecology
St Johns Institute of Medical Sciences, Bengaluru
Consultant
Department of Obstetrics and Gynecology
Cloudnine Hospital
Bengaluru, Karnataka, India

Narendra Malhotra
MD FICOG FICMCH FRCOG FICS FMAS AFIAP
Past President, FOGSI
Professor, Dubrovnik International University, Croatia
Vice-President, World Association of Prenatal Medicine
President, ISPAT, 2017-19
Managing Director
Global Rainbow Healthcare
Agra, Uttar Pradesh, India

Neharika Malhotra Bora
MD(Obs/Gyne) FICMCH FMAS
Infertility Consultant
Rainbow IVF Hospital
Agra, Uttar Pradesh, India

Nozer Sheriar MD DNB FICOG FCPS DGO
Past Secretary General, FOGSI
Past Chairperson, MTP Committee, FOGSI
Past President, Mumbai Obstetric and Gynecological Society
Aviva Clinic for Women, Mumbai
Consultant
Department of Obstetrics and Gynecology
Breach Candy, Hinduja Healthcare Surgical and Holy Family Hospitals
Mumbai, Maharashtra, India

Nuzhat Aziz DGO DNB
Head
Department of Obstetrics and Gynecology
Fernandez Hospital
Hyderabad, Telangana, India

PK Sekharan
Past Vice-President, FOGSI
Past President, Kozhikode Society
Former Professor and Head
Department of Obstetrics and Gynecology
Medical College, Kozhikode
PVS Hospital
Kozhikode, Kerala, India

P Lekshmi Ammal MS (OBG)
Senior Consultant
Department of Obstetrics and Gynecology
SUT Hospital
Thiruvananthapuram, Kerala, India

Padmalatha Venkataram
MBBS FRCOG(UK) MRCPI(Dublin)
Past President of BSOG
Lead Consultant
Department of Obstetrics and Gynecology
Rangadore Memorial Hospital
Bengaluru, Karnataka, India

Pallavi Chandra MS
Consultant
Department of Obstetrics and Gynecology
Fernandez Hospital
Hyderabad, Telangana, India

Pratima Mittal MD FICOG FICMCH PGDHHM
Past Vice-President, FOGSI
Professor and Consultant
Department of Obstetrics and Gynecology
Vardhman Mahavir Medical College and Safdarjung Hospital
New Delhi, India

Prerna Keshan MBBS DGO FOGSI
Affiliated Training in Laparoscopy, Infertility and USG
Consultant and Infertility Specialist
Department of Obstetrics and Gynecology
Aditya Diagnostics and Hospitals
Tinsukia, Assam, India

Priyanka Dilip Kumar MBBS DNB
Obstetrician and Gynecologist
Reproductive Medicine Specialist
Department of Obstetrics and Gynecology
Anugraha Nursing Home
Bengaluru, Karnataka, India

Purnima Kishore Nadkarni
MBBS MD FCPS FICOG
Workshop Coordinator for West Zone, FOGSI
Infertility and IVF Specialist, Endoscopist
Director of Nadkarni Group of Hospitals – Killa Pardi, Vapi, Valsad and Surat
Gujarat, India

Rajneet Bhatia
Clinical Associate
Department of Obstetrics and Gynecology
Hinduja Healthcare Surgical Hospital, Mumbai
Aviva Clinic for Women
Mumbai, Maharashtra, India

Rishabh Bora MD(Radiodiagnosis)
Consultant Radiologist
Director
4D Life Care
Global Rainbow Healthcare
Agra, Uttar Pradesh, India

Sabaratnam Arulkumaran PhD DSc FRCS FRCOG
Past President, FIGO
Foundation Professor
Department of Obstetrics and Gynecology
University of Nicosia
Nicosia, Cyprus

Sadhana Gupta
MS (Obs & Gyn) MNAMS FICOG FICMU FICMCH
Vice President, FOGSI, 2016
FOGSI Representative to SAFOG, 2018-20
Chairperson, Safe Motherhood Committee, FOGSI, 2011-13
Senior Consultant Obstetrician and Gynecologist
Jeevan Jyoti Hospital and Medical Research Center
Jeevan Jyoti Test Tube Baby Center
Gorakhpur, Uttar Pradesh, India

Sanjay Gupte MD DGO FICOG LLB FRCOG
Past President, FOGSI
Secretary General, World Gestosis Organization
FOGSI Representative to FIGO
Director
Gupte Hospital and Center for Research in Reproduction
Pune, Maharashtra, India

Saswati Sanyal Choudhury
MD FICOG FICMCH FIAOG
Chairperson, Medical Education Committee, FOGSI
Associate Professor
Department of Obstetrics and Gynecology
Fakhruddin Ali Ahmed Medical College
Barpeta, Assam, India

Savvas Argyridis
Associate Professor
Department of Obstetrics and Gynecology
University of Nicosia, Nicosia
Consultant Obstetrician and Gynecologist
Archbishop Makarios Hospital
Nicosia, Cyprus

Sheeba Marwah
MBBS DNB(Obs/Gyne) CIMP CCOB(ICOG) Fellowship
Assistant Professor
Department of Obstetrics and Gynecology
Vardhman Mahavir Medical College
and Safdarjung Hospital
New Delhi, India

Sheela V Mane MBBS MD FICOG FICMCH
Past President, BSOG
Vice-President, FOGSI, 2014
Chairperson, Safe Motherhood Committee, FOGSI, 2008-11
Former Professor
Department of Obstetrics and Gynecology
DNB Faculty
KC General Hospital, Bengaluru
Senior Consultant
Anugraha Nursing Home
Bengaluru, Karnataka, India

Shivaram Chandrashekar MBBS DCP MHA
Editor-in-Chief
Global Journal of Transfusion Medicine
Consultant
Transfusion Medicine
Manipal Hospitals
Bengaluru, Karnataka, India

Shobha N Gudi MD DNB FICOG CIMP
Past President, BSOG
Chairperson, Family Welfare Committee, FPGSI
Professor and Head
Department of Obstetrics and Gynecology
St Philomena's Hospital, Bengaluru
Consultant
Manipal Sagar and Excel Care Hospitals
Bengaluru, Karnataka, India

Sitalakshmi Subramanian
MBBS DCP DNB (Pathology) PhD (Pathology)
Professor and Head
Department of Transfusion Medicine
and Immunohematology
St John's Medical College
Bengaluru, Karnataka, India

Srimathy Raman MD (OBG) FRCOG CCT (UK)
Consultant
Department of Obstetrics and Gynecology
Rangadore Memorial Hospital
Bengaluru, Karnataka, India

Srinivas Krishna Jois
MS (OBG/Gyne) DGO DNB MNAMS PGDMLE (NLS) FICOG MRCOG (UK) MA
Associate Professor and Unit Chief
Department of Obstetrics and Gynecology
Bangalore Medical College and Research Institute
Bengaluru, Karnataka, India

Suchitra N Pandit
MD DNB FRCOG (UK) FICOG DFP MNAMS FICMCH B Pharm
President, FOGSI, 2014
Consultant and Director
Department of Obstetrics and Gynecology
Surya Group of Hospitals
Mumbai, Maharashtra, India

Swati Bhargava MS (Obs & Gyne)
Assistant Professor
Department of Obstetrics and Gynecology
MGM Medical College
Indore, Madhya Pradesh, India

V Rajasekharan Nair MD DGO
Former Professor
Department of Obstetrics and Gynecology
Senior Consultant
Sree Uthradom Thirunal Hospital
Thiruvananthapuram, Kerala, India

Vidya A Thobbi MBBS MD FICOG
Professor and Head
Department of Obstetrics and Gynecology
Al-Ameen Medical College
Vijayapura, Karnataka, India

Vidya Bhargavi
Junior Consultant Interventional Radiologist
Department of Interventional Radiology
HCG Hospital
Bengaluru, Karnataka, India

Vidya V Bhat
MBBS MD DNB MNAMS FICOG
President, BSOG, 2012-13
Joint Secretary, FOGSI, 2013
Director
Gynecologic-Endoscopic Surgeon and IVF Specialist
Radhakrishna Multispeciality Hospital and IVF Centre
Bengaluru, Karnataka, India

VP Paily MD FRCOG
Past President, KFOG
Senior Consultant
Department of Obstetrics and Gynecology
Rajagiri Hospital
Kochi, Kerala, India

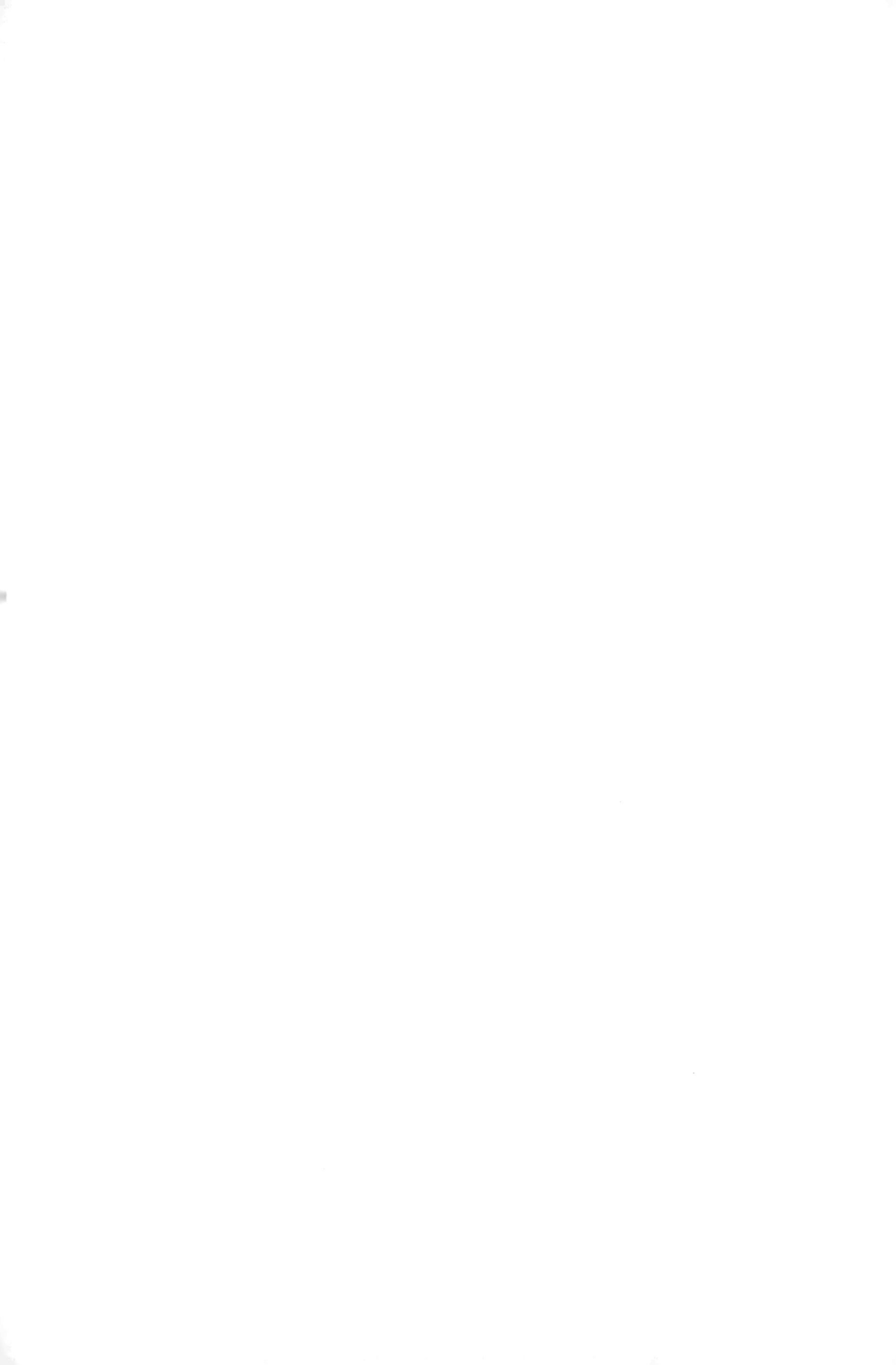

Foreword

Obstetric hemorrhage is a very debated and discussed subject. No matter how much we are prepared, it falls short of optimal care to reduce the attendant maternal mortality and morbidity. Such as the complex nature of obstetric hemorrhage and the varied way in which it can complicate a case.

This book encompasses all aspects of obstetric hemorrhage. The topics are exhaustive and have been written by the experts in the field. The book also covers topics of blood transfusion and interventional radiology. All the chapters have been written keeping in mind the current concepts and recent developments.

I would like to congratulate the editors Dr Sheela V Mane and Dr Shobha N Gudi on building up this novel idea and putting it into perspective. This book will be a very useful guide for students and clinicians.

CN Purandare
MD MAO(IRL) DO RCPI(DUB) DGO DFP
FRCOG(UK) FRCPI(IRL) FACOG(USA) FICOG FICMCH FAMS PGD MLS(LAW)
President, FIGO 2015-18
President, FOGSI 2009-10
Senior Consultant Obstetrician and Gynecologist
Dean of the Indian College of Obstetricians and Gynecologists
Emeritus Editor for the Journal of Obstetrics and Gynecology of India

Foreword

It gives me great pleasure to write the foreword for the book on *Obstetric Hemorrhage: Evidence-based Management and Recent Advances*.

I think the editors Dr Sheela V Mane and Dr Shobha N Gudi have done a wonderful job in conceptualizing the contents and selecting the authors. We at Federation of Obstetric and Gynaecological Societies of India (FOGSI) are working toward women empowerment. In fact the theme of my presidential year 'We for Stree' is well supported and enriched by this endeavor.

The responsibility lies on each and every obstetrician to act fast in cases of obstetric hemorrhage and prevent mortality and further morbidity. There are excellent directives in the book for capacity building and skill enhancement. We hope that the book will reach all the members of our fraternity and that their patients will greatly benefit from it.

Nandita Palshetkar
MBBS MD FCPS FICOG FRCOG (HON)
President, FOGSI 2019
Director, IVF and Infertility at Fortis Bloom IVF Center
Professor, Department of Obstetrics and Gynecology
DY Patil Medical College, Navi Mumbai, Maharashtra, India
Teacher, FNB Course at Lilavathi Hospital

Foreword

Obstetric hemorrhage contributes to 30% of child birth related to 300,000 global maternal mortalities. Morality is the tip of the iceberg whilst morbidity is much greater. From recent studies, it is clear that the incidence and severity of obstetric hemorrhage is on the increase. Understanding the various etiologies, basic pathophysiology, increasing evidence-based practice and recent advances in management of obstetric hemorrhage provide us the possibility to devise the best prevention and management strategies.

The editors Dr Sheela V Mane and Dr Shobha N Gudi are well-known for their passionate commitment to reduce maternal mortality due to postpartum hemorrhage (PPH). For decades, they have been advocates, teachers and trainers to reduce and if possible eliminate maternal deaths due to PPH. Now they deserve our congratulations for bringing out the excellent book '*Obstetric Hemorrhage: Evidence-based Management and Recent Advances*' which covers bleeding from early pregnancy like that related to termination of pregnancies and ectopic pregnancy to antepartum hemorrhage due to abruption and placenta previa to PPH due to various causes.

The book is well laid out into five sections. The chapters in the different sections cover the technical, nontechnical and organizational skills and requirements needed to 'eliminate' morbidity and mortality related to obstetric hemorrhage. The authors are well-renowned for expertise in the area in which they have contributed the chapter. I would encourage practicing clinicians and researches to read the book and recommend libraries and delivery units to have a copy of the book for quick reference.

Yours sincerely,

Sabaratnam Arulkumaran PhD DSc FRCS FRCOG
Past President, RCOG 2007-10
Past President, BMA 2013-14
Past President, FIGO 2012-15

Preface

Mothers continue to die due to preventable causes because societies are yet to realize that their lives are worth saving. Today we are in the era of preventive obstetrics, where there is no role of maternal mortality or major morbidity due to preventable causes like obstetric hemorrhage. Worldwide, hemorrhage remains a major cause of maternal death—it is estimated that between one-quarter and a half of preventable maternal deaths are secondary to hemorrhage especially in the developing world. Treatment is delayed by failure to recognize major obstetric hemorrhage. The physiological changes of normal pregnancy mask the clinical presentation of hypovolemia and delays the presentation. The thought for initiating contributions to compile this book has been the overwhelming concern among health providers that all obstetricians do not have adequate skills for control of hemorrhage, transfer of critically ill mothers are suboptimal and infrastructural deficiencies have a profound impact on the outcome for the mother and the fetus.

We conceptualized this book 18 months back and now finally at the threshold of All India Congress of Obstetrics and Gynaecology (AICOG) 2019, we find ourselves ready to showcase the sincere efforts of the contributors who have not only tirelessly worked to submit the manuscripts in time but also shared their invaluable experience. We thank them sincerely for accepting their assignments and writing such wonderful chapters.

We thank our families, peers and friends for being there for us throughout the editorial and working process for this book lending us their unconditional moral support.

We are convinced this book will help consultants, postgraduates and obstetric intensivists in updating their knowledge and skills.

Sheela V Mane
Shobha N Gudi

Acknowledgments

We are deeply indebted to all our contributors for dedicating their time and sharing their experience for this book. We thank the hospital authorities who provided us the clinical material and infrastructure and the patients who provided us the information needed to write these texts.

We would like to thank Shri Jitendar P Vij (Group Chairman), Mr Ankit Vij (Managing Director), Mr MS Mani (Group President), Ms Chetna Malhotra Vohra (Associate Director—Content Strategy), Ms Pooja Bhandari (Production Head) and Nikita Chauhan (Senior Development Editor) of Jaypee Brothers Medical Publishers, New Delhi, India, for facilitating the editorial process.

Contents

SECTION 1: DEMOGRAPHY, CLINICAL GOVERNANCE AND AUDIT

1. **Postpartum Hemorrhage in Third World: A Review of Clinical Management Strategies** — 3
   Sadhana Gupta, Mousumi Das Ghosh

2. **Postpartum Hemorrhage: Setting Criteria for Clinical Audit** — 12
   V Rajasekharan Nair, P Lekshmi Ammal

3. **Safety in the Labor Ward** — 21
   Nuzhat Aziz, Pallavi Chandra

4. **Clinical Governance: Standard Operating Procedure for Obstetric Hemorrhage** — 31
   Muralidhar V Pai

5. **The Obstetric High-dependency Unit: Need of the Hour** — 35
   Sanjay Gupte, Girija Wagh

6. **Obstetric Hemorrhage: Prevention and Management (Golden Hour)** — 42
   MB Bellad

7. **Assessment of Blood Loss** — 60
   BS Susheela Rani

8. **Massive Obstetric Hemorrhage and Role of Blood Transfusion in Management** — 65
   Alpesh Gandhi

SECTION 2: HEMORRHAGE IN EARLY PREGNANCY

9. **Physiological and Anatomical Changes in Pregnancy Relevant to Hemorrhagic Shock** — 75
   Shobha N Gudi, Priyanka Dilip Kumar

10A. **Preventing Hemorrhage in Ectopic Pregnancy** — 87
   Vidya V Bhat, Bhavana Girish

10B. **The Dreaded Miscarriages: Incomplete and Septic Abortions** — 97
   Vidya A Thobbi

10C. **Abnormal Placentation in Early Pregnancy** — 107
   Mala Arora, Isha Wadhawan

10D. **Bleeding in Gestational Trophoblastic Disease** — 119
   PK Sekharan

10E.	Ectopic Pregnancy in the Cervix *Purnima Kishore Nadkarni, Manisha Singhal*	123
10F.	Postabortion Hemorrhage *Nozer Sheriar, Rajneet Bhatia*	131

SECTION 3: ANTEPARTUM HEMORRHAGE

11A.	Imaging in Antepartum Hemorrhage *Narendra Malhotra, Amitha Indersen, Prerna Keshan,* *Neharika Malhotra Bora, Rishabh Bora, Jaideep Malhotra*	143
11B.	Surgical Challenges in Placenta Previa *Suchitra N Pandit, Swati Bhargava*	154
11C.	Abruptio Placentae *Saswati Sanyal Choudhury*	162
11D.	Rupture Uterus: The Catastrophe Compendiously Summarized *Pratima Mittal, Sheeba Marwah*	171
11E.	Expectant Management of Placenta Previa *Gomathy Narayanan, Narayanan R*	180
11F.	Morbidly Adherent Placenta (Placenta Accreta Spectrum): Prearm and Perform *VP Paily*	184

SECTION 4: POSTPARTUM HEMORRHAGE

12A.	Golden Hour Concept and First Response *Sheela V Mane, Garima Kachhawa, Asmita Kaundal*	193
12B.	Atonic Postpartum Hemorrhage *Srinivas Krishna Jois*	203
12C.	Traumatic Postpartum Hemorrhage *Padmalatha Venkataram, Srimathy Raman*	218
12D.	Secondary Postpartum Hemorrhage *Jyothika A Desai, Ashakiran T Rathod*	225
12E.	Vascular Interventions in Postpartum Hemorrhage *Indusekhara S, Vidya Bhargavi*	230
12F.	Newer Approaches in Management of Postpartum Hemorrhage *Savvas Argyridis, Sabaratnam Arulkumaran*	239

SECTION 5: CRITICAL SITUATIONS

13A. Disorders of Hemostasis in Pregnancy 249
Sitalakshmi Subramanian

13B. Peripartum Hysterectomy 259
Ashis Kumar Mukhopadhyay

13C. Disseminated Intravascular Coagulation in Obstetric Hemorrhage 265
Anahita Chauhan, Madhva Prasad

13D. Massive Transfusion Protocol: Role of Component Therapy 276
Shivaram Chandrashekar

Index *287*

Section 1: Demography, Clinical Governance and Audit

- **Postpartum Hemorrhage in Third World: A Review of Clinical Management Strategies**
  Sadhana Gupta, Mousumi Das Ghosh
- **Postpartum Hemorrhage: Setting Criteria for Clinical Audit**
  V Rajasekharan Nair, P Lekshmi Ammal
- **Safety in the Labor Ward**
  Nuzhat Aziz, Pallavi Chandra
- **Clinical Governance: Standard Operating Procedure for Obstetric Hemorrhage**
  Muralidhar V Pai
- **The Obstetric High-dependency Unit: Need of the Hour**
  Sanjay Gupte, Girija Wagh
- **Obstetric Hemorrhage: Prevention and Management (Golden Hour)**
  MB Bellad
- **Assessment of Blood Loss**
  BS Susheela Rani
- **Massive Obstetric Hemorrhage and Role of Blood Transfusion in Management**
  Alpesh Gandhi

Chapter 1

Postpartum Hemorrhage in Third World: A Review of Clinical Management Strategies

Sadhana Gupta, Mousumi Das Ghosh

■ INTRODUCTION

Any pregnant woman who will deliver is at risk of postpartum hemorrhage (PPH).[1] Worldwide, PPH is the major cause of maternal mortality, contributing to 25% of 300,000 maternal deaths each year.[2] The disease burden makes it a global priority. However, women in third world countries have higher morbidity and mortality compared to those in developed world.[3,4] The main reason being "too little, too late", which means patients do not get the right treatment (oxytocics, fluids, and blood) at the appropriate time. The suffering is due to poverty, gender inequality, and limited access to health care. These causes delay in decision to seek treatment, delay in reaching the healthcare facility due to lack of transport, road conditions and delay at the hospital due to poor health infrastructure, incorrect treatment, and excess workload.[5] The fifth Millennium Development Goal (MDG-5) by the United Nations failed to achieve reduction of maternal deaths. The maternal mortality ratio (MMR) of India has fallen from 750 in the 60s to 400 in the 90s and 130 in 2014–2016. About 20% of maternal deaths happen in India in spite of having only 16% of world population.[5] Most of these deaths occur within first 4 hours of delivery reflecting the importance of third stage of labor.[1] To achieve the sustainable development goal by 2030, increased access to quality maternal care before, during, and after childbirth should be targeted.[6]

■ POSTPARTUM HEMORRHAGE

It is defined as blood loss more than 500 mL in vaginal birth and 1 L in cesarean section. Clinically, any blood loss that can produce hemodynamic instability should be considered as PPH.[7] Primary PPH occurs within first 24 hours of birth and uterine atony is the most common cause. Secondary PPH occurs between 24 hours of birth and 6 weeks postpartum. The causes are retained products of conception, infection, or both.[7] The incidence of PPH is less after vaginal birth (2–4%) compared to cesarean section (6%).[5]

■ ETIOLOGY[7]

The causes of PPH are classified as per mnemonic, the four Ts.
1. *Tone*: This can be uterine atony/distended bladder
2. *Trauma*: Uterine, cervical, or vaginal injury
3. *Tissue*: Retained placenta or clots and abnormal placentation
4. *Thrombin*: Pre-existing/acquired coagulopathy.

Tone and trauma contributes to 70% and 20%, respectively.

DIAGNOSIS

Postpartum hemorrhage can happen without warning. Hence, prompt diagnosis by monitoring blood loss after delivery and vitals is the key for successful management. Quantitative methods to assess blood loss are more accurate and preferable compared to visual estimation. This can be done by weighing pads and sponges before and after blood soakage. Use of underbuttock graduated drapes also helps in quantitative assessment.[3]

Absorbent delivery mats, which can hold 500 mL of blood is being used in many countries.[4] The ordinary plastic bag (24 inches × 16 inches) used by shopkeepers can be developed into PPH bag (designed by WHO) which is cheap, easily available, and can be disposed after use.[8] Clinical markers (signs and symptoms) depend on amount of blood loss and her pre-existing condition. Symptoms of hypovolemia like giddiness, weakness, palpitations, sweating, restlessness, confusion, and signs like hypotension, tachycardia, oliguria, and falling oxygen saturation should be monitored. Tachycardia is an early sign and shock is a late sign.[9] Often mother experiences hypotension only after significant blood loss of more than 1,500 mL. Obstetric shock index (OSI) can be used to identify significant blood loss. This is defined as heart rate divided by systolic blood pressure and ranges between 0.7 and 0.9. Values more than 1 is an indicator for estimating blood loss and need for blood transfusion.

MANAGEMENT

A number of national and international organizations have developed and updated guidelines for the prevention and management of PPH. All healthcare facilities should have protocols based on these with local modifications as necessary.[4]

Stay Prepared

The strategy is to stay prepared to handle hemorrhagic emergencies. Protocols and algorithms should be available, displayed in labor room and audited from time to time to ensure that the practices are evidence based. The preparedness to face emergencies should be tested periodically through simulation-based team training (PPH drills). Drills identify the weaknesses and strengths and hence improve teamwork and coordination among staff.[4] Randomized controlled trials of teamwork training report increase in knowledge, practical skills, communication, and team performance.

Maintenance of obstetric hemorrhage carts or boxes is another strategy to ensure preparedness as all the drugs and surgical instruments are in one place which saves time (Table 1).[4]

Management of Postpartum Hemorrhage

Management includes a range of medical, mechanical, temporizing, and surgical procedures.[4] The critical steps are communicate (for help), resuscitate (assess blood loss and replace with fluids and blood), investigate (cause of bleeding), initiate uterotonics, and ligate the great arteries.[10]

Medical Management (Uterotonics) (Table 2)

For management of PPH, oxytocin is the first choice. It acts on the smooth muscle of the upper segment of uterus and contracts it rhythmically, constricts blood vessels, and decreases blood flow through the uterus.[7] Intravenous (IV) infusion facilitates steady flow and a sustained effect. The effect can be stopped within 1 hour of discontinuing IV infusion.

Ergometrine is the second line of treatment. It acts on the smooth muscle of

TABLE 1: Postpartum hemorrhage box.

Emergency obstetric kit developed by the Safe Motherhood Committee of FOGSI, 2010.

IV cannula	Gray #1
	Green #1
Blood sample bottles	Pink #1
	Blue #1
	Red #1
Syringes	10 mL #4
	5 mL #2
	2 mL #4
Plaster to fix the cannula	1
Catheter	1
Urobag	1
Distilled water 10 mL	1
Infusion set	1
Blood set	1
Sterile gloves	1 pair
Cotton swabs	
Pair of scissors	1
Ringer lactate	1
3 way connection	1
Oxygen face mask	1
PPH drug kit	
Oxytocin	5 amps
Methylergometrine (methergine)	2 amps
15-methyl-PGF2α (prostodin)	2 amps
Misoprostol 600 μg	1 tab
Instruments and supplies	
Large speculums	3
Sponge holding forceps	4
Condom tamponade	
Uterine pack	6 cm wide and 3 meter (2 in No.)

(FOGSI: Federation of Obstetric and Gynaecological Societies of India; IV: intravenous; PGF2α: prostaglandin F2α; PPH: postpartum hemorrhage)

both upper and lower segment of uterus and contracts tetanically.[11] There is increased frequency of retained placenta requiring manual removal. Also maternal adverse effects are higher.

Prostaglandin is the third line of treatment. Misoprostol may also be considered as third-line drug because of low cost, easy storage, and ease of administration compared to prostaglandin.[11] There is a quick response with oral and sublingual administration but tapers fast. Vaginal or rectal administration have slower onset but prolonged effect.[1] Ministry of Health and Family Welfare (MoHFW), India recommends Misoprostol as second-line treatment after oxytocin.[12]

A key factor in third world countries is the continued preference for home deliveries, which are often attended by family members or unskilled birth attendants. Therefore, integrated interventions that inform women and the surrounding community on birth preparedness and possible risks, and train providers in high-quality antenatal services ensuring timely detection and management or referral of high-risk obstetrical cases are essential for getting women the care they need in emergency situations.[12] The MoHFW, Government of India has taken a policy decision to identify mothers who may have home delivery and distribute Misoprostol tablets in advance by Accredited Social Health Activists (ASHAs).[12,15] The woman has to take one tablet of Misoprostol (600 mg) orally just after delivery of the baby and before the placenta comes out.[15] ASHA/Auxiliary nurse midwife (ANM) sensitizes the key decision makers of the pregnant household for timely referral through preidentified transport for helping women access the services available as and when required. This takes care of the first two delays that cause maternal death.

TABLE 2: Drugs used in atonic postpartum hemorrhage.[11,13,14]

Drug	Dosage	Contraindications	Adverse effects
Oxytocin	10 IU IM or 5 IU slow IV push or 20–40 IU/L IV fluid infusion	Rare, hypersensitivity to medication. Do not give as IV bolus	Overdose can cause water intoxication
Ergometrine/methylergometrine	0.2 mg IM can repeat every 2–4 hours maximum of 5 doses (1 mg) in 24 hours	Hypertension, pre-eclampsia, cardiovascular disease, hepatic or renal disease, patients with HIV on protease inhibitors	Nausea, vomiting
15-methyl prostaglandin F2α Carboprost	0.25 mg IM, repeated every 15 minutes, maximum 2 mg	Asthma	Fever, headache, chills, nausea, vomiting, diarrhea, bronchospasm
Misoprostol Prostaglandin E1	600–1,000 mg One time	Rare, hypersensitivity to medication	Pyrexia, shivering

(HIV: human immunodeficiency virus; IM: intramuscular; IV: intravenous)

Storage of uterotonics: Both oxytocin and methylergometrine are stored at 2-8°C. Oxytocin is preferably refrigerated, but it may be stored at room temperature up to 3 months. Misoprostol is packed in aluminum blister and stored at room temperature in a closed container.[7]

Fluids and blood transfusion: Resuscitation during PPH includes restoring both blood volume and oxygen carrying capacity. Two wide bore intravenous lines should be established and blood sample drawn for diagnostic tests (full blood count, coagulation screen, urea, and electrolytes) and crossmatching minimum of 4 units blood. General practice is to start with IV fluids followed by packed cells and coagulation factors. Warmed fluids reduce the risk of coagulopathy.[9] Preferably isotonic crystalloids are used in place of colloids.[10,12] Fluid replacement corrects hypovolemia but aggravates dilutional coagulopathy. This leads to academia and hypothermia. Crossmatched blood is the best fluid to replace and early transfusion leads to better outcome. A high concentration of oxygen should be administered.

Monitoring pulse rate, blood pressure, oxygen saturation, and urine output is the cornerstone of management. Record chart of fluid balance, blood, blood products, and procedures helps in management. Delivery of any drug to the uterus, especially intramuscular (IM) will be compromised by poor circulation, therefore fluid resuscitation should be effective.[9] Ratio of fresh frozen plasma (FFP) and red blood cells (RBCs) at 1:1 or 1:2 improves survival.[4] Fibrinogen levels should be maintained between 100 mg/dL and 200 mg/dL and the fall seen in severe PPH is corrected with cryoprecipitate transfusion.[4]

Massive postpartum hemorrhage: This is defined as the loss of more than 2,500 mL of blood and is associated with massive blood transfusion, need for obstetric hysterectomy, and critical care. This leads to increased morbidity and mortality. Main therapeutic goal is to maintain hemoglobin > 8 g/dL, platelet count > 75,000/mL, prothrombin < 1.5 × mean control, activated prothrombin time < 1.5 × mean control, and fibrinogen > 1.0 g/L.[14]

Role of Tranexamic acid: The World Maternal Antifibrinolytic trial (WOMAN trial) was a randomized, double-blind, and placebo-controlled study with a clinical diagnosis of PPH, recruiting over 20,000 women (regardless of mode of birth). The trial authors concluded that early use (within 3 hours) of IV Tranexamic acid reduces maternal death due to PPH, and that early treatment has more favorable outcome.[16,17]

Mechanical and Temporizing Methods

If uterotonics fail to arrest bleeding, mechanical methods need to be considered.[7] Although atonicity is the major cause of PPH, other causes (three of four Ts) must be ruled out. They include:
- Bimanual compression of the uterus (external or internal)
- Aortic compression
- Hydrostatic intrauterine balloon tamponade
- Uterine packing
- Use of an antishock garment for the treatment of shock or transfer to another level of care, or while waiting for laparotomy
- Compression sutures.

Uterine massage: Uterine massage is recommended by the WHO and International Federation of Gynecology and Obstetrics (FIGO) for treatment of PPH based on "low cost and safety".[18]

Bimanual compression: In bimanual compression, one hand is inserted deep into the vagina and rotated either clockwise or counterclockwise against the cervix and uterus that is being firmly grasped by the abdominal hand. The advantage of this technique is that it can be applied by midwives also and training requirements are minimal.[19]

Aortic compression: Aortic compression is a simple technique which does not prevent or delay any other steps. Blood pressure is kept higher, blood is prevented from reaching the bleeding area in the pelvis, and volume is conserved.[7]

Uterine packing: Gauze soaked with 5,000 units of thrombin in 5 mL of saline inserted from one cornu to the other with ring forceps serves as tamponade to control bleeding.[13] Careful count is documented and checked during removal and antibiotic coverage is useful. This is not recommended by WHO due to the potential risks.

Balloon tamponade: The various types of balloons used are Foley's catheter, Rusch balloon, Bakri balloon, Sengstaken-Blackmore esophageal catheter, and sterile glove and condom. If bleeding is controlled after tamponade, it is a positive test and a negative test indicates that bleeding is persisting despite tamponade and may be coming from a genital tract trauma. Cases with negative balloon tamponade test need immediate surgical interventions.[14]

One can use Foley's balloon catheters filled to 75 cc or 100 cc in each instance. Despite being designed for a 30 mL capacity, larger volumes up to 150 mL can be reached before the catheter bursts.[19] In the absence of urinary catheters, a condom can be inserted into the uterus on a straight catheter, inflated with 200–500 mL of normal saline according to need and tied off with silk so as to facilitate retention into the uterus. A balloon tamponade alone is successful in 77.5–88.8% or more cases, thus avoiding further surgical treatment.[7]

Nonpneumatic antishock garment: The nonpneumatic antishock garment (NASG) is a first-aid compression garment device used in obstetric hemorrhage and shock. It looks like the bottom half of a wetsuit, cut into segments. This helps in transportation of a patient to a hospital or overcoming delay in obtaining blood and definitive treatment. The unique garment permits perineal access so that operative procedures can be accomplished.[19] It acts by decreasing blood flow to the pelvis and maintaining circulation of the core organs—heart, lungs, and brain.

WHO and FIGO recommend use of NASG.[4] It is easy to use and a short training is enough for nonmedical personnel.

Referral transportation—quick initial assessment and referral: A functional referral system with teamwork between referral levels will be effective to achieve goals in third world countries. Initial assessment should be done, assessment of CAB (circulation, airway, and breathing), IV fluids started along with oxytocin infusion, bladder catheterized and uterine massage/bimanual uterine compression/aortic compression and balloon tamponade considered before transferring with ongoing uterotonic infusion.

During transporting a woman who is bleeding, a skilled health worker should accompany her.[12] The woman should be kept warm with legs elevated to improve blood circulation to vital organs if NASG is not available. Uterine massage should be continued with bimanual uterine compression.

There should be unified record system and a protocol-based referral.[12]

Surgical Methods

A fifth T is added along with four Ts of etiology to emphasize the importance of theater and surgery in managing all patients of PPH.[20]

It is advisable to start with uterotonics, and then gradually step up to invasive procedures. Compression sutures and vascular ligation may be tried. Senior obstetrician should be involved, when available. In cases of massive PPH, early decision for hysterectomy should be taken.[7]

Vascular ligation: The aim of vascular ligation in atonic uterus is to decrease the pulse pressure and thereby reduce blood supply to the uterus.[13] The median success of vascular ligation is 92%.

- Bilateral uterine artery ligation (O'Leary sutures)—first-line approach
- Utero ovarian ligament ligation—second-line approach
- Internal iliac artery ligation requires a retroperitoneal approach.

Knowledge of pelvic anatomy and course of great vessels and ureter is needed. This dampens the pulse pressure and transforms the pelvic arterial system into a venous like system losing the trip hammer effect of arterial pulsations facilitating hemostasis.[10]

Widely used uterine compression suture is B-Lynch. This is placing a "belt and suspenders" on the body of the uterus, whereby the fundus is compressed and held in a compact position.[19] The intervention is ideal after a cesarean section when a hysterotomy wound exists on the anterior uterine surface. Other techniques like Cho multiple square suture and Hayman have been described. All these techniques have equal efficacy, approximately 60–75%.[13]

Nausicaa compression suture has been recently published to be useful in placenta accreta spectrum (PAS) and other causes of severe PPH.[21] This preserves fertility and avoids extensive surgery in cases of PAS without parametrial invasion.

Hysterectomy: Emergency postpartum hysterectomy is the definitive treatment when conservative therapies have failed. It causes permanent loss of reproductive function and postpartum depression. However, when needed, early decision saves lives.

Radiological Methods

This technique is used before surgical intervention in a hemodynamically stable patient with active bleeding.[1] Percutaneous transcatheter arterial embolization is performed by interventional radiologists and needs special set up, which is available in limited centers. The advantage is that it is fertility preserving. After fluoroscopic identification of bleeding vessels, they are sealed with absorbable gelatin sponges, coils or microparticles.[13]

Hematoma at catheterization site, technical difficulty in accessing the uterine arteries, infection, uterine ischemia requiring hysterectomy, and radiation hazards are the problems encountered.[8]

TRAUMATIC POSTPARTUM HEMORRHAGE

Injury to the genital tract is suspected when bleeding persists in spite of a well-contracted uterus. This may be spontaneous or iatrogenic (manipulations used to deliver the baby). Patient has to be shifted to operation theater and trained assistants are needed for adequate exposure and identification of the bleeding points. Good lighting, effective pain relief, and proper positioning is essential.[8]

There can be vulvar and paravaginal hematomas in lower genital tract and broad ligament and retroperitoneal hematomas adjacent to the uterus.[8] Lower genital tract hematomas will need evacuation with layer closure followed by vaginal packing. Upper genital tract injury will need laparotomy and surgical therapy.

SECONDARY POSTPARTUM HEMORRHAGE

This occurs in 1% of pregnancies. Most common cause is retained products of conception with or without infection.[13] Diagnosis can be confirmed by ultrasound. Uterine tenderness and low grade fever may be present.

Treatment should be focused on etiology and includes uterotonics and broad antibiotic coverage. Uterine curettage may be needed after diagnosis of retained products. Often small amount of tissue may be removed, but effective enough to control bleeding promptly. These patients may require hysterectomy if uncontrolled bleeding, hence should be counseled before initiating any operative procedure.[13]

TO DECIDE WHEN TO START TREATMENT

Early and proactive treatment has the best outcome and prevents coagulopathy.[2] In Benedetti classification, alert line is when there is blood loss of 500–1,000 mL and no clinical signs of cardiovascular instability. Observation and staying prepared for resuscitation is advised. However, action line which calls for full protocol to resuscitate, monitor, and arrest bleeding is with blood loss more than 1,000 mL or clinical signs of shock.[22]

AFTER CARE

Continued care of woman over next 24–48 hours is essential. The aim is to maintain systolic blood pressure of at least 100 mm Hg and a stabilizing heart rate (90 beats/min).[7]

Secondary sequelae from hemorrhage include adult respiratory distress syndrome, shock, disseminated intravascular coagulation, and acute renal failure.[13] These women are at risk of anemia. Hence, iron supplements should be given for at least 3 months.[7] It can also lead to lactation failure. Late sequelae are infertility and pituitary infarction (Sheehan's syndrome).

Interestingly, there are increased chances of recurrence of PPH in future pregnancies.[18] The incidence and volume of blood loss are also proportionate to number of episodes in previous pregnancies.

THE INDIAN SCENARIO

India is emerging as the leading economy in the world and global power, yet we are losing mothers to a cause, PPH which is not only preventable but also treatable even in low resource settings.[8] Efforts have been made by Government of India to reduce maternal deaths like training of doctors and paramedical staff [Emergency Obstetric Care (EmOC), Basic EmOC (BEmOC), and skilled birth attendant (SBA)] and promotion of institutional deliveries under various schemes (Janani Suraksha Yojana and Janani Shishu Suraksha Karyakram). WHO and FIGO supports community-based Misoprostol distribution by health worker.[4] MoHFW, Government of India has introduced home distribution of Misoprostol to pregnant women who may have home deliveries by ANMs and ASHAs.[15]

Federation of Obstetric and Gynaecological Societies of India (FOGSI) in collaboration with MSD for Mothers and Jhpiego implemented a 3-year program (2013–2016) aimed to increase access to high impact, evidence-based antenatal, intrapartum, and immediate postpartum care to mothers by leveraging the enterprise of private sector providers in Uttar Pradesh and Jharkhand. In the second phase, FOGSI has developed 16 core clinical standards and Manyata is a stamp of quality which ensures the best clinical practices for safer experience of mothers during childbirth. Jhpiego is providing the technical support for this quality improvement implementation.[23] After five rounds of assessments, 122 out of 140 participating facilities achieved a 70% score or better, compared to only 3% of facilities at baseline.[23]

KEY MESSAGES

- Any pregnant woman who will deliver is at risk of PPH. This can be prevented by overcoming the three delays and by preparedness of the center to handle hemorrhagic emergencies.
- The critical steps are **C**ommunicate (for help), **R**esuscitate (assess blood loss and replace with fluids and blood), **I**nvestigate (cause of bleeding), **I**nitiate uterotonics, and **L**igate the great arteries.
- Conservative measures to be tried first, rapidly moving if these do not work to more invasive procedures. Along with four Ts of etiology, fifth T (Theater) is emphasized in managing patients.
- Early and proactive treatment prevents adverse outcomes and saves lives.
- Postpartum hemorrhage is a preventable and treatable disease, even in low resource settings.
- *Will, Skill, and Drill* of every health worker and obstetrician will overcome all hurdles.

HAEMOSTASIS is a pneumonic used in the series of sequential steps taken to control postpartum hemorrhage.

H Ask for Help
A Assess vitals, blood loss, and resuscitate
E Establish etiology and treat accordingly
M Massage uterus
O Oxytocin infusion and medical management
S Shock garment and shift to higher center/theater
T Tamponade balloon
A Apply compression sutures—B-Lynch or modified
S Systematic pelvic devascularization (uterine, ovarian, and internal iliac)
I Interventional radiologist—uterine artery embolization
S Subtotal or total hysterectomy.

REFERENCES

1. Leduc D, Senikas V, Lalonde AB, et al. Active management of the third stage of labour: Prevention and Treatment of postpartum haemorrhage. J Obstet Gynaecol Can. 2009; 31(10):980-93.
2. Kerr RS, Weeks AD. Postpartum haemorrhage: a single definition is no longer enough. BJOG. 2017;124(5):723-6.
3. Lockhart E. Post partum hemorrhage: a continuing challenge. Hematology Am Soc Hematol Educ Program. 2015;2015:132-7.

4. El Ayadi AM, Robinson N, Geller S, et al. Advances in the treatment of postpartum hemorrhage. Expert Rev Obstet Gynecol. 2013; 8(6):525-37.
5. Devi K, Singh L, Singh M, et al. Postpartum hemorrhage and maternal deaths in North East India. Open J Obstet Gynecol. 2015;5:635-8.
6. World Health Organization. (2017). World Health Statistics 2017: Monitoring health for the SDGs. [online] Available from https://www.who.int/gho/publications/world_health_statistics/2017/en/ [Last accessed July, 2019].
7. FIGO Guidelines. Prevention and treatment of postpartum haemorrhage in low resource settings. Int J Gynaecol Obstet. 2012;117:108-18.
8. Pankaj Desai, Atul Munshi. FOGSI Focus, 2007.
9. PPH Prevention and Management. Clinical Practice, Auckland Guideline, 2015.
10. Pandit SN, Khan RJ. Prevention and management of PPH. [online] Available from https://www.fogsi.org/wp-content/uploads/2015/05/pdf/editor/dr_reshma_pai/3.pdf [Last accessed July, 2019].
11. World Health Organization. (2009). WHO guidelines for the management of postpartum haemorrhage and retained placenta. [online] Available from https://www.who.int/reproductivehealth/publications/maternal_perinatal_health/9789241598514/en/ [Last accessed July, 2019].
12. Ministry of Health and Family Welfare. Guidance note on prevention and management of postpartum hemorrhage. Maternal Health Division, Ministry of Health and Family Welfare; 2015.
13. Shields LE, Goffman D, Caughey A. ACOG practice bulletin: Clinical management guidelines for obstetrician-gynecologists. Obstet Gynecol. 2017;130(4):e168-86.
14. Reddi Rani P, Begum J. Recent advances in the management of major postpartum haemorrhage–A review. J Clin Diagn Res. 2017; 11(2):QE01-QE05.
15. NRHM. (2013). Operational guidelines and reference manual for advance distribution of misoprostol to prevent postpartum haemorrhage during home births. [online] Available from http://www.nrhmorissa.gov.in/writereaddata/Upload/Documents/Operational%20Guidelines%20and%20Reference%20Manual%20for%20Misoprostol%20for%20PPH-Nov.%207,%202013-final.pdf [Last accessed July, 2019].
16. FOGSI. (2014). Consensus statement for prevention of PPH. [online] Available from https://www.fogsi.org/wp-content/uploads/2015/11/pph.pdf [Last accessed July, 2019].
17. The Lancet. WOMAN: reducing maternal deaths with tranexamic acid. Lancet. 2017;389(10084):2081.
18. Association of Ontario Midwives. (2016). Postpartum hemorrhage: Clinical Practice Guideline No. 17. [online] Available from https://www.ontariomidwives.ca/sites/default/files/CPG%20full%20guidelines/CPG-Postpartum-hemorrhage-PUB.pdf [Last accessed July, 2019].
19. Louis K, Mahantesh K, Christopher B-L. Postpartum hemorrhage: prevention and treatment. J Obstet Gynecol India. 2008; 58(5): 392-8.
20. RANZCOG. (2017). Management of Postpartum Haemorrhage (PPH). [online] Available from https://ranzcog.edu.au/RANZCOG_SITE/media/RANZCOG-MEDIA/Women%27s%20Health/Statement%20and%20guidelines/Clinical-Obstetrics/Management-of-Postpartum-Haemorrhage-(C-Obs-43)-Review-July-2017.pdf?ext=.pdf [Last accessed July, 2019].
21. Shih JC, Liu KL, Kang J, et al. 'Nausicaa' compression suture: a simple and effective alternative to hysterectomy in placenta accreta spectrum and other causes of severe postpartum haemorrhage. BJOG. 2019;126(3): 412-7.
22. Coker A, Oliver R. Definitions and classification. In: B-Lynch C, Keith L, Lalonde A, Karoshi M (Eds). A Comprehensive Textbook of Postpartum Hemorrhage, 2nd edition. Duncow: Sapiens Publishing; 2006.
23. MSD for Mothers, JHPIEGO, FOGSI. Lessons learned from a quality improvement program for private maternity care facilities in India. [online] Available from https://www.merckformothers.com/docs/White_Paper_Merck_for_Mothers.pdf [Last accessed July, 2019].

Chapter 2

Postpartum Hemorrhage: Setting Criteria for Clinical Audit

V Rajasekharan Nair, P Lekshmi Ammal

INTRODUCTION

Between the year 1990 and 2015, there was a 44% reduction in the global maternal deaths but we find that even now around 3,03,000 women die annually due to childbirth-related problems.[1] It is also well-known that 99% of these deaths are occurring in resource poor countries. A closer look at the proximate causes of maternal deaths, one could find that obstetric hemorrhage is the leading cause of maternal mortality as well as serious morbidity. Atonic postpartum hemorrhage (PPH) tops the list of causes, accounting to 10–35% of maternal deaths. Gaps in data collection, poor quality of service, and human resource constraints are the major contributory factors to high maternal mortality rates.

PROCESS OF CLINICAL AUDIT

Clinical audit exercises are necessary for refinements in the patient care in any given scenario, irrespective of the country or facility. It is a continuous process, where standards are set, implemented, and analyzed over a time frame to bring in fresh changes or corrections for improving the clinical care of a particular condition or disease. This whole process is called the audit cycle. With reference to PPH the following observations can be made:

Two types of audit process may be employed in this situation:[2]

1. *Event audit:* Involve auditing of maternal death or morbidity by methods such as verbal autopsy, confidential enquiry, facility-based audit, or near miss reviews. These audits attempt a comprehensive assessment of a sentinel event, be it death or morbidity.
2. *Clinical audit:* It is a structured peer review, which focuses on specific issues of a clinical problem, and is an essential part of quality assurance.[3]

Out of the many types of clinical audits, criteria-based clinical audit acts as a tool for measurement of quality. Criteria-based clinical audit has been defined as a quality improvement process that seeks to improve patient care and outcomes through systematic review of care against explicit criteria and finally improvement in the care. To achieve a reduction in maternal mortality ratio (MMR), interventions as suggested by national and international guidelines exist. These are formulated by competent bodies like World Health Organization (WHO), Royal College of Obstetricians and Gynaecologists (RCOG), International Federation of Gynecology and Obstetrics (FIGO), Federation of Obstetric and Gynaecological Societies of India (FOGSI), etc. and systematic review of various studies by Cochrane database. It has been recognized that limiting healthcare activities to passive dissemination of guidelines alone is insufficient to improve standards of care to desired levels. These disseminations should be supplemented by clinical audits done in obstetric care hospitals and have been shown to improve outcomes in terms of reduction on morbidity and mortality.

Criteria-based clinical audit essentially involves five steps:
1. Establish criteria for good practice.
2. Documenting base line data by observing the current practice through staff questionnaire, patient case records, labor room registers, and discharge summaries.
3. Give a feedback regarding the observations and make a local target (through educational meeting ideally).
4. Implement changes in the existing practice as desired in the newly drawn up protocols or guidelines.
5. Reevaluate the changes made in the practice and give a feedback. Compare it with the baseline data and do the impact evaluation.

The last step is very important to validate the improvements made by the audit and that closes the loop of one cycle of criteria-based clinical audit. In the absence of baseline data, the final conclusion will be unsatisfactory. Criteria-based clinical audit can make measureable positive impacts varying from minimal to moderate. The focus of criteria-based clinical audit generally is on a specific topic. In this context, it will be obstetric hemorrhage. Setting the criteria is a very important step and is the cornerstone for the improvement in care we are targeting.

Criteria are systematically developed statements that can be used to assess the healthcare services and outcomes. They should be:
- Evidence-based (preferably locally generated)
- Easily achievable and measurable
- Should be locally relevant
- Should not be conflicting with national and international recommendations.

Since PPH is the most common entity contributing to the highest percentage of maternal mortality and near miss cases, the criteria can be narrowed to this single entity. It is essential to have definitions, which specify how each case and its severity is assessed. We can arrive at working definitions where the essential features are distinguished from additional features.

Observations from a study conducted in Netherland bring out few important lacunae in maintaining quality of care in the scenario of obstetric hemorrhage, which is applicable to our settings also.
- Failure to document antenatal risk factors
- inadequate knowledge or awareness of guidelines
- Failure to monitor vital signs
- Nonsystematic approach in carrying out different steps in management of PPH
- Delay in treatment and poor team work.

SETTING UP CRITERIA FOR CLINICAL AUDIT IN OBSTETRIC HEMORRHAGE

Obstetric hemorrhage is an ideal situation for clinical audit as it has all the prerequisite components for an effective clinical audit.
- Obstetric hemorrhage is the major killer of mothers worldwide. It has the highest case fatality rate.
- Obstetric hemorrhage can be clearly defined and identified in case records, labor room registers and discharge summaries making it easier to collect and analyze data.
- It is an important cause for "near miss" cases also.
- Availability of sound research evidence and strong support from review of literature makes it an ideal subject for criteria-based clinical audit.

SETTING STANDARDS FOR STRUCTURED AUDIT IN POSTPARTUM HEMORRHAGE

Maternal survival can clearly be attributed to the quality of care she receives during all the phases of pregnancy. The modern day concept of quality originates from Donabedian's classical proposal of the triad of structure, process, and outcome in evaluating the quality of healthcare.[4] Quality is an attribute of care. It neither has an accepted standard definition nor has standard tools to measure. It is diverse and multidimensional, but can be simply stated that quality is "doing the right thing, rightly, and right away" Unfortunately in our undergraduate and postgraduate training, the importance of the quality component is not getting enough thrust. Generally, one has to depend on sources like International (WHO) and National guidelines, Cochrane database for developing the quality of care. Unfortunately, locally made protocols and guidelines are sparse and when available are based on limited institutional data. The publication from Kerala Federation of Obstetrics and Gynaecology titled "Why mothers die" is an exception because the data generated from the state is used for the analysis and formulation of recommendations.[5]

To assess quality of care, three components have to be taken care of, viz. structure, process, and outcome.
1. *Structure* refers to the facilities, equipment, and human resources to carry out the proposed type of care.
2. *Process* refers to the management and care delivered.
3. *Outcome* is the result of the process and indicates the quality of care delivered finally.

Out of the above three components, process is the most difficult to assess and measure and is the best indicator to know whether medicine is properly and effectively practiced. Monitoring and evaluating the care given will be a significant step to give an insight into deficiencies in clinical practice and the necessary corrective measures. In this regard, clinical audit gains significance.[6]

STANDARDIZATION OF TOOLS FOR AUDIT OF POSTPARTUM HEMORRHAGE

Table 1 shows few criteria and standards that can be adopted in clinical audit in obstetric hemorrhage, after taking into consideration the current practices, local needs, as well as constraints like human resource or infrastructure deficiencies.

Any number of criteria listed in Table 1 can be selected for the audit process. Limiting to four or five criteria will be convenient to the practicing clinician.[7-13] The more the number, the more it becomes cumbersome and fallacies set in. The selected key interventions can be designated as the quality standards for that audit purpose. To give an example, one may select fourth stage maternal deaths as an area of audit. In our studies, we find that around 10% of deaths are due to PPH during fourth stage of labor. By mere observation and early minimal interventions, we may be able to bring down these maternal deaths. But standards have to be clearly laid down like how you are going to observe these women, how often, etc. to get the desired measurable outcome.

Outcome Measures

Several outcome measures can be selected for each clinical audit situation depending on the criteria and standards set. Amount of blood loss, drop in hematocrit, development of hypotension or shock, units of blood and blood products transfused, development of multiorgan dysfunction, severe acute maternal morbidity (SAMM), or maternal death may be considered for outcome measure. To give an example, if the audit criterion is efficacy of intravenous oxytocin in reducing third stage complications, one may fix the amount of blood loss as an outcome measure. Secondary outcomes such as incidence of retained placenta can also be considered.

TABLE 1: Criteria and standards for clinical audit in obstetric hemorrhage.

No.	Criteria	Process
1.	Anemia is a well-known antenatal risk factor for PPH, since it predisposes to atonicity and decreases the tolerability to blood loss. Hb status should be known of all patients going into labor Ensure that hemoglobin is above 10 g in all parturients	Hemoglobin status of all parturients should be known prior to delivery. If not done recently, at the time of intravenous cannulation a sample of blood should be taken for hemoglobin estimation
2.	The incidence of adherent placenta is increased with increasing rate of cesarean section. Adherent placenta is a very significant antenatal risk factor for major obstetric hemorrhage, near miss cases, and maternal mortality	Use ultrasound imaging for all pregnant women with previous cesarean section at 32 weeks to determine the placental site and presence of invasion
3.	Identification and referral of gravidas with antenatal risk factors like placenta previa as it greatly increases the risk of subsequent PPH	• Refer pregnant women with placenta previa to an institution where blood and blood products are easily available for confinement • If adherent placenta is suspected, MRI may be considered in appropriate cases • If it is adherent placenta on the scar, refer to institutions where clinicians are familiar with management of such cases
4.	Active management of third stage of labor decreases blood loss by 50–70%. Oxytocic agents administered during child birth are responsible for this beneficial effect. Oxytocin is the drug of choice when compared with other oxytocic agents	At the time of delivery of anterior shoulder or within 1 minute of the birth of the baby, all laboring women should receive 10 units of oxytocin intramuscularly. In cesarean section as well as vaginal delivery 5 units oxytocin diluted in 5 mL of normal saline be preferably given as a slow IV bolus dose. This should be followed by IM administration of 10 units of oxytocin
5.	Genital trauma is to be excluded early in all parturients developing PPH before continuing with medical management. It is a good practice to do the same in all women who had instrumental deliveries	All labor suites should have dedicated sets for vaginal as well as cervical inspection. Two long-bladed sims speculum along with three pairs of sponge holding forceps must be readily available in a sterilized pack (cervical inspection sets)
6.	The most common cause of primary PPH is uterine atony. Intravenous oxytocin infusion is the drug of choice for the primary treatment	All women with atonic PPH should receive oxytocin infusion (20 units in 500 mL of crystalloids at the rate of 125 mL/hr
7.	*Add on oxytocics*: If bleeding is not controlled with oxytocin alone, addition of other oxytocic agents is found to be useful in reducing bleeding.[2,13]	If bleeding is not controlled and if the woman is not a hypertensive, administer injection ergometrine 0.25 mg IV or IM Injection prostaglandin F_2 alpha, 250 µg s/c is administered (repeated at 15 min interval for up to 8 doses maximum) Misoprostol 800 µg may be given S/L
8.	Early use of tranexamic acid in PPH, within 3 hours of birth of the baby reduces severity and mortality associated with PPH	Tranexamic acid 1 g IV in normal saline to be given over 10 min, in women with postpartum hemorrhage in addition to the standard care

Contd...

Contd...

No.	Criteria	Process
9.	Surgical interventions are to be instituted soon once medical measures fail. Delay in control of bleeding leads to irreversible multiorgan dysfunction and increased mortality Balloon/condom tamponade is the first-line intervention in women with uterine atony as the major cause of PPH, especially in low resource settings	Once bleeding continues in spite of medical measures, condom tamponade should be used without undue delay
10.	Hemostatic suture techniques are effective in controlling the bleeding and reducing the maternal mortality	Ongoing PPH— resort to laparotomy, proceed with hemostatic sutures or step wise devascularization Ensure personnel trained in such procedures
11.	Retained placental tissue constitutes a risk factor for PPH and leads to atonicity of uterus	All women with continued bleeding not responding to medical management should undergo without much delay exploration of uterine cavity to rule out retained placental bits or lobes. On site ultrasound examination may also be useful in such cases
12.	Lack of optimal care, following moderate or severe PPH leads to increased maternal mortality. All patients with major PPH should be managed in high dependency unit (HDU) or intensive care unit (ICU)	Treat women with moderate or severe PPH in HDU or ICU for adequate care Ensure minimum standards for the above mentioned care available in the institution
13.	Visual estimation of blood loss is notoriously inaccurate in assessing the severity of PPH and hence clinical signs and symptoms should be monitored for the same	Women with excessive blood should be monitored continuously with pulse, BP, respiratory rate, and urine output measurement to assess the severity of hemorrhage
14.	Visual assessment of blood loss is inaccurate	Use preweighed drapes and swabs for vaginal delivery and C-section. Weigh these after delivery to estimate blood loss
15.	Along with oxytocics and other methods to arrest bleeding, rapid intravascular volume replacement is the cornerstone for successful resuscitation of women with PPH	Secure two intravenous access with number 14 G cannula for all bleeding women in the postpartum period for rapid crystalloid infusion and later for blood should the need arise
16.	Rapid intravenous replacement by warmed clear fluids is recommended till cross-matched blood is made available	In all women with PPH administer, normal saline 2 L followed by 1.5 L of warmed colloid over a period of 1 hour (if blood is not ready)
17.	Blood transfusion is the lifesaving measure in obstetric hemorrhage (Green-top Guideline 47) There is an unavoidable delay in screening and cross-matching blood for transfusion. Such delays and nonavailability of cross-matched blood lead to ischemic irreversible multiorgan dysfunction and maternal death Blood bank/storage facility in all delivery points	Identify source for blood and blood products with estimated delay
18.	DIC can be a cause as well as effect of obstetrical hemorrhage. All women who are suffering from obstetrical hemorrhage should be screened for coagulation failure	Send blood at the initial venepuncture itself for bedside clotting test or coagulation profile

Contd...

Contd...

No.	Criteria	Process
	A bedside clotting test may be done initially. If facilities are available do further coagulation assays	
19.	Blood component therapy is instituted as per the coagulation parameters or transfusion protocol	Ensure protocol for blood component therapy Start 12–15 mL/kg body weight of fresh frozen plasma (FFP) after 4 units of RBC, if APTT > 1.5 transfuse FFP at a rate >15 mL/kg body weight Transfuse cryoprecipitate when fibrinogen is less than 2 g/L Transfuse platelets when platelet count is less than 75×10^9/L
20.	Many women slip into irreversible shock due to undetected hemorrhage in fourth stage of labor (3–4 hr immediate postpartum)	Define fourth stage. All parturients are to be monitored every 30 minutes with pulse, BP, height of fundus, and inspection of episiotomy meticulously. Look for expressed clots per vaginum also

(DIC: disseminated intravascular coagulation; Hb: hemoglobin; IM: intramuscular; IV: intravenous; MRI: magnetic resonance imaging; PPH: postpartum hemorrhage; RBC: red blood cell)

RELEVANCE OF QUALITY STANDARDS IN CLINICAL AUDIT: THE KERALA EXPERIENCE

Instead of incorporating all dimensions of PPH in the clinical audits, selected cardinal events can be picked up to monitor the quality of patient care. For example, the pivotal point in the management of third stage is whether the parturient received the recommended dose of oxytocin at the defined time. Such an approach was beneficial in bringing down the morbidity from PPH and eased the process of clinical audit as we are looking at specific standards in patient care. Observations of confidential review of maternal deaths (CRMD) in Kerala, reveal that 30% of maternal deaths are due to two conditions, viz. PPH and hypertensive disorders of pregnancy.[5] Based on these findings, we went ahead with development of five quality standards for each of these conditions, which are measurable in any clinical settings. This exercise was done by the Kerala Federation of Obstetrics and Gynaecology with governmental support and collaboration with the NICE international, UK. In fact, these quality standards are widely disseminated and practiced by all facilities conducting deliveries. The five quality standards, we are recommending for prevention and early treatment of PPH, are given in Table 2. These are endorsed by the Government of Kerala as standard practice guidelines.

There has been definite decrease in the incidence of third stage complications following the introduction and dissemination of quality standards.[14] The need for blood transfusion, incidence of obstetric hysterectomies, etc. decreased. A short-term observation shows a precipitous decrease in the deaths following adherent placenta with the new strategy. In Kerala, there is early indication that PPH is being pushed back from its prime position to second or third position as a causative factor in maternal mortality.

Ethical Issues Involved in Clinical Audit

Whenever an audit is designed, the rights of the clients should be kept in mind. It may not be possible to get consent of the patient in

TABLE 2: The five quality standards for PPH practiced in Kerala.

Quality standard (criteria)	Process, indicators	Outcome measure
All women delivering, should receive a bolus dose of IV oxytocin within 1 minute of delivery of the baby (CS also) Additional oxytocic, if necessary	• 5 units oxytocin, diluted in 5 mL saline, over 1 minute • Evidence of oxytocin supply, fridge, and personnel • Provisions for blood loss measurements • Documented in labor room register.	• Reduction in blood loss following delivery/CS • Reduction in need for blood transfusion, HDU admissions, hysterectomy, etc.
Following delivery, all women should be observed for 2 hours with half hourly pulse, BP, uterine height, uterine consistency, and vaginal bleeding	• Personnel to observe • Stamp or records denoting the observations	Reduction in fourth stage deaths as evidenced by monthly or annual statistics
All women having excessive bleeding following delivery, should be resuscitated with rapid infusion of crystalloids Blood and blood components to be given as per requirement	• Secure 2 separate Intravenous access line with 14 G cannula • Availability of normal saline/crystalloids • Blood and blood products	Reduction in number of women with severe acute morbidity (shock, anuria, and multiorgan dysfunction)
All women having moderate-to-severe PPH should be treated in an HDU/ICU	Shift all postpartum patients treated for PPH to HDU/ICU	Reduction in mortality or SAMM
Prior CS gravidas should have an ultrasound scan around 32 weeks to rule out placenta previa Suspected cases of accrete should be referred to specified institutions	• Designated institutions with trained personnel in dealing with such cases • Other specialists • Aortic clamps, common iliac artery clamps • Blood, components	Reduction in morbidity or mortality from adherent placenta

(BP: blood pressure; CS: cesarean section; HDU: high dependency unit; ICU: intensive care unit: PPH: postpartum hemorrhage; SAMM: severe acute maternal morbidity)

all situations, but confidentiality should be maintained to the fullest extent possible.[15] The data collected should be specific for the purpose and should not contain personnel identity such as name, hospital number, etc. The data should be processed quickly and should not be preserved indefinitely once the pooled results are ready. In designing and implementing clinical audits, all the stakeholders are involved, preferably the patient and relatives wherever permissible.

■ NEAR MISS AUDIT

Maternal near miss (MNM) audit has been found to be an excellent form of clinical audit in midwifery practice. The added advantage over maternal death review is that, the survivor telling the story and sharing her experience will add to the content of the audit process. 1-year pilot study of near miss cases from five Government medical colleges was conducted in Kerala during the year 2017–18 (unpublished results), which yielded useful results which were complementary to the information gained from the CRMD, an ongoing maternal death audit process in Kerala. The most important cause of MNM continues to be hemorrhage, followed by sepsis and hypertension. Results point to the fact that our efforts at treating obstetric hemorrhage is finding good success, but the efforts to prevent and treat sepsis and hypertension have to be augmented still further.

GOOD PRACTICE POINTS

- Clinical audit is a necessary tool for healthcare improvement.
- It is relevant at all levels of healthcare institutions.
- Clinical audits should be designed with specific objectives, defining clear standards.
- Clinical audits in PPH improve the quality of maternity care.
- Too many objectives can adversely affect the outcomes.
- All stakeholders should be involved, if possible patients and relatives.
- There must be robust systems for data collection and handling.
- Maternal near miss reviews supplement the mortality reviews.

CONCLUSION

The millennium development goal (MDG) 5 has failed to achieve the desired target of reducing MMR by 75% in 2015. This calls for intensive efforts to revisit the preventable causes maternal mortality and the lacunae in obstetric healthcare delivery in our country. An important contributor to the high maternal mortality rates in developing countries is the poor quality of obstetric care. In spite of the availability of several guidelines for management of obstetric conditions including PPH the compliance seems to be poor. In short, there exists a quality gap between guidelines and its actual implementation. Clinical audits continue to be an important component of healthcare quality improvement. Only through systematic audits, these gaps can be narrowed down resulting in improved quality of obstetric care and better management of obstetric emergencies. A giant leap is necessary in the quality of obstetric services in our country to realize the Sustainable Development Goals (SDGs) in the field of maternal health. It is really heartening to note that the whole concept of maternal death audit is transforming into one of Maternal Death Surveillance and Response (MDSR) ushering in an important change in our outlook on maternal health.

REFERENCES

1. World Health Organization. WHO fact sheet 2015, Trends in maternal mortality 1990-2015, WHO/RHR/15.23. [online] available from: https://www.who.int/reproductivehealth/publications/monitoring/maternal-mortality-2015/en/ [Last Accessed July, 2019].
2. Shaw CD. Criterion-based audit. In: Smith R (Ed). Audit in Action. London: British Medical Publishing Group;1992. pp. 122-8.
3. Graham WG. Criteria based clinical Audit. Best Prac Res COG. 2009;23:375-85.
4. Ayanian JZ, Markel H. Donabedian's lasting framework for healthcare quality. N Eng J Med. 2016;375:205-7.
5. Paily VP, Ambujam K, Thomas B. Why Mothers die. Trissur, Kerala: Kerala Federation of Obstetrics & Gynaecology; 2012.
6. Dupont C, Deneux-Tharaux C, Touzet S, et al. Clinical audit: a useful tool for reducing postpartum haemorrhage. Int J Qual Health Care. 2011;23(5):583-9.
7. Begley CM, Gyte GML, Devane D, et al. Active versus expectant management for women in the third stage of labour. Cochrane Database Syst Rev. 2015;13:CD007412.

8. Weeks A. The prevention and treatment of PPH. What do we know where do we go to next? BJOG. 2015;122:202-12.
9. Silver RM, Landon MB, Rouse DJ, et al. Maternal morbidity associated with multiple repeat cesarean deliveries. National institute of Child Health and Human Development Maternal—Fetal Medicine Units Network. Obstet Gynecol. 2006;107:1226-32.
10. Novikova N, Hofmeyr GJ, Cluver C. Tranexamic acid for preventing postpartum haemorrhage. Cochrane Database Syst Rev. 2015;16(6): CD007872.
11. Mavrides E, Allard S, Chandraharan E, et al. Prevention and management of postpartum haemorrhage. BJOG. 2016;124:e106-49.
12. Committee Opinion No. 529: Placenta accrete. Obstet Gynecol. 2012;120:207-11.
13. WOMAN Trial Collaborators. Effect of early tranexamic acid administration on mortality, hysterectomy and other morbidities in women with postpartum haemorrhage (WOMAN); an international, randomized double-blind, placebo controlled trial. Lancet. 2017;389: 2105-16.
14. Paily VP, Ambujam K, Rajasekharan Nair V, et al. Confidential Review of maternal deaths in Kerala: a country case study. BJOG. 2014; 121(Suppl 4):61-6.
15. Soliman A. Principles of methodical design of clinical audit. Arch Med. 2018;10(2):2.

Chapter 3

Safety in the Labor Ward

Nuzhat Aziz, Pallavi Chandra

■ INTRODUCTION

Childbirth is a complex process. The place of childbirth, the labor and delivery (L and D) unit becomes the most vital area for all mothers going through pregnancy. The work in this area is unique. With the majority of workload being unplanned, unpredictable workload makes the L and D a unique place to work in, compared with other high-paced, high-risk areas, such as the operation theaters (OTs). The team here deals with complexities of obstetric care, where the risk factors change their profile rapidly, where emergency responses are expected to be prompt and precise and where errors can lead to major catastrophes. Requirement for appropriate communication and coordination between multidisciplinary teams adds to the complexity. Promoting safety in intrapartum period is the basic central concept of designing an L and D unit.[1] Safety is the condition of being protected from danger, risk or injury. Promotion of safety starts with the design of a unit and ends with periodic accreditation and assessment of each of its processes.

■ DESIGNING FOR SAFETY

The design of an L and D aims to provide patient satisfaction, creating a home-like environment, which may be converted to an intensive care facility, as and when the need arises. The variables that are taken into consideration into the layout and design are the planned number of deliveries per month, the bed strength, workflow design, the dimensions of each room, concept of triage, high dependency unit (HDU), emergency OT, neonatal resuscitation area, the equipment, lighting solutions, storage, workstations, waste management (dirty utility) and toilets. Workflow pattern should start from an emergency entry point to obstetric triage which then leads to L and D or emergency OT or HDU or antenatal ward (Figs. 1 and 2). This triaging concept allows the L and D area to receive only those who need its services. The Emergency OT should be a part of the L and D complex to allow rapid category 1 cesarean sections (CSs). The recommendations by the Government of India mandate the presence of HDU for all and an obstetric intensive care unit (ICU) if the number of deliveries exceed 500 per month.[2] If the workflow of a unit has the concept of a first stage room (as is found in places with high volumes), then it has to be different from HDU. The risk categorization at admission into low- and high-risk pregnancy also enables appropriate allocation of resources. The criteria for HDU and ICU admissions allow appropriate monitoring of these women and thus promote safety.[2] The checklist for designing an L and D complex is shown in Tables 1 and 2.

■ IDEAL BED STRENGTH FOR SAFETY

The overloading of a system with volumes exceeding its capacity is the most common reason for failure of safety processes. The bed strength of L and D is dependent on

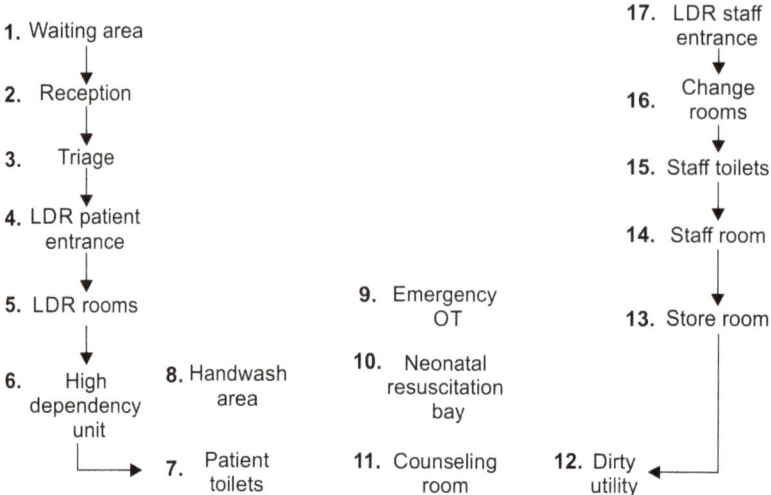

Fig. 1: Workflow design for labor, delivery and recovery (LDR).

1. Waiting area
2. Reception
3. Triage
4. LDR patient entrance
5. LDR rooms
6. High dependency unit
7. Patient toilets
8. Handwash area
9. Emergency OT
10. Neonatal resuscitation bay
11. Counseling room
12. Dirty utility
13. Store room
14. Staff room
15. Staff toilets
16. Change rooms
17. LDR staff entrance

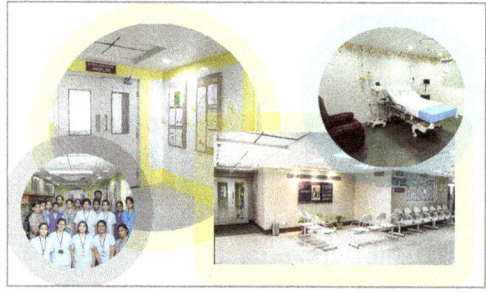

Fig. 2: Labor and delivery complex.

the projected number of deliveries that are expected to take place in that unit. The birth volume in a birthing unit is linked to the admission rate, vaginal birth rate, emergency CS rate and the average duration of stay for vaginal delivery or a CS. The formula used to calculate the number of labor, delivery, and recovery (LDR) beds required is as follows: The number of LDR rooms = Projected LDR events × ALOS/365 × occupancy rates.[3] Projected LDR events are vaginal births and emergency cesareans that go from the labor ward; ALOS is the average length of stay in days, usually taken as 12 hours or 0.5 days. For example, a hospital with 3,600 deliveries a year with 30% CS rate will have 2,400 vaginal births and 600 emergency giving 3,000 LDR events per year.

Number of LDR rooms = 3,000 × 0.5/365 × 0.75 = 5.49 or 6 LDR rooms complex. Safety of maternity care in an institute is through designing for a specific projected number and then defining your limits of booking.

DESIGNING EACH LDR ROOM FOR SAFETY

The changing perspectives on birthing have changed the birthing room—LDR to a focus on more emphasis on mobility, concealment of all equipment behind panels, which can be taken out if needed. Complete emergency care would require gas lines, delivery bed, operative light source, emergency equipment to monitor mother and fetus and local storage. Addition of railings for support, Rebozo, birthing balls, a shower area, a water tub for hydrotherapy or water birth are optional but very useful to the woman to maintain mobility and upright positions. The storage of all equipment, drugs, instruments, bed sheets, sterile trays in the same room allows easy access in times of emergency (Fig. 3).

CHAPTER 3: Safety in the Labor Ward

TABLE 1: Checklist for designing an L and D complex for 3,000 births per year.

LDR complex
- Waiting area for patients
- Reception for labor ward complex
- Two entrance—for patients and for staff with access doors
- Staff entrance leading to:
  - Change room for staff, with lockers
  - Change room for doctors, with lockers
  - Toilet
  - Dirty utility room
  - Store
  - Delivery (LDR) rooms—6 in number
    - Ideal size 15 × 17 feet
    - With attached bathroom
    - Ceiling mounted light
    - Oxygen/suction lines
  - Neonatal resuscitation bay
    - For two resuscitation trolleys
    - Parking one trolley
  - Labor ward trolley parking area
  - Equipment bay
    - For crash cart
    - For charging and parking equipment
    - Refrigerator
  - Working station for labor ward
    - Sitting and standing platforms
    - 3 computer terminals with printer
    - With pin board for notices
    - Nursing call system
    - Pneumatic system
    - Cabinets for storage
    - Below and above the working area
    - Reading lights in the working area
    - Phone lines—3
  - Wash area (surgical hand scrub)
  - Patient display board for 6 delivery rooms
  - High dependency unit/induction room
    - Beds—6 in number
    - Oxygen and suction lines
    - Nursing station
    - Storage
    - Wash basin for washing hands
    - Patient display board
    - Ultrasound, crash cart and CTG machine parking area
    - Toilet for patients
  - Doctors lounge
    - A table with 8 chairs
    - A couch to sleep

Contd...

Contd...

LDR complex
  - Labor ward (LW) handover board
  - With toilet
  - Microwave, refrigerator, tea, coffee trays
  - Lockers
- Staff lounge
  - A table with 8 chairs
  - A couch to sleep
  - Notice board
  - With toilet
  - Lockers
- Counseling room leading to patient entry/exit door

Maternal and fetal monitoring equipment can be either wall mounted or on trolleys. Panels can be used for concealment of equipment to promote a concept of home-like room, without any medical equipment. Good visualization is paramount for rapid control of traumatic hemorrhage. A ceiling-mounted light has more advantages than a movable or a wall-mounted source. A checklist for equipment in an LDR room is given in Table 3.

EQUIPMENT FOR SAFETY

The L and D should be equipped with all monitors required for maternal and fetal monitoring, for a low-risk mother has a transition to a high-risk zone suddenly. The electrical power supply needs may vary and needs to be thought of before planning the infrastructure of L and D. The LDR and HDU beds require at least 6 plug points, three each of 5 and 15 amps, with one or two having a connection to the uninterrupted power supply (UPS) source. The equipment which are commonly used in L and D requiring an electrical power supply are delivery bed, infusion set, maternal multiparameter monitor, cardiotocography machine, ultrasound machine if needed. The ultrasound machine is a very essential safety tool that must be present in all L and D units

TABLE 2: Components of LDR, triage and HDU as a checklist.

	Triage	LDR complex	HDU
Reception	Yes	Yes	
Toilet for patients family	Yes	Yes	
Nursing station	Yes	Yes	Yes
Trolley and wheelchair parking	Yes	Yes	
Triage rooms/beds	3	6	4–6
Toilets for patient use	Yes	Yes	
Staff room with toilet	1	1	
Counseling room	Yes	Yes	
Crash cart parking area	Yes	Yes	Yes
Storage room	Yes	Yes	Cabinets
Plug points for each bed	6	6	6
Handwash area	Wash basin	Scrub area	Wash basin
Equipment bay	Yes	Yes	Yes
Dirty utility	Yes	Yes	

(LDR: labor, delivery and recovery; HDU: high depending unit)

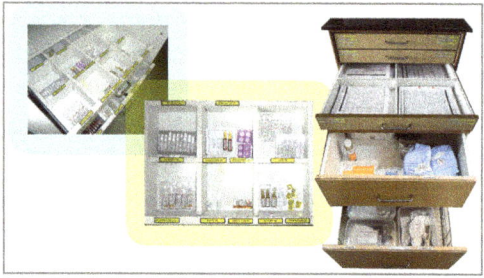

Fig. 3: Storage and signage in each labor, delivery, and recovery (LDR) room.

as it aids in rapid decision making. Most of the electrical equipment require charging and need a storage place which is designated by the term equipment bay with multiple electrical sockets of different amps. Standby equipment is sometimes designated as equipment library, to be utilized by all departments across the hospital, a concept of safety.

EMERGENCY KITS FOR SAFETY

A toolkit has all the required equipment, drugs and disposables in a single box or tray for a management of a specific condition or a procedure. Obstetric emergencies require prompt and quick response to prevent a catastrophe. Being prepared for an emergency with all the instruments needed for that emergency is very helpful. For example, a cervix exploration set has required instruments, to visualize, hold the cervix and suture the tear. A postpartum hemorrhage (PPH) tray similarly has all equipment required in the management of PPH, including Vacutainers for blood samples, drugs and documentation sheets (Fig. 4). The toolkits that should be present in the L and D are a delivery tray or set, PPH tray, eclampsia tray, cervix exploration set, anal sphincter injury repair set, Foley catheterization set, and postpartum intrauterine contraceptive device (PPIUCD) tray. The contents of these sets have to be verified and replaced on a daily basis which is recorded as a log for verification. A vaginal pack, sterile, autoclaved is always kept for emergency use along with a

TABLE 3: Checklist for planning each LDR.

Individual LDR room planning

Major requirements:
- Labor and delivery bed
- Good light source—ceiling light
- Recliner/chair for patients attender
- Stool for doctors/nurses
- Trolley in LW
- CTG machine
- Handheld Doptone
- Wash basin with elbow operated arm
- Cabinet—topmost draw and baskets below
- Cabinet to hold linen for the room

Minor equipment:
- BP apparatus
- Stethoscope
  Infusion pump
  Patient board, with pen stand
- Partogram board
- CTG board to display
- Clock
- Handrub on the wall
- Paper towel stand
- Sharps container
- Clock
- Dustbin
- Thermometer

Cabinet tray to have space for:
- Aprons, disposable sheets
- Gloves
- Foley catheter, urobag
- Venflon, swabs and stickers
- Drugs—to stock for immediate use
- ARM hooks
- Syringes
- Sterile sets—speculums, one delivery set, one epidural set
- Foley catheterization set

Plug points:
- Bed
- CTG machine
- Infusion set
- Two or three extra points—ultrasound machine, multiparameter monitor

Oxygen and suction lines

Bakri balloon.[4-6] The crash cart is mandatory in the labor ward and in the triage. The crash cart requires a disposable scalpel blade for a perimortem CS if needed.

STAFFING FOR SAFETY

Presence of a consultant 24 × 7 has been proven to be one of the factors that improve safety in L and D units. It facilitates confidence, earlier decision making, and promotes vaginal birth. The staffing again depends on the projected number of births. The nurses or midwifery staffing is planned with a concept of providing 1:1 care in LDR and 1:2 in the HDU. The working hours should be reviewed and most optimal shift hours chosen to avoid fatigue. Errors are most often reported in night within a 24-hour shift system. A labor ward coordinator should be supernumerary to the staff not be responsible for patient care directly, with a role to coordinate the systems in labor ward.[7]

TRAINING AND CERTIFICATION FOR SAFETY

Training of the team and assessment of the skills are a vital part of improving safety in labor wards. Multidisciplinary training may help better coordination in a crisis. Teams that work together should also have training and drills together, in the place of work rather than offsite. The mandatory and optional certifications can be decided by the team. Training needs have to be identified, and training opportunities provided. We have included basic life support, obstetric emergencies, perineal repair, electronic fetal monitoring and basic surgical training as mandatory. Growth assessment protocol (GAP) by perinatal institute, Birmingham also has now been added to basic prerequisite for working in obstetrics department. Training is one aspect; assessment is another part of making sure the team is geared up to dealing with emergencies. Simulation-based training and assessment should be the way forward for making obstetric emergencies safer for our mothers.[8]

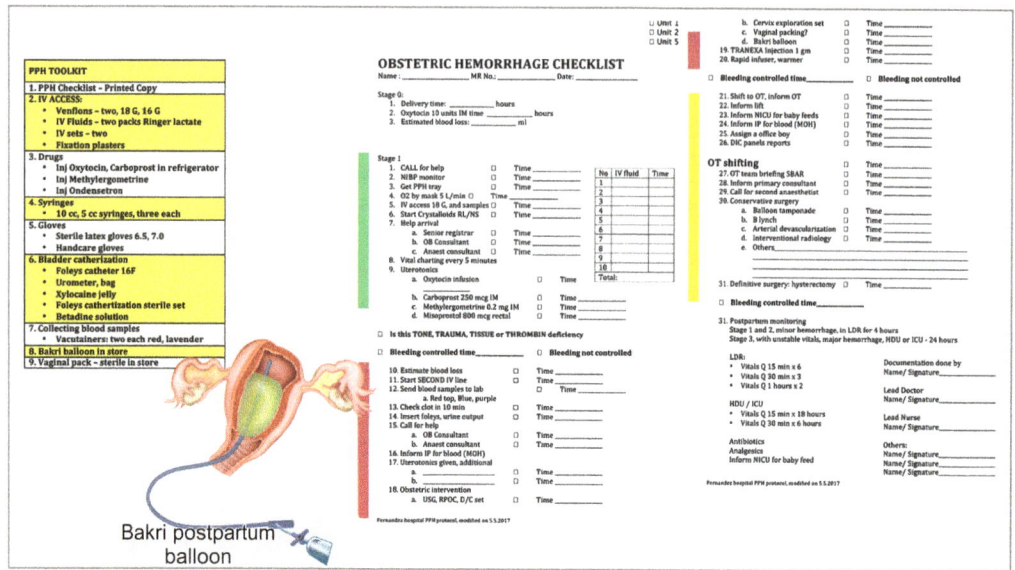

Fig. 4: Postpartum hemorrhage (PPH) toolkit and checklist.

■ INFECTION CONTROL SYSTEMS IN THE LABOR WARD

The process of cleaning, disinfecting, maintenance of hygiene in the labor ward is of paramount importance. The handwashing or hand disinfection policy needs an L and D design to promote these practices with a wash basin, surgical handwash, placement of hand rubs at strategic locations. Audits to ensure the control of hospital-acquired infection rates with a hospital infection control committee help to keep the processes under check.[9]

■ SIGNAGE FOR SAFETY

Appropriate signage for all storage, drugs, equipment and documentation sheets (see Fig. 3). Any person coming to the labor ward for the first time should be able to navigate and be able to access the required item. Induction to the labor ward policies, and crash cart, obstetric emergencies trays, and code blue policies has to be done.

■ OBSTETRIC HANDOVER BOARD

Shift handovers serve to ensure continuity of care between one group of healthcare providers and another; they involve changes in numbers, seniority and experience of staff and represent the formal transfer of responsibility and accountability from one team of health workers to another. Obstetric handover board can be designed and individualized for every unit updated at regular intervals (Fig. 5). This board can be kept in the staff lounge or in the working station, taking care to maintain patient confidentiality.

■ COMMUNICATION, TEAMWORK FOR SAFETY

One of the major reasons for errors and mismanagements is poor or lack of communication. It may be lack of communication within a team, or between different teams, or from one handover to another. A structured handover, an accepted method of communicating [situation, background,

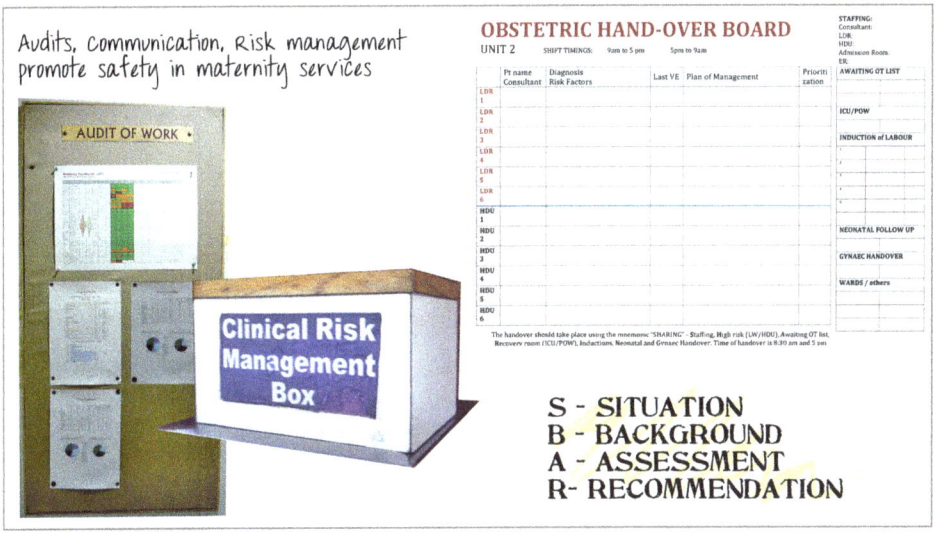

Fig. 5: Audits, handover board, clinical risk management (CRM), communication in L and D complex.

assessment, and recommendation (SBAR)], or a formatted method of writing notes [subjective, objective, assessment, and plan (SOAP)] are ways to ensure a high quality of standards with uniformity.[10,11] Promoting team building exercises, improving teamwork is an important aspect of safety.

ALARMING AND ALERTING SYSTEMS

Hospital emergency alerting systems have code blue for resuscitation, pink for baby alert amongst many others including fire and disaster. Standardized color codes are preferred and announced over the public address system, with a predesigned rehearsed response. There has been a recommendation to use plain language instead of color coding, which was found to increase the levels of stress in the response team. When the L and D has a special need for an urgent CS, an alerting system between the OT, anesthesia and neonatal teams is required. It can be a color code over the public addressing system or a separate sound and light alarm system. The advantage of this alerting pathway is the removal of human response, telephone delays, and communication errors. We use a red light with alarm for category 1 cesarean (urgent) and a yellow one to call for category 2 cesareans [the National Confidential Enquiry into Patient Outcome and Death (NCEPOD) classification of urgency of cesareans][12] as shown in Figure 6.

AUDITS, MATERNITY DASHBOARD FOR SAFETY

The quality indicators for an L and D unit can be divided into workforce, maternal and fetal morbidity, mortality related or can be process-related complaints. The indicators can be added by the team, for example surgical site infection rates, or breastfeeding at birth, to allow an audit cycle coming into play for this parameter. Display of results to the team allows each one to become a part of the quality improvement program (Fig. 5). The Obstetric Dashboard concept was first presented by the Royal College of Obstetricians and Gynaecologists and has since been adapted and modified by many.[13] The concept of

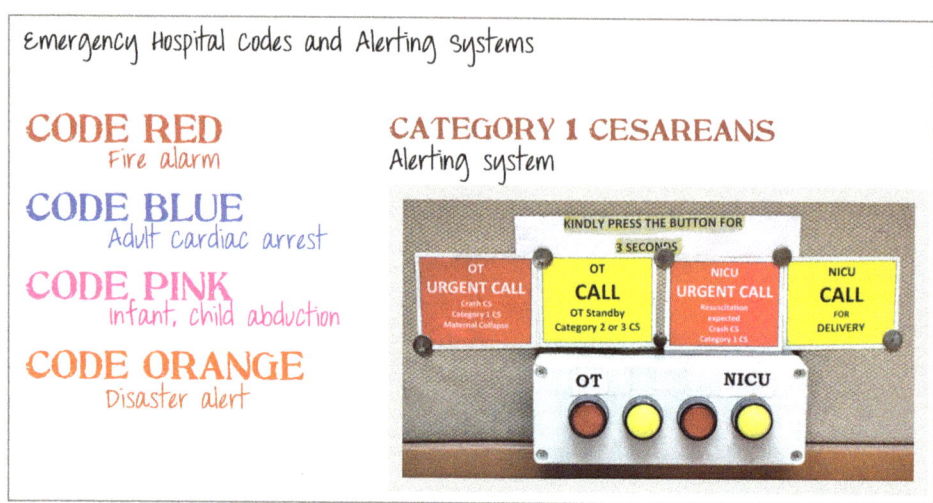

Fig. 6: Emergency codes and alerting systems.

green, amber and red coding for each of the indicators allows a color-based attention to the indicators which need urgent attention.

CHECKLISTS FOR SAFETY

The number of diagnosis, the pathways, and emergency responses is so varied and so many that it is humanly impossible to memorize and reproduce them when needed. It is also a known human factor that we are not at our best when we find ourselves in a stressful situation. Checklists are very helpful to ensure that no step is omitted and to ensure all steps are done in a particular order.[5] The checklist can be with a verbal prompt in emergencies such as PPH (see Fig. 4). Checklists are also an excellent tool to document the events that have taken place, a tool of medicolegal importance. The checklists commonly used in obstetrics are the WHO childbirth checklist, PPH, eclampsia, shoulder dystocia, adherent placenta, obstetric anal sphincter repair or to document events accurately like vaginal births, CSs or instrumental delivery.

CLINICAL RISK MANAGEMENT FOR SAFETY

Principles of safety also encompass strategies for identification and prevention of harm to patients; unintentional harm. Hospital systems can expose patients to a multitude of errors; a human error or a process or a system error. Errors are an effect of consequences rather than causes and need to be minimized by placement of systems which ensure that errors are prevented. Clinical risk management (CRM) system ensures there is an open and free environment of reporting of errors or deviations from protocol and adverse outcomes. Anonymous reporting through slips and boxes placed in all nursing stations have been a very good feedback system for us for many years (see Fig. 5). The reporting should be acknowledged and appreciated for CRM leads to improvement of processes and rectifies errors. CRM committee is a multispecialty management team which then disseminates the learning points to the team.[14]

BACKUPS

It is better to have a backup plan B if the initial plan A fails. It is the team leader or coordinator's responsibility to have backups planned and available when needed. Unavailability was found to be one of the factors quoted in adverse outcomes. It may mean backup of beds, staff, equipment, electricity or expertise. Safe places have backups and emergency exit plans.

MIDWIFERY TEAM AS SAFETY PRINCIPLE

Improving safety in our maternity services is the only way to improve the maternal mortality and morbidity. Teams with midwifery services are much safer that those without. Midwifery services have been shown to have a major impact on reduction of morbidity.[15] Risk stratification and midwifery care for the low-risk patients allow the obstetricians to focus on high-risk pregnancies and care.

CONTINUOUS SUPPORT IN LABOR AS SAFETY FOR MOTHER

A support person in labor was designated as one of the most effective interventions in obstetric care, for improving outcomes. Not allowing a support person with a laboring mother is one of the worst practices that have to be addressed and eradicated as a priority. The supporting person is an advocate for the mother's safety and promotes respectful care. The evidence for having a birth partner or support person is overwhelming and cannot be ignored.[16]

WHAT IS A SAFE LABOR WARD? CONCLUSION

A woman entering the L and D is apprehensive, hopes to birth without any medical interventions, expects to be respected, cared for and monitored for any deviation from the normal. The care we provide should be woman centered, respecting her culture, preferences and choices. Maternity care should be safe, and capable of dealing with the most adverse complication that may arise for her or her baby.

REFERENCES

1. Royal College of Obstetricians and Gynaecologists, Royal College of Midwives, Royal College of Anaesthetists, Royal College of Paediatrics and Child Health. Safer Childbirth: Minimum Standards for the Organisation and Delivery of Care in Labour. London: RCOG Press. 2007.
2. ICU and HDU guidelines. National Health Mission. Ministry of Health and Family Welfare, Government of India; 2016.
3. Department of Defense Space Planning Criteria. Chapter 420: Labor and Delivery/Obstetric Units. 2015.
4. LAQSHYA. Labour room quality improvement initiative. National Health Mission. Ministry of Health and Family Welfare, Government of India. 2017.
5. World Health Organization. WHO Safe Childbirth Checklist Implementation Guide: Improving the Quality of Facility-based Delivery for Mothers and Newborns; 2015.
6. Vencken P, van Hooff M, van der Weiden R. Cardiac arrest in pregnancy: increasing use of perimortem caesarean section due to emergency skills training? BJOG. 2010;117: 1664-5.
7. National Institute for Health and Care Excellence. Safe midwifery staffing for maternity settings. NICE guideline; 2015.
8. Royal College of Obstetricians and Gynecologists. Labour Ward Solutions. Good Practice No. 10; 2010.
9. World Health Organization. Trends in maternal mortality: 1990–2008, estimates developed by WHO, UNFPA, UNICEF and the World Bank, Geneva; 2010.

10. Achrekar MS, Murthy V, Kanan S, et al. Introduction of situation, background, assessment, recommendation into nursing practice: a prospective study. Asia Pac J Oncol Nurs. 2016;3(1):45-50.
11. Manning ML. Improving clinical communication through structured conversation. Nurs Econ. 2006;24(5):268-71.
12. Royal College of Obstetricians and Gynaecologists. Classification of Urgency of Caesarean Section: A Continuum of Risk. Good Practice No. 11; 2010.
13. Chandraharan E, Arulkumaran S. The role of clinical dashboards in improving patient care: experience with the 'maternity dashboard'. Ceylon Med J. 2016;61:83-5.
14. Farokhzadian J, Dehghan Nayeri N, Borhani F. Assessment of clinical risk management system in hospitals: an approach for quality improvement. Glob J Health Sci. 2015;7(5):294-303.
15. Horton R, Astudillo O. The power of midwifery. Lancet. 2014;385:1075-6.
16. Bohren MA, Hofmeyr GJ, Sakala C, et al. Continuous support for women during childbirth. Cochrane Database Syst Rev. 2017;7:CD003766.

Clinical Governance: Standard Operating Procedure for Obstetric Hemorrhage

Muralidhar V Pai

■ POSTPARTUM HEMORRHAGE

Preamble

Postpartum hemorrhage (PPH) is still the leading cause of maternal death in both urban and rural India. Quantitatively, it is defined as bleeding from the genital tract after the delivery of the baby, in excess of 500 mL, after vaginal delivery and 1,000 mL, and after cesarean delivery. Qualitative definition is more important in day-to-day practice, as it is difficult to measure the exact amount of bleeding all the time and everywhere. Qualitatively, PPH is one which pushes the patient into shock. However, one should not wait till she goes into shock. In fact, the aim of every obstetrician should be to prevent the PPH. Once PPH occurs, it should be managed swiftly and aggressively else it can be life threatening. The definition obviously includes third stage bleeding due to retained placenta and bleeding after the delivery of placenta due to any reason such as atonicity, inversion, trauma, coagulation failure, or combination of all. Hence, the standard operating procedure (SOP) should address all these issues.

The SOP cannot be same at different levels of care; for example, at primary care level, for that matter even at secondary care level, the aim is quick assessment, initiation of treatment, and transferring the patient to tertiary care as early as possible. Whereas at tertiary care level, it is more of definitive management including intensive care unit (ICU), if needed. The different levels of care of SOP are shown in Flowchart 1 as an algorithm.

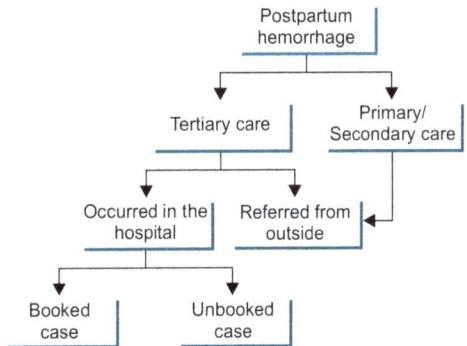

Flowchart 1: Levels of care.

Standard Operating Procedure Primary or Secondary Care Level

- *Anticipation:* PPH can occur in any lady, especially high-risk women, hence, it is prudent to anticipate it and be prepared to prevent or tackle it.
  - Anticipate PPH in grand multi, anemic patients (multiple pregnancy and placenta previa should not be handled at this level).
  - If blood group and type and recent hemoglobin (Hb) of the patient are not known, draw blood for the same as soon as the patient comes in labor. Send for typing and cross matching.
  - It is always better to have an intravenous (IV) line ready, even if IV fluids are not given during labor, as it is difficult to insert the line when PPH occurs and veins are collapsed.
- *Prevention*: Follow principles of active management of third stage of labor:

- Administer 10 units of oxytocin intramuscularly, either at the time of delivery of the shoulder or within 1 minute of the delivery of the baby.
- Perform controlled cord traction as the signs of separation of cord appear (if placenta is not separated start 5 units of oxytocin infusion. If placenta is not delivered despite waiting for 30 minutes diagnose. Retained placenta and refer to tertiary care center).
- Massage the uterus.
- *Treatment:* Despite active management of third stage, if PPH occurs:
  - Quickly assess the pulse and BP and make sure that the patient is not collapsed.
  - Quickly assess if it is due to atonicity or trauma or both.
  - Next steps should be simultaneously and not one after another even though they are given in different bullets.
  - If uterus is atonic:
    - Continue massaging the uterus, one may even try bimanual compression of the uterus.
    - Administer 0.2 mg of ergometrine intramuscular (IM) (may repeat every 15 minutes up to a maximum of 5 doses) or injection PGF2α 250 μg IM (may repeat every 15 minutes to a maximum of 8 doses). Ergometrine and PGF2α may be given alternatively every 15 minutes.
    - Insert 600 μg misoprostol per rectally, if available.
  - If there are any obvious vaginal or cervical tears, start suturing them promptly.
  - Run the IV fluid fast.
  - Second line may be started to transfuse blood products, if available.
  - Insert an indwelling Foley's catheter to measure the urine output.
  - Meanwhile inform nearby tertiary care hospital about the case and ask them to be prepared to receive the patient.
  - If all pharmacological methods fail, any of the following methods may be adopted to transfer the patient to tertiary care hospital:
    - Packing the uterus with sterile roller gauge or a towel.
    - Condom catheter or Bukri balloon.
    - Pneumatic suits, if available may be applied.
  - It is better, if a medical staff or nurse accompanies the patient to tertiary care hospital.

Standard Operating Procedure Tertiary Care Level

Whether the PPH occurs in a booked or unbooked case at tertiary care hospital, the SOP from 1 to 3 hours is same as in primary or secondary care level. The additional steps of management in such cases and cases referred from primary/secondary care hospital after initial management include the following:

- If the patient is collapsed:
  - Summon emergency "Code Blue" (in Manipal) and initiate CPR and shock the patient with automated external defibrillator (AED) as required.
  - Keep intubation and central line set ready for team Code Blue to perform intubation and secure central line as necessary.
  - Call the blood bank and initiate massive transfusion protocol.
  - Inform ICU or critical care medicine department and reserve a bed and ventilator for the patient and shift the patient to ICU as early as possible for ionotropic and/or ventilator support.

CHAPTER 4: Clinical Governance: Standard Operating Procedure for Obstetric Hemorrhage

- Seek consultation from transfusion medicine (for blood component therapy), nephrology (for dialysis), and cardiology as the case demands.
- If the patient is relatively stable:
  - Consider emergency uterine artery embolization and prepare the patient accordingly.
- If the patient is neither collapsed nor stable and continues to bleed:
  - If it is a case of retained placenta—consider manual removal placenta under deep general anesthesia by an experienced obstetrician and once complete removal is performed start pharmacological therapy for atonic PPH.
  - If it is a case of inversion of uterus consider manual replacement or hydrostatic method in labor room itself, if such simple methods do not work, consider replacement in OR under anesthesia.
  - If there are vaginal or cervical lacerations, extension of episiotomy and suspected scar rupture, patient is explored in OR under anesthesia and dealt appropriately.
  - If it is a case of atonic PPH, patient is shifted to OR for exploratory laparotomy after proper counseling and informed consent. At laparotomy one of the following may be performed:
    - Stepwise devascularization
    - One of the restrictive stiches such as B lynch suture
    - Internal iliac ligation
    - Peripartum hysterectomy.
- It is important to keep the communication on with the patient and patient relatives at every step and informed consent to be taken for all procedures.

ANTEPARTUM HEMORRHAGE

Preamble

Antepartum hemorrhage (APH) is a potential cause of maternal death whether it is due to placenta previa, abruption placenta, or indeterminate cause. While there is scope for conservative management in cases of hemorrhage due to placenta previa and indeterminate causes, there is no waiting in cases of abruption, placenta as it is a progressive condition, which can be fatal to both fetus and mother. Ideally, all cases of APH should be managed at tertiary care hospital only. The SOP at tertiary care hospital is as follows:

Placenta Previa or APH due to Indeterminate Causes

- Admit the patient and preferably keep the patient in the hospital once the patient presents with APH.
- Determine the type/degree of placenta previa and rule out adherence.
- All major degree placenta previa are for elective cesarean delivery at term, the exact timing depends upon the fetomaternal condition.
- Placenta increta and percreta are preferably managed by elective cesarean section (classical) and hysterectomy in current practice.
- Minor degree previa or others with minimal bleeding are managed conservatively.

Abruptio Placenta

Obstetric management:
- Ascertain the grade of abruption:
  - If it is grade 3 where mother is in danger and usually fetus is dead contemplate immediate delivery:
    - If she is in established labor, one may go ahead with artificial rupture of membrane (ARM) and oxytocin.

- If she is not in labor and cervix is unfavorable, even cesarean delivery is justified for dead baby to save the mother.
- Simultaneous resuscitation of patient with blood component therapy and ICU care as required.
• If mother is stable and fetus is in distress:
  - Immediate cesarean delivery would save the fetus and mother.
• If mother is stable and fetus is not in distress:
  - If she is in labor or having favorable cervix one may induce (ARM + oxytocin) and deliver.
  - If cervix is not favorable or if uterus does not respond to oxytocin then cesarean delivery is prudent to save both fetus and mother.
  - Hysterectomy is indicated only if there is Couvelaire uterus, which is refusing to contract even after delivery.

Maternal resuscitation:
• It goes without saying this should be performed simultaneously with obstetric management and includes similar principles as management of PPH.
  - If patient is collapsed:
    - Summon emergency "Code Blue" (in Manipal) and initiate CPR and shock the patient with AED as required.
    - Keep intubation and central line set ready for team Code Blue to perform intubation and secure central line as necessary.
    - Call the blood bank and initiate massive transfusion protocol.
    - Inform ICU or critical care medicine department and reserve a bed and ventilator for the patient and shift the patient to ICU as early as possible for ionotropic and/or ventilator support.
    - Seek consultation from transfusion medicine (for blood component therapy), nephrology (for dialysis), and cardiology as the case demands.
  - If patient is not collapsed:
    - Send blood for grouping and cross matching, CBC, coagulation profile, and other investigations as necessary [renal function test (RFT), liver function test (LFT), and platelets].
    - Secure IV lines or central lines as per the need of the situation start IV fluids while waiting for blood components to arrive.
    - Transfuse blood components in consultation with transfusion specialists.

5
Chapter

The Obstetric High-dependency Unit: Need of the Hour

Sanjay Gupte, Girija Wagh

INTRODUCTION

The concept of obstetric high-dependency unit (HDU) is comparatively new and has gained major significance today as high-risk pregnancies are on the rise. There are many reasons for this. Obesity epidemic, delaying pregnancies till third and fourth decade, and increased coexistence of diseases like diabetes mellitus and hypertension being some. Advances in fields of organ transplant medicine, heart surgeries, and advanced infertility treatment have added to these. In our country, basic problems like anemia and sepsis continue to persist as important contributory factors. Despite considerable progress made in maternal health, India is still lagging behind in its need for reducing maternal mortality. Activities to facilitate high-quality basic care during childbirth, timely identification and management of complications, and improved monitoring and accountability in basic and emergency obstetric care (EmOC) are important components of the strategy to reduce maternal deaths, especially the ones that can be avoided.

BACKGROUND

In the current scenario, many lacunae are perceived in the overall obstetric management. Therefore, the immediate approach to curb the maternal deaths would be to improve care during life-threatening scenarios arising out of maternal complications. These life-challenging situations, if not addressed through high-quality specialist care in resourced environments may lead to death of the pregnant women, which is preventable. This is where the role of obstetric HDU comes in. Maternal mortality is an important indicator of maternal health. Focusing on institutional delivery has substantially contributed in reducing the maternal mortality rates (MMRs), from 212 in 2007–2009[1] to 167 maternal deaths per 100,000 live births reported in 2011–2013 in a span of 5 years. However, the target for India of 140 maternal deaths per 100,000 live births, which was to be achieved by 2015 under the United Nations-mandated Millennium Development Goals, is still to be achieved. In an excellent review of maternal deaths "Why Mothers Die" meticulously documented and analyzed in the state of Kerala, it was observed that 24% of maternal deaths were as a result of multisystemic affliction and this was in association with hypertensive disorders of pregnancy. Till recent days, the major contributors to maternal deaths predominantly were hemorrhage and sepsis, but recent statewise observations have seen hypertensive disorders to be responsible, especially to the very serious irreversible multiorgan failure. The deaths due to hemorrhage, sepsis, and pregnancy-associated hypertension seem to be leading to the similar endpoint of coagulation and multiorgan failure. Also in such eventualities, it seems that there is a sudden change in events in a shorter duration needing immediate action and quality of advanced care. Looking at the quantum of the maternal deaths and the underlying cause being a complex and sudden occurring disorder like hypertension in pregnancy, HDU care seems to be the appropriate approach. Such a unit seems to be essential to those facilities, which have a good quantum of deliveries, may be more than 3,000 or so per annum. The unit will be able to cater to the level I and II care which may be necessary during the peripartum period and will be able to accommodate the delivery dynamics. The units should have an easy access to the intensive care or an intensive care unit (ICU), if necessary, for example, when a ventilatory support may be essential. Obstetricians should be trained to deal with such medical emergencies and training be offered to nurture such a special interest.[2] Maternal mortality is the penultimate eventuality but represents just the tip of the iceberg. Like the hidden part of the iceberg under the surface lies the vast quantum of those mothers who suffered serious morbidity, did not die but missed death and survived (Fig. 1). The urgent need is to address these clinical situations leading to such near-miss deaths. For every mother who dies, 20–30 more suffer severe disease and disability. Recent World Health Organization systematic review shows worldwide incidence of severe acute morbidity (SAM). SAM is a serious life-threatening pregnancy complication mandating immediate medical assistance or speciality care in order to prevent a possible maternal death. This review identified the occurrence of such SAM from 0.01% to 8.23%. The case fatality ratio was noted to be 0.02–37%.[3] Pregnancy is a dynamic condition in which the clinical situation can deteriorate swiftly, in critical scenarios. This makes the critical care in obstetrics unique. Obstetric patients are generally young and a loss is detrimental to the domestic structure. The younger women respond very well to timely treatment and this has to be delivered promptly and effectively.

THE HIGH-RISK OBSTETRICS

Incidence of high-risk pregnancy is approximately 15% in India, but every pregnant woman has a potential to develop serious life-threatening complications without any advanced warning or sometimes a little

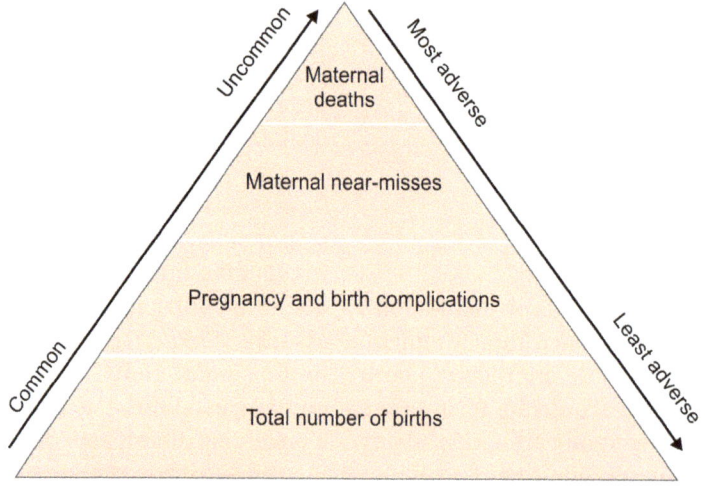

Fig. 1: The maternal safety pyramid and levels of care.[4]

warning. There are two categories of life-threatening conditions in pregnancy. The first set includes obstetric complications like postpartum hemorrhage (PPH), pre-eclampsia, eclampsia, etc. which can be managed by skilled obstetricians providing intensive obstetric care. Second set includes patients with existing comorbid medical conditions and may require multidisciplinary approach. Pregnancy has a potential of modifying the pre-existing disease, e.g. diabetes, heart disease, etc. and more so during delivery the dynamics may change suddenly. Physiological changes of pregnancy can alter the pharmacokinetics and all these can affect the fetoplacental unit and impact the fetus. The obstetric complications are further divided in two types—the first set of complications include obstetric complications like PPH, pre-eclampsia/eclampsia (PE/E), etc. which when severe, require intensive obstetric care by specially trained providers, and the second type of complications include multiorgan involvement/failure which necessitates care provision by intensivist and super-specialists such as those from nephrology, neurology, cardiology, pulmonology, and anesthesia. Critically ill pregnant mothers need a composite quality health care which will have access to all such specialty services including obstetric care complete with timely detection and prompt management. These women need 24 × 7 personalized care by skilled providers, essentially led by obstetricians or EmOC trained providers. For a small proportion of women who have progressed to a clinical condition where there is multiorgan involvement/failure, the care has to be provided in an ICU setting led by intensivists and super-specialists. For the above-mentioned conditions, there is a need for setting up specialized units for appropriate and timely care.

TYPES OF SPECIALIZED CARE UNITS

Intensive Care Unit

Intensive care unit is a specialized area of the hospital dedicated to management of critically sick patient, injuries or complications. This is that area of the facility, which is structured, equipped, and staffed in accordance and is placed in a fashion so as to be accessible to provide such a care optimally. The staff and the infrastructure are dedicated to critical care services.

Obstetric ICU is an exclusive ICU facility, which also accommodates obstetric care and is dedicated to mothers who are critically ill and have developed multisystemic abnormalities or multiorgan failure necessitating specialized care by super-specialists like intensivist/nephrologist/cardiologist, pulmonologist/endocrinologist, etc.

High-dependency Unit

High-dependency unit is a middle level infrastructure where concentrated care is offered at a level above the normal in-hospital care with close monitoring. This can be considered as an intermediate care unit between the obstetric ICU and the regular hospital care. Mothers admitted in an HDU may need an ICU if they have multiorgan serious disorder. Mothers who have been stabilized in the ICU can be observed in the HDU as a stepdown care.

THE NEED OF OBSTETRIC HDUS IN INDIA

In India, most of the public health facilities do not have a separate special care unit for high-risk pregnancies and postpartum mothers with complications. Such women are being managed in the labor room, without dedicated team(s) of competent providers and appropriately equipped facilities. To further bring down the MMR, a dedicated facility offering skill-based critical care services, with state-of-the-art infrastructure, technical support, and a team of appropriately trained professionals are the need of the hour. Life-threatening complications are a sudden occurrence during pregnancy and women are at the potential risk to do so. High-risk pregnancy contributes to 7–8% of pregnancy complications. Underlying medical conditions are identified as risk for pregnancy and can get modified to severity due to pregnancy. Likewise pregnancy can get adversely influenced by the medical condition.

Comprehensive guidelines for obstetric HDU and ICU in 2016 have been devised by the Government of India, which are worth emulating.

The HDU Concept

A dedicated area for management of high-risk antenatal, intranatal, and postnatal mothers requiring attentive monitoring is the need of the hour. The unit should be able to provide any intervention if such a need arises and should be staffed by an appropriately trained personnel. Obstetric HDU is a part of the maternity wing and located near the labor room and operation theater, for easy and prompt shifting of the patient whenever required. The guidelines recommend that mothers having complications should be universally managed in obstetric HDU; a step-down/step-up and intermediate care unit between labor room and ICU.[5] The Government of India guidelines suggest that the district hospitals catering as referral to the primary health centers (PHCs) and first referral units (FRUs) should have obstetric HDUs while hospitals affiliated to the medical colleges should have obstetric HDU as well as an obstetric ICU or ICU with beds and facilities allocated to obstetric critical care. These operational guidelines have mentioned the further dissemination of the movement of creating obstetric HDU services to the PHCs and the community rehabilitation centers (CRCs) based on the volume of obstetric services that they cater to. The patient flow should be systematic such that after initial assessment in the examination room (of triage area), if the facility is a district level, medical college or a tertiary care center, pregnancies with complications may be managed in the obstetric HDU. Facilities not equipped to deal with high-risk mothers, after triaging, the complicated cases should be closely monitored by an obstetrician or EmOC trained medical officer or transferred with stabilization and with attendance. Cases identified to be low risk after triaging, can be delivered by a skilled birth attendant (SBA) (preferably with a backup support of an obstetrician/EmOC trained medical officer). It is suggested that every medical college should have dedicated obstetric ICUs or beds earmarked/dedicated beds in their ICUs for care of obstetric cases, which have developed multiorgan failure/complications. If resources permit, it is recommended that every medical college should have at least four bedded obstetric ICU attached to the obstetric HDU. The states have the flexibility to establish more need-based obstetric HDUs/obstetric ICUs in high case load facilities, subject to fulfilling the mandated prerequisites. Even in private setups where obstetrics load is high, one should think of setting up HDUs. However, in the small private hospitals, many times there are space constraints and it is also difficult to sustain multispecialty trained staff. In these situations, tie-up for HDU or ICU care with larger local hospital is a reasonable compromise.

Mothers Requiring HDU Admission

Patients with following parameters require admission in obstetric HDU/ICU (Table 1).
- Anemia (severe) and associated complications.
- *Severe hypertension:* Systolic blood pressure (SBP) 160 mm Hg and/or diastolic blood pressure of 110 mm Hg or mean arterial pressure of 110 mm Hg or more. Women with lower blood pressures but with severe features of pre-eclampsia and eclampsia.
- Sepsis and infections.
- Obstetric hemorrhage cases including morbidly adherent placenta.
- *Organ dysfunction:* Renal failure, jaundice, hepatitis, acute respiratory distress syndrome (ARDS), and cardiomyopathy.
- Heart disease.
- Severe hyperglycemia of pregnancy and associated complications.
- Risk of thromboembolism.
- Obesity and thyrotoxicosis.
- Any other clinical situations needing close surveillance and intermediary care.
- Women receiving tocolysis, thromboprophylaxis, etc.
- Fetuses such as fetal growth restriction (FGR), macrosomia needing close surveillance and be individualized to be managed in HDU.

PROTOCOLS AND PRACTICES FOR THE HDU

It is a good practice to devise some important protocols and practices for optimum management of HDU.

Protocols
- Hypertensive crisis and eclampsia
- Hypotension especially management of hemorrhagic shock
- Tocolysis
- Primary resuscitation
- Massive transfusion protocol

TABLE 1: Indications for HDU care.

Obstetric complications	Pregnancy with medical complications
Pregnancy with severe anemia Hb < 7 g%	Pregnancy with GDM uncontrolled
Antepartum hemorrhage	Pregnancy with cardiac disease
Postpartum hemorrhage: Atonic, traumatic	Pregnancy with liver disorders
Severe pre-eclampsia, eclampsia, HELLP syndrome	Pregnancy with fever, dengue, malaria, urinary tract infection, upper respiratory tract infection, septic shock
Ruptured ectopic pregnancy	Pregnancy with pulmonary edema
Multiple gestation with complications	Pregnancy with renal disorders, ARF
Preterm labor requiring active tocolysis and monitoring	Pregnancy with acute abdomen
Postoperative patients requiring hemodynamic monitoring or intensive nursing care	Pregnancy with trauma, poisoning, asthma, H1N1 pneumonia
Any need-based admissions based upon the judgment of the obstetrician.	

(ARF: acute renal failure; Hb: hemoglobin; HDU: high-dependency unit; HELLP: hemolysis, elevated liver enzymes, and low platelet count; GDM: gestational diabetes mellitus)

- Septic shock identification and management, etc.

All these are to be managed in algorithmic fashion.

Practices

Some important practices can help increase the efficiency of the HDU care:
- Use of infusion pump
- Nonpneumatic anti-shock garments
- Subclavian vein access
- Emergency tracheostomy
- Fast-track access to critical care
- Pressure pump for fast transfusion
- Balloon tamponade for atonic PPH
- Warming blankets
- Antibiotic policy
- Fluid management
- Access to blood and component therapy.

Epidemiological evidences have revealed unequal distribution of maternal health services and outcomes. The difference is more evident in the poorer and the inaccessible parts of the country.[6] There may be an overall improvement in the maternal mortality ratios but these disadvantaged sectors could be still contributing in the same proportion and still deprived of the improvised quality of care. Comparing the outcomes within the social stratus and the communities could probably help to analyze such trends and much of the interests today seem to be focusing on such a specific analysis. In India, we have seen that economically backward states have much higher maternal mortality than most of the southern states. So in our country not only setting up HDUs is the need of the hour but while doing so we need to look at correcting the regional inequalities and choosing the right places where they will be most effective.

■ PERSONAL EXPERIENCE

The high-risk pregnancy and critical care in obstetric unit was set up in Bharati Hospital on 14th January 2019. The basic aim was to formulate a strategy to care for the high-risk mothers. In previous reviews, capacity of the system to address obstetric emergencies and resultant life-threatening complications was found to be inadequate.

The obstetric HDU has six specialized beds with multipara monitors, noninvasive blood pressure (NIBP) monitors, oxygen, and suction. Bharati Hospital is one of the few in the city of Pune to possess a dedicated obstetric HDU. Since the inception, the admissions in the HDU reached a staggering 103 within a span of 100 days. On an average,

TABLE 2: Indications of admission to HDU at our center (BHRC, Pune).

Etiologies for HDU admission	
Indications	Number of HDU admissions
Hypertensive disorders of pregnancy	63
Eclampsia	7
Dibetes	13
Cardiac disease	9
Obesity	8
Ectopic pregnancy	4
Severe anemia	12
Sepsis	5
Liver disorders HELLP syndrome	8
Abruptio placentae	11
Placenta previa	3
Postpartum hemorrhage	7
Obstetric hysterectomy	4
Acute kidney injury	4
ARDS	7
Rupture uterus	1

(ARDS: acute respiratory distress syndrome; HDU: high-dependency unit; HELLP: hemolysis, elevated liver enzymes, and low platelet count)

TABLE 3: Academic activities of the HDU at BHRC.

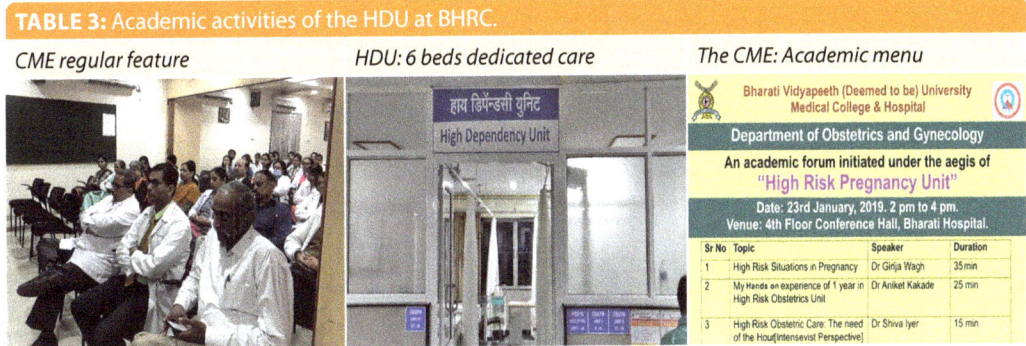

(CME: continuing medical education; HDU: high-dependency unit)

there was one high-risk mother who required HDU care and monitoring per day. 103 high-risk mothers were benefitted with the HDU services. 50 patients (48.5%) were referred from consultants and hospitals in and around Bharati Hospital. The indications for admission to the HDU are seen in the Table 2.

Hypertensive disorders in pregnancy are on the rise and the increasing need for HDU care in these needs to be registered. The unit functions as a joint activity of all the main units. It is headed by a professor and day-to-day working is managed by faculty trained in critical care in obstetrics. Fellows under the university and the Indian College of Obstetricians and Gynaecologists (ICOG) fellowship (we are the second recognized center in the country) are the other important specialized resource. Such focused and advanced approach has helped us in offering quality care, increased access for other facilities, and learning opportunities to our students and has encouraged training through fellowships. Regular continuing medical education (CME) (Table 3) for academic interaction is an ongoing feature of the HDU center and it has led to creation of newer approach to the concept of HDU.

REFERENCES

1. Registrar General of India. Special bulletin on maternal mortality in India 2007-2009. New Delhi: Office of the Registrar General; 2011.
2. Kerala Federation of Obstetrics and Gynecology (KFOG). Second report of confidential review of maternal deaths, Kerala. Why Mothers Die, Kerala 2006–2009. Kerala: KFOG; 2012.
3. Mittal P. Concept of critical care in obstetrics. Practical Approach to Critical Care in Obstetrics; 2018.
4. Ramarajan A. The obstetric high-dependency unit (HDU). Severe Acute Maternal Mortality. New Delhi: Jaypee Brothers Medical Publishers (P) Ltd; 2011. pp. 37-40.
5. NHM. (2016). Guidelines for Obstetric HDU and ICU. [online] Available from: https://nrhm.gujarat.gov.in/images/pdf/Obstetric-ICU-National-Guidelines.pdf [Last accessed July, 2019].
6. Houweling TA, Ronsmans C, Campbell OM, et al. Huge poor-rich inequalities in maternity care: an international comparative study of maternity and child care in developing countries. Bull World Health Organ. 2007;85(10):745-54.

6 Obstetric Hemorrhage: Prevention and Management (Golden Hour)

MB Bellad

A profuse hemorrhage occurring prior to or shortly after the birth of the child is always dangerous and not infrequently a fatal complication.
—*J Whitridge Williams (1903).*

INTRODUCTION

Obstetrics is a bloody business as rightly said. Following are the important causes of obstetric hemorrhage excluding accidental and incidental causes.

Obstetric hemorrhage with hypertension and infection to be one of the dangerous "triad" of maternal death causes. It also is a leading cause for admission of pregnant and postpartum women to intensive care units.

- *Bleeding in early pregnancy:* Miscarriage related, ectopic pregnancy, molar pregnancy, and others.
- *Antepartum hemorrhage (APH):* Placenta previa, abruptio placenta, and others.
- *Postpartum hemorrhage (PPH):* 4 Ts—(1) tone, (2) trauma, (3) tissue, and (4) thrombin.

Shock index (SI): Heart rate or systolic blood pressure (SBP).

This is an important that helps in the management even when the hypertensive woman who after bleeding still has normal range of blood pressure.

Shock index:
1. < 0.9 = Normal
2. 0.9–1.69 = Mild shock
3. >1.7 = Severe shock, this is a very simple and practical guide for assessment and resuscitation of shock.

BLEEDING IN EARLY PREGNANCY

Three important causes—(1) miscarriage (abortion), (2) ectopic pregnancy, and (3) molar pregnancy.

Prevention in General

Optimal age of conception plays an important role as extremes of reproductive ages are associated with increased chromosomal defects.

Preconceptional health and care: Optimal state of health at the entry of pregnancy is single important factor for good pregnancy outcome. Treatment and correction of common health conditions like anemia, hypothyroidism, hyperglycemia, and other conditions (that impair both maternal health, conception, embryo, and fetus) play an important role to ensure healthy pregnancy. Immunization against rubella is important.

To ensure good health, of women before and during pregnancy, it is important to give good health facilities and adequate nutrition to the girl child and adolescent. In government surveys, eligible couple survey should be used to ensure this.

Case Scenario 1

Miscarriage or Abortion Related

A short of amenorrhea followed by bleeding is generally the woman presents. Diagnosis is very important. If abortion or miscarriage, history, examination, and investigations like ultrasonography (USG) and beta human chorionic gonadotropin (hCG) play an important role.

Diagnosis is basically:
- *Threatened miscarriage:* Slight bleeding or spotting with short period of amenorrhea with good maternal and fetal or embryonic status. However, she needs reassurance and careful observation under supervision.
- *Inevitable miscarriage:* Short period of amenorrhea with significant bleeding may be with clots and cervical os dilated with may be products in canal, USG confirms. Assessment of blood loss by pulse, blood pressure (BP) and appearance [air hunger (breathlessness), pallor, soaked clothes] and how she has entered to the facility, i.e. walked in or brought on stretcher. Management generally includes resuscitation and completion of the process of the miscarriage.
- *Incomplete abortion:* Presents as in inevitable miscarriage with additional blood loss and with history of passage of products, generally confirmed by USG. May be woman in shock or altered vitals. Need to resuscitate with fluid and blood and complete the process of miscarriage.
- *Complete miscarriage:* Woman generally presents with short period of amenorrhea and bleeding with expulsion of products of conception with presently no active bleeding. USG is confirmative. Woman may be in shock, simultaneous resuscitation and management of shock play an important role in saving the woman.

Case Scenario 2

Unruptured Ectopic Pregnancy

Any woman of reproductive age, who presents with abdominal pain with altered menstrual pattern (not always necessary to have amenorrhea) one needs to suspect ectopic pregnancy unless proved otherwise. History of frequent blackouts suggestive of vasovagal stimulation (due to stretching of peritoneum of mesosalpinx) assists in suspecting ectopic pregnancy. Urine pregnancy test kit will help to diagnose pregnancy, USG along with beta-hCG helps in diagnosis of unruptured ectopic pregnancy. It is important to note the critical level of beta-hCG with USG (level of 1,500 mIU must visualize intrauterine pregnancy exception multiple pregnancy and molar pregnancy). Appropriate rise of beta-hCG (>66% increase in 48 hours) confirms intrauterine pregnancy, rise in beta-hCG but lesser (<66%) suggest unruptured ectopic pregnancy. Falling beta-hCG generally suggests miscarriage or missed abortion.

Case Scenario 3

Ruptured Ectopic Pregnancy

Symptoms as above along with severe abdominal pain with or without shock, usually brought by in a state of shock at times admitted in other departments. Any woman of reproductive age group married, otherwise or even tubectomized presents with severe pain abdomen one should suspect ruptured ectopic pregnancy confirm by USG along with urine pregnancy test or beta-hCG. Approach to such a woman is usually resuscitation followed by surgery (laparoscopy or laparotomy depending upon hemodynamic state).

Molar Pregnancy

History of short period of amenorrhea with hyperemesis gravidarum may be frequent bleeding or spotting episodes. The ultrasound picture in molar pregnancy typically shows a snow storm appearance. The β-hCG levels are raised. Resuscitation along with evacuation is the treatment of choice.

ANTEPARTUM HEMORRHAGE

Bleeding per vagina during pregnancy after the period of viability till the onset of labor (before labor). Two important causes that affect the condition of the mother and the baby are abruptio placenta and placenta praevia. Other causes like vasa previa and circumvallate placenta are rare but not significantly associated with maternal condition.

Case Scenario 4

A gravida 3 para 2 living 2 presents with (24–36 weeks amenorrhea) 28 weeks of pregnancy with bleeding per vagina. No history of pain in abdomen. On examination, her general condition is good, uterus is nontender and relaxed, and fetus is in good condition.

Another case may present in a state of shock with above period of gestation without pain in abdomen.

Placenta Previa

Diagnosis generally based on clinical history and examination, confirmed usually by ultrasonography. Usually, history of early pregnancy bleeding favors the diagnosis. Generally, first bout of bleeding is not significant but can be, called as warning hemorrhage. At times, the bleeding is severe and put both mother and fetus in jeopardy. Generally, expectant line of management is given in a woman where the maternal and fetal condition is good, preterm pregnancy with normal fetus (without lethal anomaly) in a center where 24 hours emergency service including blood transfusion is available.

When the bleeding is severe generally resuscitative measures and surgical interventions are taken. Resuscitative measures are described later (Annexure-1).

Case Scenario 5

A primigravida presents with (24–36 weeks amenorrhea) 28 weeks of pregnancy with bleeding per vagina, with history of pain in abdomen, and with loss of fetal movements.

On examination, her general condition depends upon the amount of blood loss and her blood pressure depends upon amount of blood loss and prior blood pressure. In such situations, SI helps as the woman may be in shock yet BP may be in normal range.

Abruptio Placenta

This is another important cause of APH and is dangerous for both fetus and matter. Generally, there is an associated risk factor in the form of hypertension. SI generally helps to know even when the blood pressure is in normal range (generally woman may be hypertensive prior to this episode). The duration between the onset of abruption and delivery is directly proportional to the morbidity and mortality. Earlier the delivery, better the prognosis. History examination and investigations including USG help in the diagnosis and management. Differentiation between the two conditions *(placenta previa and abruptio placenta)* is essential for the management. Resuscitation along with coagulation status is important along with renal condition. Management includes prompt resuscitation and earlier delivery with the close monitoring on the coagulation and renal function.

Case Scenario 6

A gravida 3, para 2, living 2 delivered in a primary health center and started bleeding per vagina.

POSTPARTUM HEMORRHAGE

No woman is immune to PPH. This is one of the important causes of maternal mortality and morbidity with interval between the occurrence and death is 2 hours. Hence, prevention diagnosis and prompt treatment/referral are essential to prevent morbidity and mortality.

Prediction

- *Antenatal*: Age—>35 years, Asians, BMI—>27, diabetes, macrosomia, multiple pregnancy, fibroids, APH, previous history of PPH, previous lower segment cesarean section (LSCS), adherent placenta, and placenta previa.
- *Intranatal*: Induced labors—>18 hours, prolonged labor, labor analgesia, GA V/s spinal, instrumentation, LSCS—more bleeding in emergency than elective, big baby and manipulations, vaginal delivery—instrumental and with episiotomy—more bleeding.

Prevention

Actually, this starts antenatal period itself (to improve the health status and recognize high risk factors, *although in two-thirds PPH occurs in low risk women*). Treatment and prevention of anemia is important. Recognition of adherent placenta by ultrasonography is also an important component.

All deliveries by skilled birth attendants in hospitals, use partogram to prevent prolonged labor, follow active management of third stage of labor (AMTSL) in every delivery.

Components of AMSTL

- Administer uterotonic (oxytocin-10 IU) as early as possible (within 1 min)—intramuscularly
- Clamp the cord after cessation of pulsations in healthy newborn—delayed clamping of the cord
- Controlled cord traction with the onset of uterine contraction
- Examination of the placenta to ensure its completeness
- Palpate the uterus periodically (at every 10-15 minute) to ensure contracted and retracted uterus for at least 2 hours
- Close observation of the woman at least 2-4 hours after vaginal delivery and up-to 24 hours following operative delivery.

Diagnosis of PPH

Diagnosis mainly clinical, usually *PR BP*, by the time signs appear 25%, blood loss has occurred (Annexure 2). Diagnosis can be assisted by keeping the used gauze and mops/BRASS-V Drape (Fig. 1). Close observation—as slow trickling is highly dangerous.

Close Watch on the Blood Loss

Visual estimation is poor. Calculation of blood loss can be done from soaked mops/gauzes, Clothes (standardized visual estimation) or BRASS-V Drape. Monitor the pulse and BP closely—the change in the vital signs indicates already significant blood loss, which is most common.

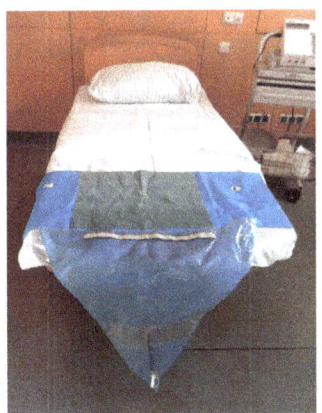 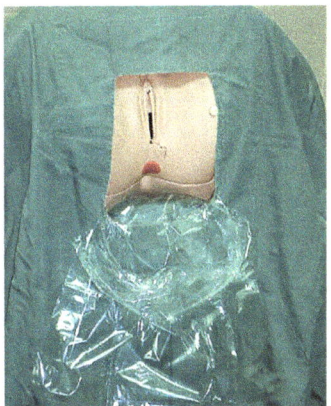

Fig. 1: BRASS-V Drape.

Measure Blood Loss—Drape

Helps early identification—timely intervention.

How to Recognize?

Appearance of clinical signs indicates >25% blood loss (Tables 1 and 2).

What is PPH?

Volumetric > 500 mL,
Hemodynamic change: pulse and blood pressure.
Change in hematocrit: > 10%,
Blood loss: > 500 mL—PPH,
> 1000 mL—severe PPH,
1,500 mL—LSCS.

How to Classify the PPH?

- *Primary (<24 hours):* Tone—70-80%, trauma—10-20%, tissue—9-10%, and thrombin—<1%
- *Secondary (>24 hours):* Uterine infection, retained placental fragments, and abnormal involution of placental site.

Principles to Prevent PPH Morbidity and Mortality

Anticipate PPH in every woman in labor, all deliveries with skilled birth attendant, uterotonics in third stage, IV access and blood samples, and blood group must be known; keep emergency tray (crash kit) and team involvement.

TABLE 1: Stages of shock.

Classification	Stage 1	Stage 2	Stage 3	Stage 4
Blood loss (% volume lost)	10–15	15–30	30–40	>40
Conscious state	Alert, mild thirst	Anxious and restless	Agitated or confused	Drowsy, confused or unconscious
Respiratory rate	Normal	Mildly elevated	Raised	Raised
Complexion	Normal	Pale	Pale	Marked pallor or gray
Extremities	Normal	Cool	Pale and cool	Cold
Capillary refill	Normal	Slow (>2s)	Slow (>2s)	Minimal or absent
Pulse rate	Normal	Normal	Elevated	Fast but thready
Systolic blood pressure	Normal	Normal	Normal or slightly low	Hypotensive
Urine output	Normal	Reduced	Reduced	Oligoanuric

TABLE 2: Modified early obstetric warning score.

	Score						
	3	2	1	0	1	2	3
Respiratory rate (bpm)		<8		9–18	19–25	26–30	>30
Pulse rate (bpm)	<70	<40	40–50	51–100	101–110	111–129	>129
Systolic blood pressure (mm Hg)		71–80	81–100	101–164	165–200	>200	
Diastolic blood pressure (mm Hg)				<95	95–104	>105	
Conscious level	Unresponsive	Responds to pain	Responds to voice	Alert	Irritated		
Urine hourly (mL/h) or in 24 h	0	<30 (<720 mL)	<45 (<1000 mL)	>45 (>1000 mL)			

Source: Dr R Jones, Consultant Anesthetist, Royal Berkshire Hospital, UK

How to Approach?

Evaluation, diagnosis, resuscitation, and management must occur simultaneously.

How to Diagnose?

Find the cause and to assess the condition, per abdominal examination, presence or absence—well contracted and retracted uterus, proper blood-loss estimation/assessment is the key. Exploration with good light and assistant for traumatic PPH, and bedside sonography to look for retained products. Placenta, pulse, blood pressure, respiratory rate, and extremities.

Fluid Therapy

Initially, start preferably *two IV* lines with wide bore cannulae (16 or 18) (Fig. 2) draw blood for investigations, NS, RL (crystalloids), and later colloids, till the blood is available with uterotonic drugs, blood, and other blood components (Figs. 3 to 6). The team must have their defined roles, e.g. management, record keeping, monitoring, drugs and fluid records, counseling/consenting, transport arrangements, blood and other components records, etc.

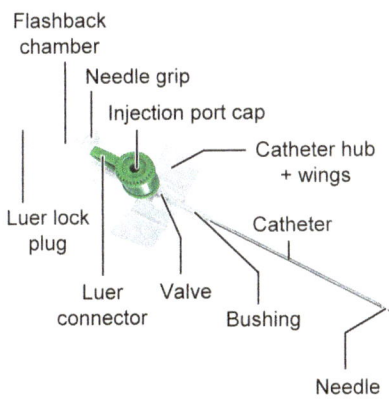

Color	Gauge	Flow/Rate mls/min	Type of infusion
Orange	14	343	• Rapid blood transfusion • Emergencies
Gray	16	196	• Rapid blood transfusion • Emergencies
Green	18	90	Blood produces, medicines, fluids
Pink	20	61	General crystalloid use
Blue	22	36	Pediatrics, oncology

Fig. 2: IV cannulae: Gauge and low rate.

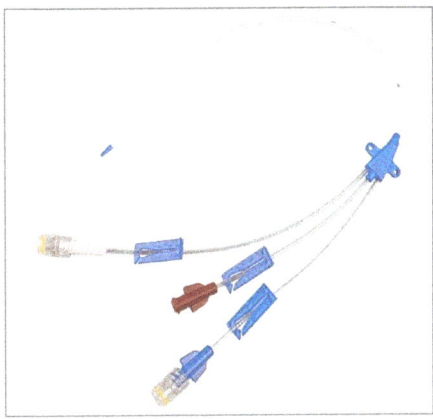

Fig. 3: Central venous catheters.

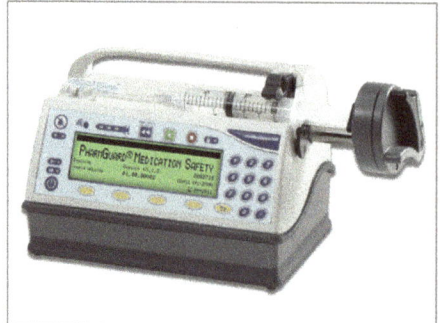

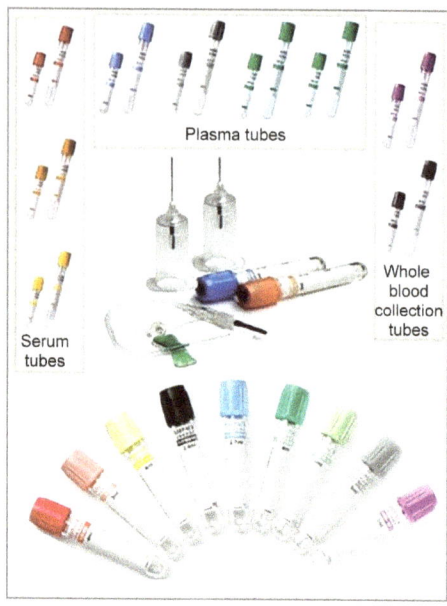

Fig. 6: Blood collection vacutainer and tubes.

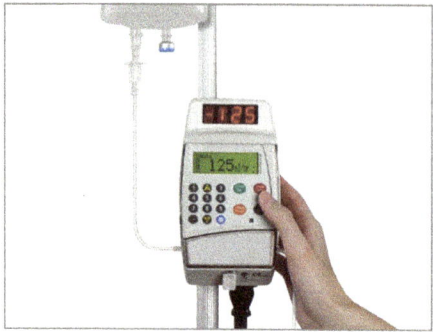

Fig. 4: Infusion syringe pump.

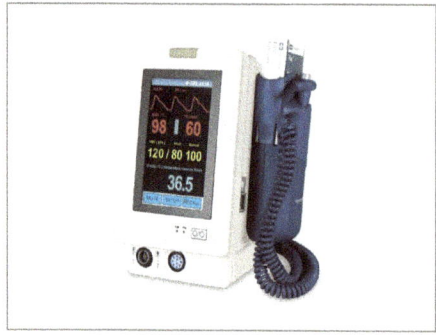

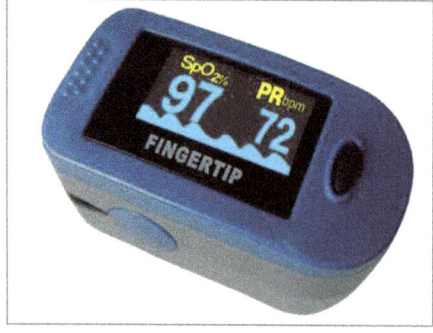

Fig. 5: Noninvasive BP monitoring.

Oxytocin—First-line Drug

First-line drug, nonapeptide, secreted—posterior pituitary, oxytocin receptors—increase last 9 weeks of pregnancy, dose—20 IU/1,000 mL, 10 mL/min till contracts there after 1–2 mL/min. Maximum up to 40 units in 24 hours, routes—IV, IM—10 IU, storage—up to 15–25°.

Direct IV is not advisable—hypotension and vomiting (though two RCTs have proved contrary), have been reported with doses of more than 40 IU. This occurs due to water intoxication effect, and saturation of all the oxytocin receptors.

Dose 20 units intravenous drip, side effects are minimum, injection oxytocin IM 10 units (AMTSL), onset-immediate, duration-20 minutes, side effects—hypotension, antidiuresis, caution—cases with cardiac failure and prone for pulmonary edema (Fig. 7).

Oxytocin Analog—Carbetocin

Carbetocin-1987: Long acting (half-life—40 min), quick onset of action (uterus contacts

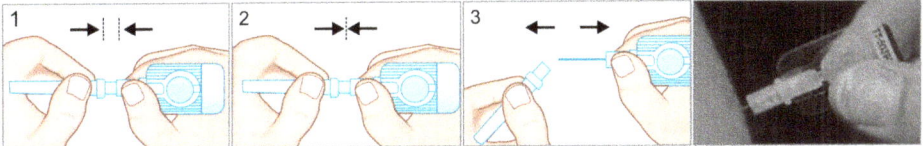

Fig. 7: Uniject—preloaded.

within 2 minutes) with IM/IV, optimal dosage—100 µg, as effective as syntometrine (oxytocin 5 IU +0.5 mg ergometrine), less side effects, expensive, and not available in India.

Recent World Health Organization (WHO) trial (CHAMPION trial) showed that carbetocin is not inferior to oxytocin for prevention of PPH (<500 mL). However, the sample size was inadequate for 1,000 mL blood loss (NEJM June 27th, 2018).

Syntometrine (Oxytocin 5 IU +0.5 mg Ergometrine)

More effective than either oxytocin or methergine alone, more side effects, carbetocin is superior but costly, more commonly used in europe.

Methylergometrine

Intravenous/IM 0.2 mg can be repeated up to five times at interval of 30 min; cannot wait for 2.5 Hours for completion, onset—3-5 min—IM and 1 min for IV, duration—>3 hours, IM and 45 min—IV, more side effects—nausea, vomiting, and hypertension; needs refrigeration (2-80°C), contraindications—hypertension, cardiac disease, etc.

PGF2α (Carboprost)—IM Only

Strong uterotonic, IM 250 µg can be repeated up to eight doses, every 15 minutes—please note the duration required. More side effects—shivering, nausea, vomiting, diarrhea, abdominal cramps, and avoid in asthmatics (bronchospasm), role of intramyometrial use—in shock as peripheral circulation is poor.

Misoprostol (PGE 1 Analog)

Oral/vaginal/sublingual/rectal are accepted routes of administration and have proved to be effective against placebo (Lancet Oct-2006), and are less effective than injectable uterotonics, oral—rapid onset but short lasting. More side effects, vaginal—slower onset, sustained, and longer effect, sublingual—400-600 µg quickest of all routes, more side effects, rectal—least absorbed, can be kept at room temperature.

Misoprostol

Dose 400-1,000 µg (safety margin high), can be given safely in asthmatics and MI, must be tried before surgical intervention is attempted. For prevention—400-800 µg orally immediately after clamping and cutting the cord has been recommended in places where injectables are not feasible.

Crash Kit: Every One with Patient

Brannula (16, 18, 20), bulbs—grouping and cross matching, venesection set, syringes/gloves, roller gauze/mops, sticking plaster, scissor, Foley's catheter, drip sets, IV Fluids—RL, DNS, haemaccel, intubation materials, oxytocin, misoprostol, PGF2 alpha, methergine, oxygen with mask, hydrocortisone deriphyllin, atropine, $MgSO_4$, nifedipine/labetalol, calcium gluconate, adrenaline, noradrenaline, dopamine, dobutamine, and *central line set-in higher centers where experts are available (Fig. 8)*.

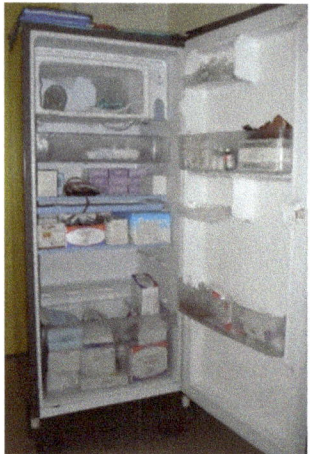 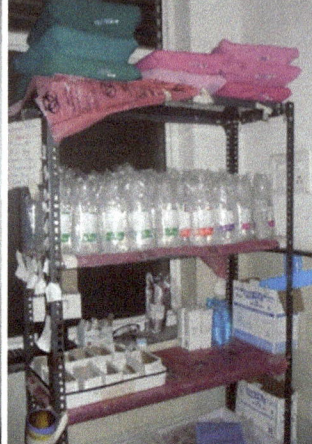 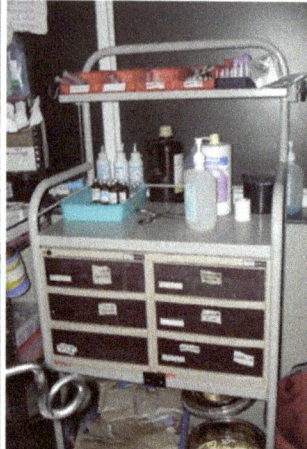

Fig. 8: Crash kit in labor room.

Sequential Action for Patients with Postpartum Hemorrhage

Identify cause—palpate abdomen to note uterus, measures for hypovolemia—IV line (blood drawn), IV oxytocin (20 IU/1,000 mL), methergine/PGF2α/misoprostol. If no response prepares for surgical treatment, other causes—traumatic and retained bits.

Management of Atonic PPH

The AMTSL for prevention—palpate abdomen examination—diagnosis, start two IV line (draw the blood) with IV fluids and with 20 units oxytocin in 1000 mL, additional uterotonics, keep watch on the blood loss, to avoid shock, act before the clinical signs appear (<25% blood loss), 90% of atonic PPH is usually controlled with these measures, further management is surgical.

Further Management

Time interval from onset of PPH to death is 2 hours; hence diagnosis, referral, and management must be on time to save the life. At periphery-arrangements for transfer must begin earlier.

What to do in the Transition Period?

Transition period (from periphery to referral hospital and in the hospital from decision to actual surgical intervention). Maintain hemodynamics, i.e. blood pressure to be maintained.

How to Refer?

To proper place—place where equipped provider and blood, with Foot end elevated, With IV drip and drawn blood samples (for grouping and cross matching) accompanied by paramedical staff with emergency drugs. Prior information to the place of referral about the blood group of the patient with a note (diagnosis and treatment given, attenders—young adults for blood, if possible). After applying noninflatable antishock garment (NASG) (Figs. 9A and B).

Role of the following procedures:
- Uterine tamponade with balloon condom catheter (Figs. 10A and B), uterine packing, many use these with broad gauze/mops no clear evidence.
- Bimanual compression and aortic compression—usually for short time.

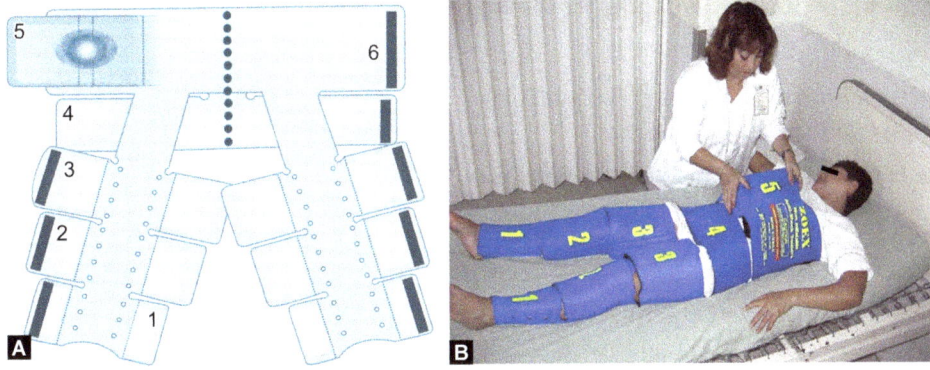

Figs. 9A and B: Noninflatable antishock garment.
Courtesy: Suellen Miller et al.

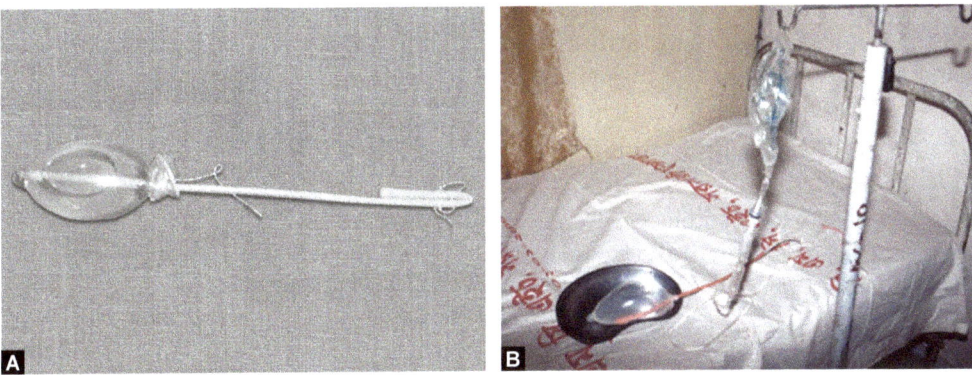

Figs. 10A and B: Balloon condom catheter.
Courtesy: Saiba Akhtar et al.

Medical Management

Intravenous line with normal saline (NS) or ringer lactate (RL), oxytocin first-line of drug—effective and no side effects, methylergometrine—effective but more side effects need refrigeration, PGF2α Injectable, IM only, more side effects, avoid in asthmatics and cardiac patients (MI); misoprostol—specially sublingual must be attempted before surgical treatment, medical management is effective in most of the cases of atonic PPH.

Traumatic

Diagnosis—palpate the uterus (contracted and retracted), explore, usual—perineal (including para urethral), vaginal, and cervical; prerequisites are must for identifying these. Involve team, correct suturing is important. At times, needs exploration under anesthesia, colporrhexis, and suspected rupture uterus—laparotomy; maintain hemodynamics during exploration.

Delay is Dangerous

The passage of time is likely to increase the complexity of any given case because continuous bleeding, not appropriately and adequately controlled on a timely basis, invariably leads to coagulopathy.

Pregnancy is a hyper coagulable state.

Role of Blood Transfusion and Component Therapy

Routine vigorous administration of crystalloids leads to *dilutional coagulopathy*.

What is new? Hemostatic resuscitation, no role for whole blood transfusion.

Hemostasis Monitoring

Prothrombin time (PT), activated partial thromboplastin time (aPTT), and international normalized ratio (INR)—poor predictors for transfusion requirements.

What is new...Thromboelastograph.
- Both the reaction time/clotting time and the alpha angle reflect the activity of clotting factors.
- Maximum amplitude correlates with platelet function.
- Velocity at which the amplitude decreases correlates with fibrinolytic activity (Figs. 11 and 12).

Blood product required to rise the fibrinogen by 1 mg/dL:
1. *Fresh frozen plasma (FFP):* 4 units (1,000 mL).
2. *Cryoprecipitate:* 13 units (260 mL).
3. *Fibrinogen concentrate:* 2 g (100 mL) (Fig. 13).

Massive Transfusion Protocol

	PRBC	FFP	Platelets	Cryoprecipitate
1	6 units	6 units	6 units	10 units
2	6 units	6 units		20 units
3	Recombinant activated Factor VII (40 µg/kg)			

Criteria for Administering rFactor VII a

rFVII: Before administration, patient should ideally have a platelet count 50,000/mm^3, fibrinogen 50–100 mg/dL, temperature 32°C, pH 7.2, and normal ionized calcium.

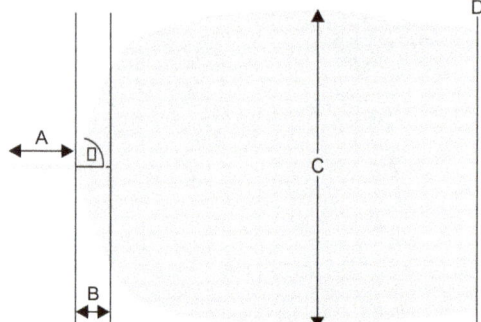

Fig. 11: Thromboelastograph.

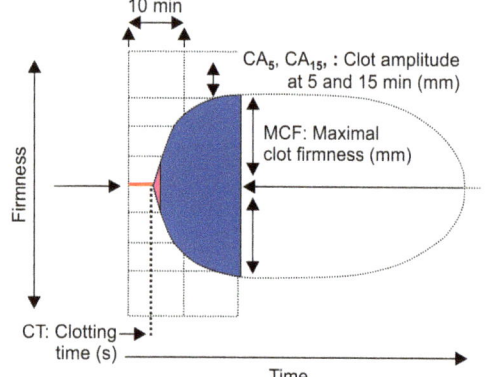

Fig. 12: Thromboelastograph signature waveform.

Retained Tissue

Examination of placenta/USG, antibiotics, evacuation with or without USG guidance, and adherent placenta needs special attention. Appropriate treatment must be given along with the resuscitation simultaneously.

Secondary PPH

Retained bits of placenta, infection, treatment: antibiotics and evacuation, and resuscitation with blood and blood products.

Summary

- Prevention is the key
- Close watch on blood loss is the key factor

CHAPTER 6: Obstetric Hemorrhage: Prevention and Management (Golden Hour)

Consider activation of an MT protocol when patient actively bleeding and any of the following:
Systolic blood pressure < 90 mm Hg
Ph < 7.1
Base deficit > 6 mEq/L
Temperature below 34°C
INR > 2.0
Platelet count <50,000/mm^3

	PRBC	FFP	Platelets	Cryoprecipitate
Round 1	6 units	6 units	6 units	10 units
Round 2	6 units	6 units		20 units
Round 3	Recombinant activated factor VII (40 µg/kg)			

Once activated, the blood bank will send 6 units of PRBC, 6 units of FFP, 6 units of platelets, and 10 units of cryoprecipitate. After this, if the patient remains bleeding (the protocol has cryoprecipitate. The latter product is given in order to elevate the fibrinogen level since the next step of the protocol is to administer recombinant activated factor VII. At any point, if the patient's hemorrhage stops, the blood bank should be notified so that the protocol can be terminated.
If bleeding persists, the sequence is started again.
(FFP: fresh frozen plasma; INR: international nomalized ratio; MT: massive transfusion; PRBC: packed red blood cells.)

- Oxytocin first-line of drug—effective and least side effects
- Methylergometrine—effective but more side effects need refrigeration (2–8°C)
- PGF2α IM, more side effects, avoid in asthmatics, smokers, and cardiac patients
- Misoprostol—specially sublingual must be tried
- Medical management is effective in most of the cases.

Conclusion: PPH BY PPH

- *Prediction:* Risk factors prevention—AMTSL, examination placenta
- *Prepare:* Team, uterotonics, IV line, transport, referral, and blood
- *Handle:* First medical, usually effective in most, failure needs proper maintenance of hemodynamics followed by surgical treatment by equipped providers. Blood components play an important role in reducing morbidity and mortality.

"Women are not dying because of a disease we cannot treat. They are dying because societies have yet to make the decision that their lives are worth saving".
—Mamoud Fathalla

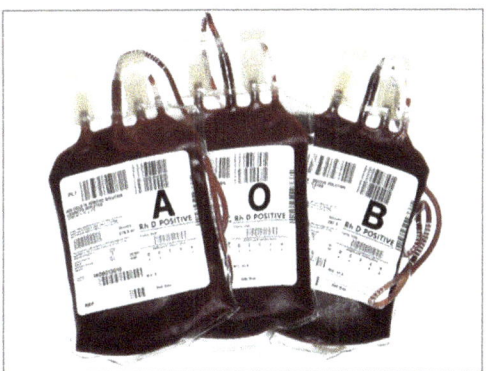
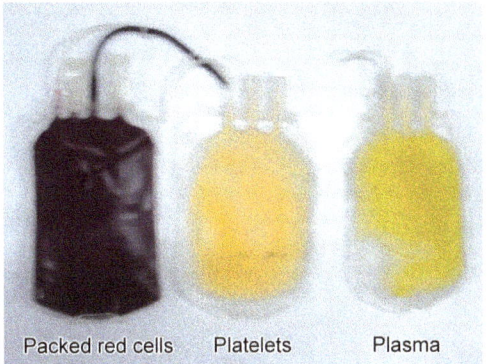

Packed red cells   Platelets   Plasma

Fig. 13: Blood component therapy.

President of the International Federation of Gynecology and Obstetrics (FIGO), World Congress, Copenhagen 1997.

ANNEXURE-1

Approach to Hemorrhagic Shock (Source: Shock in Obstetrics, Workshop Manual)

29th KSOGA Conference, Bagalkot—the conference where the manual was released.

The management of shock including hemorrhagic is a team (together everyone achieves more) approach. It is important to call for help whoever is closed by till the concerned specialists/personnel arrive.

Fundamental Principles

Team leader—takes the important decisions and assigns responsibilities to other members, who promptly follow with discussions. This team approach helps in proper diagnosis, investigations, and treatment as well as for monitoring.

A Quick Assessment of Patient

Shock is defined as the syndrome initiated by acute hypoperfusion, leading to tissue hypoxia, and vital organ dysfunction. It is a systemic disorder affecting multiple organ systems. Shock in a pregnant woman differs in two important aspects:
1. Normal physiologic changes
2. Mother and fetus—both vulnerable.

Hence, simultaneous assessment and management of the mother and fetus is important.

Hypovolemic shock: Characterized by decreased circulatory volume. Hemorrhagic (most common cause) (Table 3).

Primary Survey

Mother first:
- Airway
- Breathing
- Circulation.

Suspect shock when:
- Air hunger
- Diminution of vision
- Restlessness or decreased consciousness
- Low blood pressure
- Rapid weak (thready) pulse
- Pallor
- Cold clammy sweaty extremities
- Decreased urine output.

TABLE 3: Hemorrhagic shock—estimation of blood loss based on patient's initial presentation for a 70 kg person.

	Class 1	Class 2	Class 3	Class 4
Blood loss (Ml)	Up to 750	750–1500	1500–2000	>2000
Blood loss (% blood volume)	Up to 15 %	15–30%	30–40%	>40%
Pulse rate (bpm)	<100	100–120	120–140	>140
Systolic blood pressure	Normal	Normal	Decreased	Decreased
Pulse pressure	Normal or increased	Decreased	Decreased	Decreased
Respiratory rate	14–20	20–30	30–40	>35
Urine output (mL/h)	>30	20–30	5–15	Negligible
Mental status	Slightly anxious	Mildly anxious	Anxious and confused	Confused and lethargic
Initial fluid replacement	Crystalloid	Crystalloid	Crystalloid and blood	Crystalloid and blood

Management

- Have a protocol for the management of shock (hemorrhage)
- Call appropriate members
- Alert blood transfusion services
- Initial priority (H), A, B, C:
  - Hemorrhage control
  - Airway control
  - Breathing support
  - Circulatory support
- Fluid resuscitation
- Blood transfusion or massive transfusion
- In case of PPH, management of cause.

Stepwise initial resuscitation steps.

Investigations to be Sent

- Complete hemogram [hemoglobin (Hb), white cell count (WBC), platelets, PS study, etc.]
- Cross matching
- Liver function test (LFT), lactate dehydrogenase (LDH), renal function test (RFT)
- Coagulation profile (CT, BT, PT, aPTT, INR)
- Arterial blood gas (ABG) and serum electrolytes, if needed
- Urine analysis
- Blood collection
- Plain sample (Fig. 14)
- Blood grouping and cross matching
- LFT, LDH, blood urea, serum creatinine, S. electrolytes

Commonly Used Anticoagulants

- Ethylenediaminetetraacetic acid (EDTA) (Fig. 15)
- Trisodium citrate (Fig. 16)
- Heparin:
  - Ethylenediaminetetraacetic acid:
    - *Mechanism of action:* Chelation of calcium
    - *Inversions:* 8–10
    - *Recommended concentration.*
  - K2EDTA—1.5 mg/mL of blood:
    - *Uses:* CBC, reticulocyte count, ESR, TC, and DLC
    - *Disadvantages:* Cannot be used for coagulation tests.

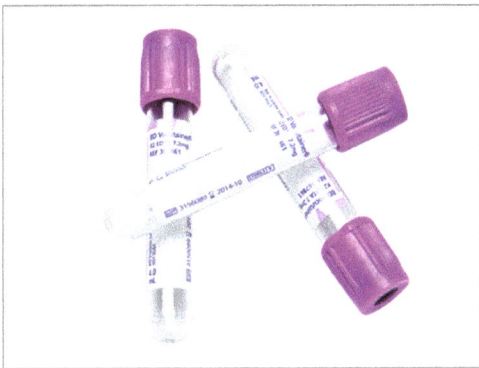

Fig. 15: K2 EDTA vacutainers.

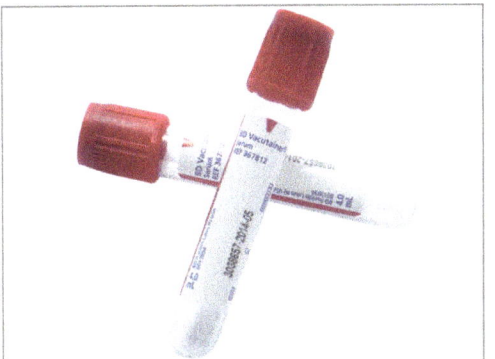

Fig. 14: Plain sample for serum vacutainers.

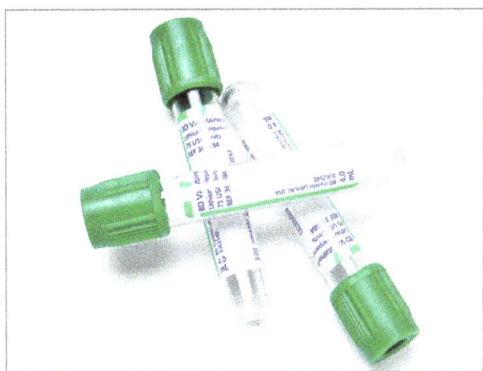

Fig. 16: Citrate vacutainers.

Can cause pseudothrombocytopenia on analyzer.
- Trisodium citrate:
  - Anticoagulant of choice—coagulation studies
  - Chelation of calcium
  - *Sodium citrate:* 3.2% solution
  - Inversions—3-4.

Uses

- 1 part sodium citrate added to 4 parts whole blood—erythrocyte sedimentation rate (ESR) by Westergren method.
- 1 part sodium citrate added to 9 parts whole blood—coagulation profile
- D-dimer
- Heparin:
  - Prevents coagulation by enhancing the activity of antithrombin III.
  - *Concentration:* 15-20 IU/mL of blood.
  - Inversions: 5-10.
  - Used for ABG analysis.

Time of Testing

- Ideally tests should be done immediately after blood is collected
- *Within 2 hours:* Coagulation studies and platelet count
- *Within 3 hours:* ESR
- *Within 24 hours:* Red blood cell (RBC), WBC count, packed cell volume (PCV), hemoglobin, and reticulocyte count.

Arterial Blood Gas

Blood gas analysis, also called arterial blood gas (ABG) analysis, is a test which measures the amount of oxygen (O_2) and carbon dioxide (CO_2) in the blood, as well as the acidity (pH) of the blood.

Blood is usually withdrawn from the radial artery as it is easy to palpate and has a good collateral supply.

The patient's arm is placed palm-up on a flat surface, with the wrist dorsiflexed at 45°. A towel may be placed under the wrist for support.

The puncture site should be cleaned with alcohol or iodine, and a local anesthetic (such as 2% lignocaine) may be infiltrated.

The radial artery should be palpated for a pulse, and a preheparinized syringe with a 23 or 25 gauge needle should be inserted at an angle just distal to the palpated pulse.

A small quantity of blood is sufficient. After the puncture, sterile gauze should be placed firmly over the site and direct pressure applied for several minutes to obtain hemostasis.

pH	7.35–7.45 (7.4)
PaO_2	80–100 mm Hg
$PaCO_2$	35–45 mm Hg (40)
HCO_3^-	22–26 mmol/L (24)
Base excess	−2– +2 mmol/L

Rule to be applied when compensation has occurred:

Condition	pH	CO_2
Respiratory alkalosis	↑	↓
Respiratory acidosis	↓	↑
Metabolic acidosis	↓	↓
Metabolic alkalosis	↑	↑

Management of Circulatory Failure

IV access/IV fluid administration/pressure support (If available):
- Restore circulatory volume with NS or RL (not D5W)
- Use blood products if needed, when available.

Intravenous/Intraosseous Access

- Two large bore IVs—18G or larger, anterior cubital fossa preferred
- Shock = inadequate tissue perfusion

CHAPTER 6: Obstetric Hemorrhage: Prevention and Management (Golden Hour)

- BP is inaccurate/late indicator of shock
- Mental status/PR/capillary refilling may be better indicators of early shock
- Norepinephrine (NE) is the primary drug of choice
- Vasopressin (e.g. dopamine) only after adequate fluid volume resuscitation, and inadequate effect from NE
- Do not use IV dextrose (D5W—hypotonic) as it is a poor resuscitation fluid
- Restore intravascular volume with crystalloids (NS and LR) or colloids (blood, FFP, and albumin)
- (1-2) + L rapid IV bolus of NS
- Based on IV volume assessment (e.g. IVC measurement by US) less or no volume for heart failure patients may be required, and may require pressors
- (500-1000)+ cc colloid fluids can be used if no response to N saline
- Overall outcomes are similar with N saline versus colloid resuscitation.

Uncontrolled Hemorrhage

- Do not pop the clot:
  - Avoid over resuscitation
  - Excess fluid—increases bleeding and mortality.
- Pop the clot:
  - Dilution of clotting factors
  - Hypothermia and coagulopathy.
- Goal is to restore perfusion.
- Radial pulse present—SBP >90 mm Hg:
  - Intravenous fluid bolus may not be needed
  - Place IV line with fluid only at maintenance rate.
- Radial pulse absent—SBP <90 mm Hg:
  - 500-1,000 cc N saline/or 250-500 cc colloid
  - Repeat as needed (maximum 1,000 cc colloid).

Only administer enough IV fluid/blood to restore the radial pulse and maintain systolic blood pressure more than 90 mm Hg.

Signs of Adequate Fluid Resuscitation

- Patient looks better
- Improved BP
- Widened pulse pressure
- Decreased pulse rate
- Decreases capillary refilling time
- Resolved diaphoresis
- Improved mental status
- Improved urine output.

Blood Transfusion

- Order blood transfusions, if blood loss is ongoing and thought to be in excess or if the patient's clinical status reflects developing shock despite aggressive resuscitation.
- Whole blood should be avoided.
- Packed red blood cells (PRBCs) are initially used with other blood components.
- If coagulation test results are abnormal from the onset of PPH, strongly consider an underlying cause [abruptio placentae, HELLP (hemolysis, elevated liver enzymes, and low platelet count) syndrome, fatty liver of pregnancy, IUD, amniotic fluid embolus, septicemia, and pre-existing disorders]. Take specific steps to treat the underlying cause and the hemostatic abnormality.
- In an extreme emergency situation when blood group is unknown, group O Rh negative red cell to be given.
- Spin method for cross matching can be used in emergency.
- It is essential that regular full blood counts (FBC) and coagulation screens are performed during the bleeding episode. FFP, cryoprecipitate, and platelets should not be given on clinical suspicion alone unless there is delay in obtaining blood results.
- Infusion of FFP should be considered before 1 blood volume is lost.

In what Circumstances should Fresh Frozen Plasma and Cryoprecipitate be used?

Fresh frozen plasma (FFP) at a dose of 12–15 mL/kg should be administered for every 6 units of red cells during major obstetric hemorrhage. Subsequent FFP transfusion should be guided by the results of clotting tests, if they are available in a timely manner, aiming to maintain PT, and APTT ratios at less than 1.5 × normal.

It is essential that regular FBC and coagulation screens (PT, APTT, and fibrinogen) are performed during the bleeding episode.

Cryoprecipitate at a standard dose of two 5-unit pools should be administered early in major obstetric hemorrhage. Subsequent cryoprecipitate transfusion should be guided by fibrinogen results, aiming to keep levels above 1.5 g/L.

The FFP and cryoprecipitate should ideally be of the same group as the recipient. If unavailable, FFP of a different ABO group is acceptable providing that it does not have a high titer of anti-A or anti-B activity.

No anti-D prophylaxis is required, if an RhD-negative woman receives RhD-positive FFP or cryoprecipitate.

When should platelets be used?
Aim to maintain the platelet count above 50×10^9/L in the acutely bleeding patient.

A platelet transfusion trigger of 75×10^9/L is recommended to provide a margin of safety.

The platelets should ideally be group compatible. RhD-negative women should also receive RhD negative platelets.

What is massive transfusion?
- Replacement of >1 blood volume in 24 hours
- 10 Units transfusion in 24 hours
- > 50% of blood volume in 4 hours (Table 4).

TABLE 4: Therapy indication in massive transfusion.

Parameters	Values to aim for
Temperature	>35°
Acid base status	Ph >7.2 base excess <6, lactate <4 mmol/L
Ionized Ca	>1.1 mmol/L
Hb	This should not be used alone as transfusion trigger; and should be interpreted in context with hypodynamic status, organ and tissue perfusion
Platelets	Platelets 50×10^9L (>100×10^9L, if head injury/hemorrhage) platelet count cut off for transfusion
Intracranial hemorrhage	
Prothrombin time/ Activated plasma thromboplastin time (PT/APTT) coagulation blood tests	≤1.5 × of normal
Fibrinogen	1.0 g/L

Vasopressors

- Vasopressor therapy initially to target a mean arterial pressure (MAP) of 65 mm Hg
- Norepinephrine as the first-choice vasopressor
- Vasopressin 0.03 units/minute can be added to NE with intent of either raising MAP or decreasing NE dosage
- Dopamine as an alternative vasopressor agent to NE only in highly selected patients (e.g. patients with low risk of tachyarrhythmias and absolute or relative bradycardia)
- Low-dose dopamine should not be used for renal protection
- All patients requiring vasopressors should have an arterial catheter placed as soon as practical if resources are available.

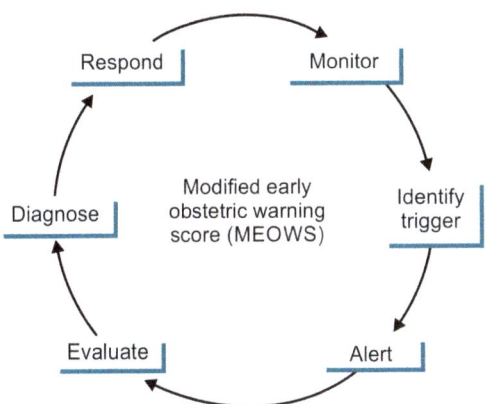

Fig. 17: Modified early obstetric warning.

ANNEXURE 2

Modified early obstetric warning score (MEOWS) (Fig. 17): It will help in timely recognition of complication which in turn will assist in the management implemented in obstetric units of hospitals in United Kingdom with improved outcomes to reduce morbidity and mortality with sensitivity and specificity of 89% and 79%. It is also incorporated in Qatar also. MEOWS can be paper-based or electronic gadget based. It also provides clarity on roles and responsibilities of staff (Clare A Cook et al. JOGNN 2014).

SUGGESTED READING

1. Arulkumaran S, Karoshi M, Keith LG, Lalonde AB, B-Lynch C. Assessing and Replenishing Lost Volume. In: Cockings JGL, Waldmann CS (Eds) A Comprehensive Textbook of Postpartum Hemorrhage, 2nd Edition. US: Sapiens Publishing; 2012. pp. 74-5.
2. Cunningham FG, Leveno KJ, Bloom SL, Dashe JS, Hoffman BL, Casey BM, Spong CY. Williams Obstetrics, 25th Edition. USA: McGraw-Hill Education; 2018. pp. 1668.
3. Huissoud C, Carrabin N, Audibert F, et al. Bedside assessment of fibrinogen level in postpartum haemorrhage by thrombelastometry. BJOG 2009;116:1097-102.
4. KSOGA Conference. Shock in Obstetrics, Workshop Manual, 29th KSOGA Conference. India: Bagalkot; 2018.
5. Nathan HL, El Ayadi A, Hezelgrave NL, et al. Shock index: An effective predictor of outcome in postpartum haemorrhage? BJOG. 2015;122(2):268-75.
6. Pacheco LD, Saade GR, Gei AF, et al. Cutting-edge advances in the medical management of obstetrical hemorrhage. Am J Obstet Gynecol.2011;205(6):526-32.

7
Assessment of Blood Loss

Chapter

BS Susheela Rani

INTRODUCTION

Blood loss in labor and delivery is inevitable. It is a part of nature. In the normal process, blood that is lost, is not associated with clinical symptoms and signs, since the mother's system is prepared to handle the loss. In certain situations, the balance is tilted. When the mother is anemic or when she has lost more than usual amount of blood, her body tries to compensate for the loss and when it is beyond its capacity to cope, she succumbs. Maternal morbidity and even mortality ensues. The key to averting this kind of situation is to be prepared and to swing into action even as hemorrhage occurs! The first step in this direction is to assess the amount of blood lost.

Studies conducted to evaluate the process of assessment of blood loss have all found that the assessment is more often inaccurate. More often than not, the blood loss is underestimated and this assessment is independent of the category of personnel doing the assessment and their seniority. The inference drawn from all these studies is that all the personnel working in the service of a pregnant woman during delivery be it in the labor room or the operation theater, should be "trained" to assess the blood loss.

Why do we need to assess blood loss?
- The moment we realize that the blood loss is more than normal, blood transfusions and other procedures required to resuscitate the mother can be started.
- Overestimation can be costly, unnecessary treatments like blood transfusions which can be risky and fluid overload.
- Underestimation on the other hand can cause delay in interventions that are required to stop the bleeding and save the woman.

METHODS OF BLOOD LOSS ASSESSMENT

This could be done by clinical methods and quantitative methods.

How do we quantify blood loss?

For many years, various studies have been conducted to find a method which was reasonably accurate, simple, and reproducible to assess blood loss. Methods included visual assessment, measuring hematocrit, gravimetric method, photometry, and various others.

Clinical Method

Blood loss is expressed as Class I to IV based on the clinical signs and symptoms (Table 1).[1] A systolic blood pressure below 100 mm Hg and pulse rate > 100 beats/min are late signs and indicate commencing failure of compensatory mechanism. When a woman has reached Class III level, all interventions need to be very quick since the progress to irreversible shock is rapid.

Therefore, it is very important to diagnose at Class I stage as further progress to Class II

TABLE 1: Classification of hemorrhage (modified from committee of trauma).

	Class I	Class II	Class III	Class IV
% Blood loss	15	20–25	30–35	40
Pulse	Normal	100	120	140
Systolic blood pressure	Normal	Normal	70–80	60
Mean arterial pressure	80–90	80–90	50–70	50
Tissue perfusion	Postural hypotension	Peripheral vasoconstriction	Pallor, restlessness, oliguria	Collapse, anuria, air hunger

and III is rapid. Changes in the vital signs and hematocrit are useful when large amount of blood is lost. Although, by themselves, they cannot be used to estimate the volume of blood lost since they are dependent on several factors. For example, a woman on beta-blockers may not show evidence of fall in the blood pressure when compared to a woman who is not.

Quantitative Methods

Photometry

A photometric technique converts blood pigment to alkaline hematin, which is then measured by a photometer.[2] Hemoglobin of the woman is first estimated using a photometer. Hemoglobin estimated from the blood collected from the woman after delivery including that extracted from the linen and sponges is estimated. The difference in hemoglobin gives the volume of blood lost. Meticulously done, this method is reliable and therefore a gold standard. However, it is neither practical nor easy to be used in the clinical settings.[3]

Radioactive Tagging of Red Blood Cells

The red blood cells (RBCs) are tagged with radioactive material and traced after delivery. The method though likely to be accurate, is not practical. Moreover, loss of RBCs from the vascular system into the interstitial tissue could wrongly be attributed to blood loss.

Visual Assessment

From good old days, blood loss has been estimated by the visual estimation across various communities. Even to this day, it is the most commonly practiced method across the world. Objectifying blood loss by visual estimation has its own limitations. The size of the sponge used to soak blood, the thickness of the sponge, the absorptive capacity and the size of the linen used, and the mixture of body fluids with the collected blood are factors, which affect the estimation. There are plenty of publications evaluating the accuracy of visual estimation. It has been found that there has been underestimation/overestimation/inconsistency in measurement in visual estimation of blood loss. Some even say that the visual assessment is so inaccurate that one should not waste precious time in visual assessment.

Quantification of blood loss by objective methods therefore becomes very important.

Direct Measurement

Measuring blood collected in bed pan, buckets, and under-buttock drapes are useful. However, pitfalls include:
- Inadequate estimation of blood lost in all linen.
- Inadequate estimation of the volume of maternal blood with placenta.
- Inadequate estimation of blood lost with amniotic fluid/urine.

- Improper transfer of blood (and therefore estimation) from collection devices to measuring devices.

Calibrated under-buttock drapes help to quantify blood loss. The Brass V under-buttock drape allows the collection of blood and body fluids into the conical receptacle which is calibrated (Figs. 1A to D). This allows direct measurement of the fluid collected within the receptacle.

Gravimetric Method

Materials soaked in blood are weighed and their original weight subtracted. The difference in weight gives the estimate of

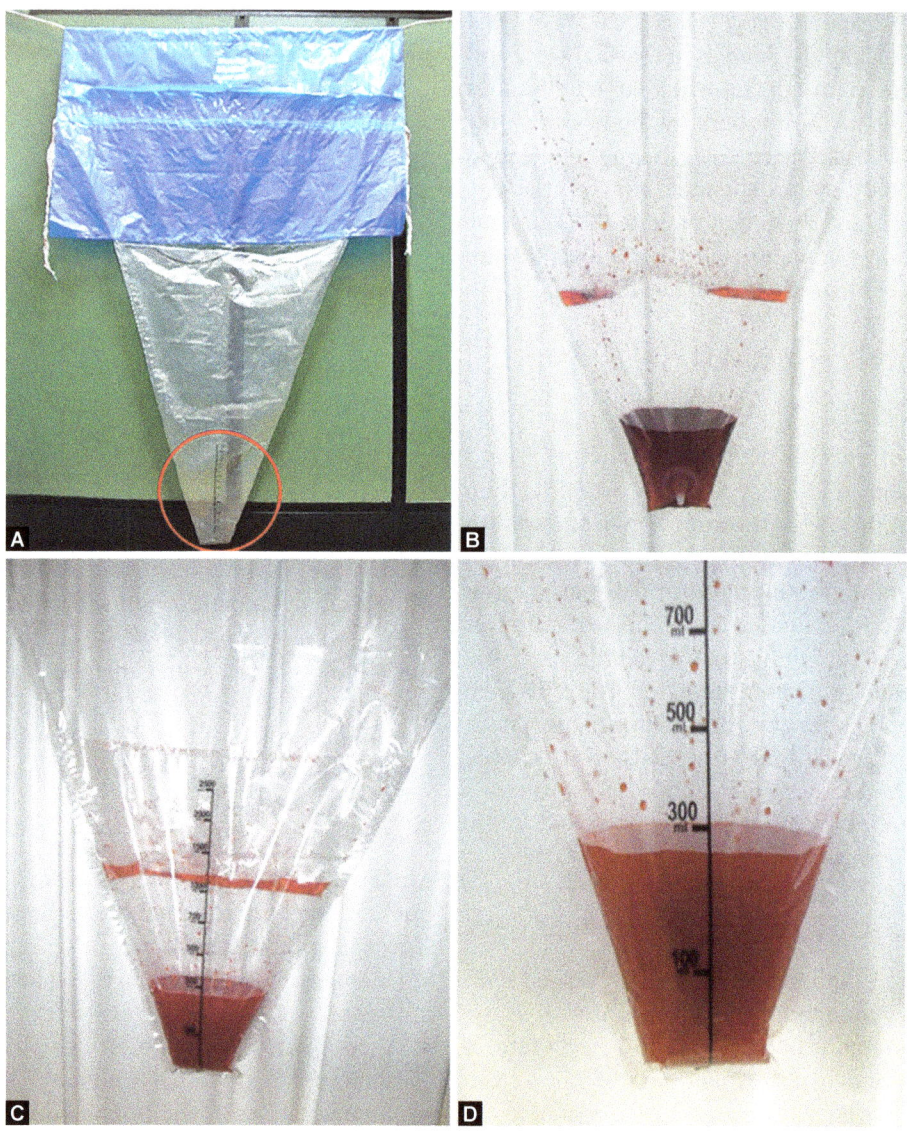

Figs. 1A to D: The Brass V drape.

CHAPTER 7: Assessment of Blood Loss

Blood soaked in linen + Blood collected in conical receptacle = Total blood loss

Fig. 2: Blood loss assessment.

blood loss (Fig. 2). The difference in gram weight is converted into milliliters.

$$1 \text{ g} = 1 \text{ mL}$$

Association of Women's health, Obstetric and Neonatal Nurses (AWHONN) has devised a method, which is useful in estimating blood loss at delivery. It is one of the most practical methods that helps in fairly accurate measurement of blood loss.[4] All that is required is calibrated under-buttock drape, measured dry weight of the sponges, and linen used during labor. Once standardized material is used, the weights can be printed and affixed on the wall of labor room and operation theaters. A scale to weigh these again after they are soaked following delivery is required. One member of the labor room team is assigned the responsibility to assess.

Quantitative blood loss assessment begins immediately after birth of the baby before the delivery of placenta.

Assessment at Vaginal Births

- Note the amount of fluid collected in the conical receptacle of the under-buttock drape or in the suction bottle if a cesarean is being done. This fluid is mostly amniotic fluid and maternal urine and feces.
- After delivery of the placenta, note the total volume of fluid collected in the conical receptacle of the under-buttock drape.
- The fluid collected in the conical receptacle after the placenta is delivered is mostly blood. Subtract the fluid volume noted *before* delivery of placenta from the fluid volume *after* the delivery of placenta. This gives the actual volume of blood lost.

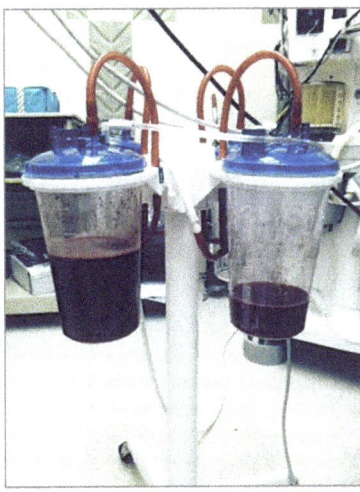

Fig. 3: Blood collected in suction apparatus.

- Weigh all blood-soaked materials and clots to determine the total volume. *1 g weight = 1 mL blood loss volume.*
- To arrive at the volume of blood lost in linen, subtract the dry linen weight from the wet linen weight.
- Add the blood volume obtained from the conical receptacle to the blood volume obtained from the soaked linen.
- This gives the total blood loss.

Assessment at Cesarean Delivery

- Once the membranes are ruptured and the amniotic fluid is drained, fluid is collected in the suction bottle (Fig. 3). After the baby is delivered the volume is noted.
- Placenta is delivered. As the surgery is completed, the volume in the suction bottle is noted again.
- The difference in the volume of fluid collected before and after delivery of the placenta gives the volume of blood in the suction bottle.
- The weights of the wet drapes are noted. The difference in weight between the wet and dry drapes gives the volume of blood lost in the linen.

- Total volume of blood lost is arrived at by adding the volume of blood in the suction bottle to the volume of blood lost in the drapes.

If an irrigation fluid is used, the volume of this fluid can come in the way of accurate estimation of blood loss. It is important to note the amount of fluid used for irrigation and subtract it in the volume of fluid collected in the suction bottle. However, it is worthwhile noting that not all of the fluid will be suctioned into the bottle. Some might remain in the tissues.

Quantification of blood loss by this method will not be exact. However, let not the good come in the way of best. Estimation of blood loss by this method is any day better than relying on visual assessment. It is simple and easy. It is not time consuming. Once it is done on a routine basis and the dry weights are available, it hardly takes a few minutes. It does not need great expertise and does not need much training. This method can be modified to local practices. For example, in many remote areas, under-buttock drapes may not be used. A bucket to collect the fluid may be used. In such cases, a second bucket replaces the first immediately after delivery of the baby. Quantification of blood loss has to be done for all deliveries since it is never possible to predict which woman has hemorrhage.

For example, nurse has noted that the collection in the bucket/drape was 100 mL before delivery (amniotic fluid, patient's urine, and very little blood). After delivery, the total volume in the bucket/drape was 700 mL. The dry weight of 5 mops was 100 g and 10 mops were used. The final weight of the mops was 575 g.

- Weight of 10 wet mops = 575 g
- Dry weight of 10 mops (100 × 2) = 200 g
- Wet weight – Dry weight = 375 mL
- Weight of blood lost in mops = 375 g
- Total volume in the bucket = 700 mL
- Volume in bucket before placenta = 100 mL
- Measured blood loss = (700 – 100) = 600 mL
- Total blood loss = Weight + Measure = 375 + 600 = 975 mL.

CONCLUSION

Assessment of blood loss is integral to prevention and management of postpartum hemorrhage (PPH). The process of measurement by AWHONN is simple, easy, and doable. It is time to adopt it in our practice.

REFERENCES

1. Committee on Trauma. Advanced Trauma Life Support Manual. Chicago: American College of Surgeons; 1997. pp. 103-12.
2. Wallace G. Blood loss in obstetrics using a haemoglobin dilution technique. J Obstet Gynaecol Br Commonw. 1967;74:64-7.
3. Mainland JF. A simple photo-electric method for the estimation of blood loss during surgery. BMJ. 1966;38:76-8.
4. Wiley Online Library. (2014). Quantification of Blood Loss: AWHONN Practice Brief Number 1. [online] Available from: https://onlinelibrary.wiley.com/doi/full/10.1111/1552-6909.12519 [Last accessed July, 2019].

8
Chapter

Massive Obstetric Hemorrhage and Role of Blood Transfusion in Management

Alpesh Gandhi

■ DEFINITION

Major obstetric hemorrhage is defined as blood loss >2,000 mL or rate of blood loss of 150 mL/minute, or 50% blood volume loss within 3 hours. It may result in a decrease in hemoglobin (Hb) >4 g/L, or an acute transfusion requirement of >4 units. Hemorrhage is a common complication of pregnancy. It further becomes complicated because of inaccuracy in determination of exact amount of blood loss.

■ CAUSES

It is the first rank direct cause for maternal mortality and morbidity in our country. There are many causes, which can lead to massive hemorrhage during pregnancy and childbirth. The most common causes are abruptio placentae, uterine atony, placenta previa, placenta accreta, retained placenta, pregnancy-induced hypertension (PIH), uterine rupture, ectopic pregnancy, coagulation disorders, birth trauma, operative trauma, amniotic fluid embolism, HELLP syndrome, etc. Pregnant women at term have hypercoagulable state caused by excess of procoagulants. Pregnancy also shares the risk of exposure to thromboplastic material from abnormal or damaged placentas as well as from labor process, which is also responsible for hemorrhage.

■ GOALS OF THERAPY

Goals of therapy for massive obstetric hemorrhage:
- To restore intravascular volume,
- To maintain tissue oxygen delivery and
- To eliminate the source of hemorrhage.

Immediately insert at least two large intravenous (IV) cannula. Take blood at the same time for urgent cross-match (type specific), full blood count (FBC) and coagulation screen. Initiate volume replacement with lactated Ringer's or normal saline. Lactate Ringer's solution, 0.9% normal saline and Plasma-Lyte A are the most commonly used crystalloid solutions. Start volume replacement with up to 1–2 L of crystalloid until blood is available. Dextran should be avoided as it may cause bleeding due to decreased platelet adhesions and dilution of clotting factors. It also interferes with subsequent cross-match. Foley's catheter (no. 16) is to be inserted to monitor urine output. Monitor central venous pressure (CVP) and arterial pressure. The recognition and removal of the underlying cause is an important part of the management of obstetric hemorrhage. To discuss medical and surgical obstetric management of massive hemorrhage, it is not the aim or scope of this chapter. Besides that the main therapeutic endeavor remains replacement of massive blood loss. Most of the places in our country, factor replacement [prothrombin complex, fibrinogen concentrate, antithrombin III (AT III), etc.] is not easily available.

ROLE OF BLOOD TRANSFUSION IN MANAGEMENT

Blood transfusion practice is an essential and important aspect of high-risk pregnancy and critical care in obstetrics. The WHO strategy emphasizes the need to reduce unnecessary transfusions for safety of blood transfusion. The improper transfusion rate is around 15–45%, either due to transfusion in nonindicated cases or to too late or too little transfusion in indicated cases. In one of the study in the countries of the South-East Asia (SEA) region, 10% of blood was utilized for surgery, 30% for obstetric cases, 24% for pediatric cases, 8% for trauma and 31% for miscellaneous cases. Obstetric cases needed blood the most (WHO, 2010).

The purpose of blood transfusion is replacement and/or therapeutic:
- To restore the intravascular volume.
- To restore the oxygen capacity of blood.
- To replace clotting factors and correction of anemia.

Indications of Blood Transfusion in Acute Blood Loss

- Estimated or anticipated blood loss >15% of total blood volume.
- Diastolic blood pressure is <60 mm Hg.
- Systolic blood pressure is decreased by >30 mm Hg.
- Oliguria/anuria.
- Tachycardia (>100 beats/minute).
- Mental status is changed.
- Shortness of breath, lightheadedness or dizziness with mild exertion.

Whole Blood and Blood Components

Approximately 350 mL/450 mL of blood is collected from a donor into a plastic bag containing an anticoagulant, which is known as one "unit" of whole blood. Whole blood can be separated into different "blood components". Types of blood components are red blood cell (RBC) concentrate (packed RBCs), platelet concentrate, fresh frozen plasma (FFP), cryoprecipitate, separated by differential centrifugation. Others include plasma proteins—intravenous immunoglobulin (IVIg), coagulation factors, albumin, anti-D, growth factors, colloid volume expanders. Apheresis can also be used to collect blood components.

It is a myth that when massive hemorrhage occurs, when patient loses whole blood only, whole blood should be given and it will take care of all. The fact is that the use of whole blood is an unscientific, inefficient, unhealthy and criminal waste of a valuable resource (WHO). Storage requirement for blood components is different. Whole blood is stored at 4–6°C, red cells at 4°C, platelets at 22–24°C (on shaker), FFP at –30°C to –40°C, cryoprecipitate is stored at –30°C to –40°C. So, when we give whole blood, FFP and cryoprecipitate had already lost its functions. Similarly, shelf-life of each component is also different. For red cells, it is 35–40 days, for FFP/CPP—1 year, for platelets—5 days, for cryoprecipitate—1 year and for white blood cells—2 days. So when we give whole blood to a patient who requires only red cells, unnecessary FFP and cryoprecipitate will be wasted which otherwise could have been separated, stored and used later on in a patient who requires it. When we compare packed red cells with whole blood, packed RBC has low volume which is good to prevent overload and has low citrate (mL), low sodium, low potassium, low ammonia and low unwanted plasma than whole blood which are responsible for more complications of blood transfusion. The whole blood is also not proper for better patient management as dose of required concentrated components, which

CHAPTER 8: Massive Obstetric Hemorrhage and Role of Blood Transfusion in Management

are low in quantity, may be useful to prevent circulatory overload, to minimize reactions and to decrease cost of management.

When acute massive blood loss occurs, it can lead to four different problems: (1) hypovolemia, (2) deficiency of clotting factors, (3) deficiency of platelets and (4) hypoxia. All these problems have different solutions and allow us for different optimum time for its correction. Plasma expanders require for hypovolemia, packed RBCs for hypoxia, FFP for clotting factors, cryoprecipitate for clotting factors deficiency and for low platelet—platelet-rich concentrate (PRC)/platelet-rich plasma (PRP) is required. We need to correct platelet deficiency as soon as possible within <1 hour, coagulation defects within 2–4 hours, hypovolemia within 6–12 hours and hypoxia within 6–12 hours.

For blood component therapy in massive obstetric hemorrhage, we should take two IV lines.

Line A	Line B
Red cells transfusions (4–6) or till Hb >9.0 g/dL	4 cryoprecipitate 4 platelets, if platelets <50 K/μL Time: 30 minutes 2–4 FFPs till prothrombin time (PT) is 6 ± control value
Time: 6–8 hours	Time: 6–8 hours (continue to monitor Hb, platelet, PT)

MTP is known as massive transfusion protocol. It is different in different institutes but it usually known as a rule of 4 or rule of 6. In patients likely to need massive transfusion, begin resuscitation with blood products as soon as possible to prevent dilution coagulopathy. Administer blood products in a ratio of *4 units of packed RBC: 4 units of FFP: 4 units of platelets: 4 units of cryoprecipitate.*

1. *Volume replacement and clotting factor correction*: FFP is used for volume expansion so that replacement of clotting factors may be started early. Generally, the initial volume required must be administered rapidly and that 600 mL to 2 L should be infused over a period of 2-4 hours. Each unit of FFP is generally contains 250 mL of volume. Until FFPs are made available, volume expander should be used.

2. *Correction of fibrinogen/platelet deficits*: Platelet count should be maintained above 50,000/μL, 1 unit of PRC raises the platelet count by 8,000–10,000/μL and accordingly platelet transfusion should be planned as soon as possible.

3. *S. fibrinogen level should be maintained above 150 mg/dL:* About 4-8 units of cryoprecipitate generally are sufficient to achieve this goal. In addition to platelets and cryoprecipitate as mentioned earlier, FFP should be continuously infused. The replacement therapy is guided by laboratory assessment. The usual trigger value for transfusion need is platelet count of 50,000/μL or less, fibrinogen <150 mg/L and prolonged PT by not more than 6 seconds.

4. *Correction of anemia (hypoxia)*: Hb should be maintained above 9.0 g/dL by transfusing red cells. One unit of red cells generally raises Hb by 1.0 g/dL. In general, once patient has disseminated intravascular coagulation (DIC), requirement of 4-6 units of red cells is usual.

5. Clinicians should consider the use of injectable tranexamic acid (0.5–1.0 g) IV, to reduce blood loss in women at increased risk of postpartum hemorrhage (PPH).

6. *Role of obstetric intervention/surgery*: Vaginal delivery makes less severe demand on the hemostatic mechanism

than cesarean section. When a coagulation defect exists, severe bleeding will occur at sites of surgical incisions and may not develop until after the operation. Therefore, in obstetric patient, extensive bleeding can occur into the abdomen from cesarean section incision on the uterus. In exceptional circumstances, when surgical intervention is being necessary, every effort should be made to correct the coagulation failure before and following operation. It is imperative to check platelet count/PT/activated partial thromboplastin time (aPTT) and fibrinogen during antenatal visit prior to delivery. Prompt reference to a hematologist is needed, if any of the above parameters are abnormal. In this attempt, quite a few abnormalities can be detected prior to labor and corrected, if possible.

7. *Follow-up treatment*: Therapy should be planned for 4–6 hours' time period. Vital sign and urine output should be monitored hourly, Hb, platelet count, PT/aPTT should be repeated to define further treatment. Once patient stabilizes these tests can be done at 12 hourly intervals and later once a day. Vitamin K, folic acid should be given to all patients.

Transfusion of FFP, platelets and cryoprecipitate should not be given only on the basis of clinical suspicion unless delay is expected in obtaining results of blood counts and coagulogram. FFP and cryoprecipitate should be ideally of same blood group of recipient. But if unavailable, FFP of different blood group can be given provided the unit does not have high anti-A or -B activity. Anti-D prophylaxis is not required if Rh D-negative women receive Rh D-positive FFP or cryoprecipitate. The platelets should ideally also be ABO group compatible. Rh-negative women should receive Rh-negative platelets. Injection anti-D will be needed if the platelets are Rh-positive and the recipient Rh-negative.

The diagnosis of DIC is made based on clinical presentation plus laboratory manifestations. Laboratory tests, which are most frequently abnormal in DIC, are platelet count, fibrin degradation product (FDP) level, PT, aPTT, and fibrinogen level. These tests show varying degree of abnormality and during early stage of DIC many of them can be normal and therefore, if DIC is strongly suspected, it is important to repeat this test 4–6 hours later. DIC should be made based on clinical presentation as well as abnormalities of the above-mentioned tests should be interpreted together and not in isolation. DIC essentially remains a clinical diagnosis.

There should be an understanding on the terminology used for blood transfusion request between blood bank staff and clinical staff to avoid any misinterpretation. Extremely urgent means blood is required within 15 minutes, very urgent means within an hour, urgent means within 2–3 hours and on the same day for during the day.

Blood transfusion can be associated with many mild to fatal complications. There is a risk of transfusion-transmitted diseases like hepatitis C, hepatitis B and human immunodeficiency virus (HIV). Disorders of excessive neutrophil function like acute respiratory distress syndrome (ARDS), transfusion-related acute lung injury (TRALI) and multiple organ failure (MOF) can occur which are fatal. Once patient is stable, the risks of transfusion far outweigh the benefits of transfusion and so transfusion should not be given.

In appropriate cases, it is advisable to keep blood ready rather than not keeping it. Separate and specific consent is to be taken for the same in advance. Prior to transfusion, we need to take written and informed consent from the patient as blood transfusion involves additional risk.

The blood bag, which is kept for more than 4 hours at room temperature or pack, which is opened or showed any sign of deterioration, should be discarded.

While choosing the donors our preference would never be 1st relation as 1st relation blood has 50% human leukocyte antigen (HLA) match white cells especially lymphocytes. These cells remain viable in recipient circulation and develop their clones of cells, produce antibodies, which act on recipient cells. Worst fatal rare complication, i.e. graft versus host disease can take place in 3 weeks times, which has nearly 100% mortality.

Whenever it is possible, fresh blood should not be used. Ultrafresh blood is the immediately unrefrigerated collected blood and fresh blood is the blood stored within 24–48 hours of collection. Any stored refrigerated blood for >6 hours, platelets lose its function. For >24 hours, all clotting factors lose their property to prevent bleeding. Before component therapy, whole blood was the principal product available and it was known that components like platelets and coagulation factors were present in full for few hours, so at that time fresh blood was justified. In fresh blood, proper screening of blood is not possible. Risk of disease transmission is more as intracellular pathogens [cytomegalovirus (CMV), human T-cell lymphotropic virus (HTLV)] can survive in leukocyte in fresh blood. *Treponema pallidum* can survive for 72–96 hours in stored blood, malarial parasite can survive up to 72 hours in stored blood. If <24 hours stored whole blood is transfused, there is risk of transmission of malaria and *T. pallidum*. This risk is eliminated if >72 hours stored blood is transfused. Fatal reactions are more with fresh blood because of presence of viable lymphocytes and granulocytes.

Cytomegalovirus screening is necessary for blood transfusion. CMV seronegative red cells and platelets should be used for CMV seronegative pregnant women but urgent transfusion should not be delayed if CMV seronegative components are not immediately available.

Use of recombinant activated factor VII (rFVIIa) may be considered for a treatment for life-threatening PPH but it is not a substitute for, nor should it delay the lifesaving procedures such as embolization or surgery, nor the transfer of a patient. Factor VIIa has a pivotal role in initiating the process of blood coagulation. The introduction of rFVIIa has stimulated interest in its use in patients with intractable bleeding despite of corrective measures such as replacement of blood components. Owing to its financial cost, limited availability and its limited use, it is advisable to keep rFVIIa in the blood bank as the stock for any bleeding emergency. The prerequisites for using rFVIIa are Hb levels should be preferably >7 g/dL, platelet levels should be >50,000/mm^3 and fibrinogen level of a minimum of 100 mg/dL, preferable >150 mg/dL, must be ensured before administration of rFVIIa. If these parameters are deranged, they must be corrected by using appropriate component therapy before rFVIIa administration. Correction of the pH to ≥7.2 is also recommended before administration of rFVIIa because efficacy of rFVIIa decreases when pH is ≤7.1. If required, bicarbonate should be given to elevate the serum pH.

Warming blood or blood products is not normally required. Usually, it is sufficient to keep patient warm during transfusion; however, when multiple units of blood are administered quickly in short time, it may become necessary or desirable to warm the blood products. Warming of blood products should be done using a device known as blood warmer that is licensed for it which has visible thermometer and audible warning alarm. It will not allow the temperature of blood to exceed more than 42°C.

Donated blood is stored in bag-containing anticoagulant citrate, which may bind with calcium in the blood and thus may deplete the concentration of free calcium in the blood. In adults, rapid liver and kidney metabolism of citrate usually prevents this complication. If more than three bags are given to a person in a row within a single day, then body may not cope up with rate of decline of free calcium in the blood. Therefore, extra calcium is to be given for that purpose. Hypocalcemia with hypothermia and acidosis is dangerous and may decrease cardiac output, causes bradycardia and dysrhythmia thus injection calcium gluconate is indicated here (WHO).

When she is on transfusion, vital signs must be taken for monitoring of a patient before the transfusion of blood products. Temperature, pulse rate, respiratory rate, blood pressure and oxygen saturation are measured in vital signs. Vital signs should be repeated at 15 minutes after infusion has started, then regularly at every 30 minutes during transfusion and at the end of transfusion. Patient should be informed of possible adverse effects because of transfusion.

The use of intraoperative cell salvage (IOCS) in obstetric practice has a limited role, owing to possibility of the risks of amniotic fluid embolism due to contamination by amniotic fluid, and of anti-D formation due to contamination by fetal blood cells. IOCS has a role in the management of patients who refuse allogenic blood transfusion and who are at risk of significant intraoperative hemorrhage (RCOG Green-top Guideline No. 47, 4 of 10).

Common Transfusion Reactions

Common transfusion reactions: It can be immune-mediated and nonimmune-mediated.

Transfusion Complications

- Acute transfusion reactions (ATRs)
- Chronic transfusion reactions
- Transfusion-related infections.

Acute Transfusion Reactions

- Hemolytic reactions [acute hemolytic transfusion reaction (AHTR)]
- Febrile reactions [febrile nonhemolytic transfusion reaction (FNHTR)]
- Mild to severe allergic reactions
- Transfusion-related acute lung injury
- Coagulopathy
- Bacteremia.

In TRALI, patient develops shortness of breath and dyspnea, mild-moderate respiratory distress, using accessory muscles, hypotension, tachycardia, no evidence of volume overload, craps bilaterally. Chest X-ray may show bilateral fluffy infiltrates. TRALI is a leading cause of transfusion-related death (30% of transfusion-related fatalities). Clinical syndrome is usually similar to ARDS. It can occur within 1–6 hours after receiving plasma-containing blood products. In management of TRALI, transfusion should be stopped immediately. It has high mortality and does not improve with diuretics, only supportive care is given, may need ventilatory support. Patient usually recovers quickly and steroids have not been shown to help.

Transfusion-associated circulatory overload (TACO) occurs up to 1% of all transfusions. Patient may develop shortness of breath and dyspnea, cough, tachycardia, hypertension, craps bilaterally, jugular vein distention (JVD) may be raised. Usually IV diuretic is given and symptoms improved due to circulatory overload. Risk is high in those who are having cardiopulmonary compromise or renal failure.

Acute hemolytic transfusion reaction occurs when incompatible RBCs are transfused. Antibodies activate the complement system and cause intravascular hemolysis. Symptoms occur within minutes of starting transfusion. This hemolytic reaction can occur with few cc of RBCs. It can happen with packed RBC, FFP or platelets. Common signs and symptoms are high-grade fever with or without chills, sudden hypotension, back pain, abdominal pain, oliguria, dyspnea, dark urine and pallor. It can be fatal. Immediately transfusion should be stopped. Blood bag with blood transfusion set is separated. IV line is maintained and NS should be started with new IV set. Try to maintain BP/pulse. Catheterization is done and diuretic is given. Blood and urine sample should be obtained for transfusion reaction workup. The remaining blood with bag and tube is sent back to blood bank. Monitor the patient for her clinical status, vital signs, renal status, coagulation status and signs of hemolysis. Patient may require hemodialysis.

Blood transfusion should never be ordered unless it is worth the risk. Blood transfusion is lifesaving but can lead to life-threatening complications. Single unit transfusion has no significant therapeutic benefit. Blood should be used only in those conditions when equally effective other alternatives cannot be used. The collected blood should be separated into different components and used in specific conditions for optimal utilization. The aim is to reduce unnecessary blood transfusions, promoting proper use of blood and its components and to minimize complications of blood transfusion. We should ensure the rational use of blood components means the right patient is getting the right product in the right amount at the right rate at the right time. All the efforts of obstetric management should be done to control hemorrhage as well as to prevent recurrence of it.

Section 2

Hemorrhage in Early Pregnancy

- **Physiological and Anatomical Changes in Pregnancy Relevant to Hemorrhagic Shock**
  Shobha N Gudi, Priyanka Dilip Kumar
- **Preventing Hemorrhage in Ectopic Pregnancy**
  Vidya V Bhat, Bhavana Girish
- **The Dreaded Miscarriages: Incomplete and Septic Abortions**
  Vidya A Thobbi
- **Abnormal Placentation in Early Pregnancy**
  Mala Arora, Isha Wadhawan
- **Bleeding in Gestational Trophoblastic Disease**
  PK Sekharan
- **Ectopic Pregnancy in the Cervix**
  Purnima Kishore Nadkarni, Manisha Singhal
- **Postabortion Hemorrhage**
  Nozer Sheriar, Rajneet Bhatia

9
Chapter

Physiological and Anatomical Changes in Pregnancy Relevant to Hemorrhagic Shock

Shobha N Gudi, Priyanka Dilip Kumar

CHANGED PHYSIOLOGY IN PREGNANCY

Pregnancy is a physiological condition but paradoxically associated with profound physiological, anatomical and biochemical changes in response to physiological stimuli provided by the fetus and placenta. These are transient effects of the gravid state beginning early, continuing throughout gestation, and completely regressing after delivery and lactation. Nature has so ordained that through these changes the mother is able to provide for the extraplacental circulation and maintains it throughout pregnancy for fetal oxygenation and nutrition. The changes also help her to sustain the inevitable blood loss during childbirth.[1,2]

Case Scenario

Case 1

Mrs A, 28-year-old primigravida, undergoes emergency lower segment cesarean section (LSCS) for severe pre-eclampsia at 38 weeks. She has atonic postpartum hemorrhage (PPH) after delivery and is managed with uterotonics. Due to nonavailability of immediate blood and blood products, crystalloids are given to maintain intravascular volume. Postoperatively she develops pulmonary edema and is shifted to intensive care unit (ICU). She requires ventilator and is in ICU for 4 days. Gradually her condition improves and she is shifted to the ward. We need to ask ourselves where we went wrong in management. This case classifies as a near miss maternal morbidity. Let us answer some questions posed in the case:

Why did she have PPH?
What was the reason to develop pulmonary edema?
Why did condition deteriorate so soon that she required critical support?

Obstetric hemorrhage remains a major cause of maternal mortality and morbidity. Shock due to obstetric hemorrhage is a situation of acute hypoperfusion, tissue and cellular hypoxia, vital organ dysfunction and eventually end organ damage. However, the management of oligemic shock in pregnancy is highly complex because of the physiological alterations. Another major challenge is that the obstetric critical care involves assessment and management of two lives, the mother and fetus, who have differing physiologic profiles.

How does nature ensure hemostasis after normal delivery?

The uterine blood flow increases from 50 mL/minute prepregnancy to 600 mL/minute at term flowing through the low pressure spiral arteries to the intervillous space. With placental separation at delivery, these vessels at the placental bed are avulsed, and hemostasis is achieved first by myometrial contraction, and then by clotting and obliteration of vessel lumens. The pelvic vasculature is highly enhanced even in the lower genital tract and the inevitable loss of blood at delivery is

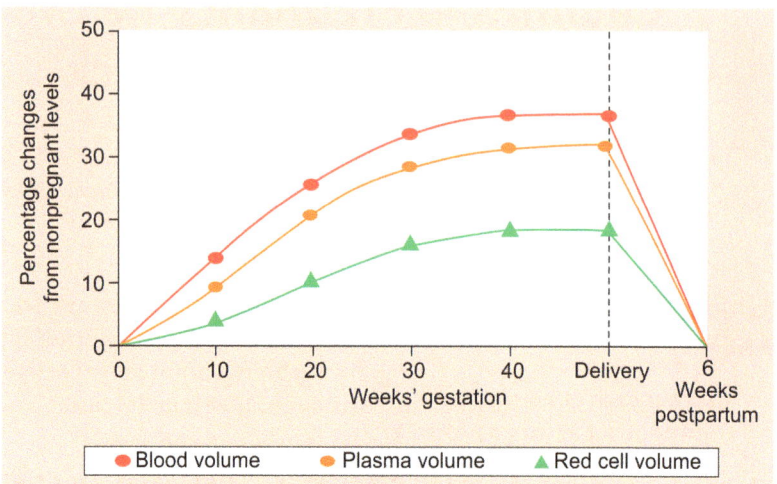

Fig. 1: Changes in hematological system.

stemmed by the hypercoagulable nature of blood in pregnancy.

Moreover, the actual blood loss is often more than is immediately apparent from the vital parameters, i.e. pulse and blood pressure (BP). The healthy pregnant woman is well able to compensate for acute loss to some extent, without overt signs or symptoms of shock due to the changes in the homeostatic mechanisms.

Changes in Hematological System

The blood volume increases, with the plasma volume rising to 40–50% and the red blood cell (RBC) mass by 20%. This differential increase leads to hemodilutional anemia of pregnancy by 32 weeks. Typically, at term the blood volume increases by 1.5 L, the volume of total body water is 6–8 L, 4 L of it is extracellular (Fig. 1).

The volume expansion is proportional to the baseline hematocrit of the subject. It is usually larger with low normal-range hematocrit (~30) and smaller with high normal-range hematocrit (~40). An anemic woman may have larger blood volume increasing the risk of cardiac failure if anemia remains uncorrected.

Average increase in multifetal gestation is 40–80%.

Average increase is less with pre-eclampsia, who have higher hematocrit and it varies inversely with severity of the disease making her more susceptible for oligemic shock with smaller amount of blood loss.

Changes in the Cardiovascular System

There is a steady increase in maternal heart rate by 12 weeks reaching 120% by 32 weeks of pregnancy. This is accompanied by increase of maternal cardiac output by 30–50%, beginning as early as 10 weeks gestation and peaks in second trimester. The cardiac output remains elevated till 48 hours after delivery (Fig. 2).

Changes in Blood Pressure

Both the systolic BP and diastolic BP decrease until mid-pregnancy, with gradual recovery to nonpregnant values by late gestation. Therefore, 130/80 mm of Hg is normal at term but not at 28 weeks and a BP of 90/50 mm of

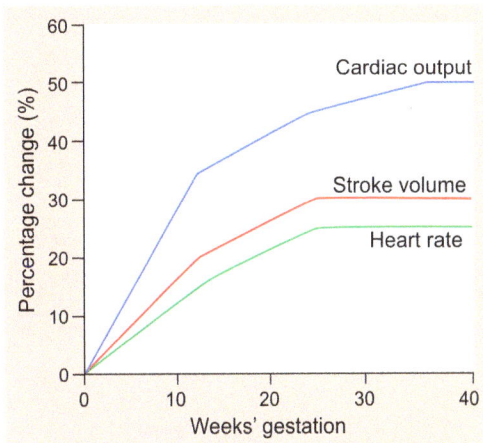

Fig. 2: Maternal cardiovascular changes.

Hg may be normal at 20 weeks not at term. The systemic vascular resistance reaches its nadir by the 24th week and progressively increases to the baseline value at term.

Challenges in Estimation of Blood Loss

It is axiomatic that a normal pregnant woman tolerates, without any decrease in postpartum hematocrit, blood loss at delivery that approaches the volume of blood that she added during pregnancy (30%). Whenever the postpartum hematocrit is lower than one obtained on admission for delivery, blood loss can be estimated as the sum of the calculated pregnancy-added volume plus 500 mL for each 3 volume% decrease of the hematocrit, so for a fall in hematocrit of 6%, 1000 mL needs to be added.

Effect of Maternal Posture on Maternal Hemodynamics

The supine position can be highly detrimental to mother and fetus with hypotension and nonreassuring fetal status.

The gravid uterus causing obstruction of venous return and peripheral pooling of blood will decrease the cardiac output, uteroplacental circulation and the systolic BP.

Intrapartum Hemodynamics

Maternal cardiovascular responses can be further modified by uterine contractions, pain, labor analgesia, surgery, and peripartum blood loss.

Cardiac output increases with each uterine contraction expressing 300–500 mL of blood. This increase is less by 11% with epidural analgesia, thereby making this analgesia suitable for women with anemia and heart disease. Approximately 500 mL of blood loss occurs with vaginal delivery and 1,000 mL with cesarean delivery beyond which the loss is defined as PPH. However, lesser amount of bleeding is tolerated in situations of low hematocrit, e.g. anemia and in situations of inadequate volume expansion, e.g. pre-eclampsia.

Changes in Clotting Factors in Pregnancy

The changes are aimed at hypercoagulable status with shortened clotting time, nature's way of protecting the mother against excessive blood loss. There is increase in fibrinogen concentration from 150–300 mg% to 450–600 mg%. There is increase in factors II, V, VII, VIII, IX, XII and other factors (Fig. 3). There is reduced platelet count due to low-grade intravascular coagulation; there is increased plasminogen activator inhibitor concentration with reduced systemic fibrinolytic capacity. The natural antithrombotics protein S, protein C, and antithrombin III are reduced, there is increase protein C resistance. These changes take 3–6 weeks postpartum to revert to normal.

Pathophysiology of Coagulopathy in Pregnancy

In normal hemostatic response to tissue injury, thrombin generation (mediated by tissue factor and activated factor VII) is

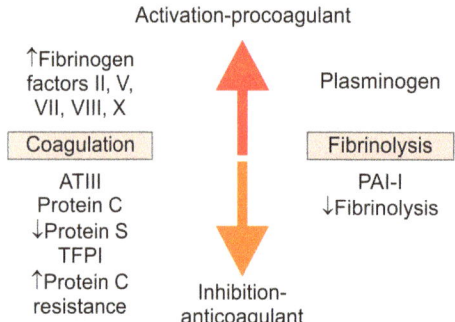

Fig. 3: Factors affecting thrombosis in pregnancy.

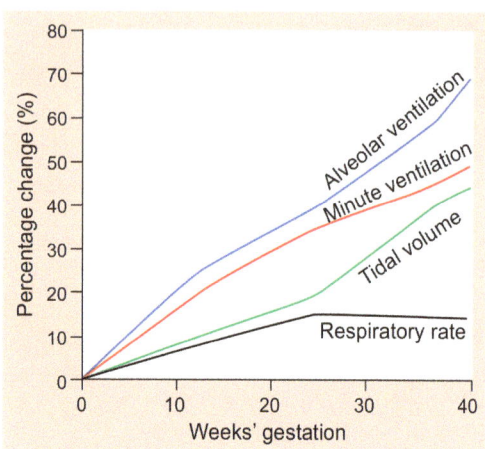

Fig. 4: Maternal respiratory changes.

localized to the site of injury. This localization of thrombin to the site of injury leads to formation of a hemostatic plug composed of platelets and cross-linked fibrin. In massive uterine hemorrhage with extensive clot formation, there is massive consumption of fibrinogen and the new clots are fibrin poor. With massive hemorrhage, there is leak of thrombin into the circulation, which binds antithrombin. Antithrombin is further diluted by infusion of crystalloids. The direct consequence of circulating thrombin, unopposed by antithrombin, is disseminated intravascular coagulation (DIC).

Respiratory Physiology

The airway mucosa in pregnancy has hyperemia, mucosal edema, hypersecretion, and increased friability. Technically classified as Mallampati grade IV airway, the most difficult one, intubation and airway management in a pregnant woman needs higher skill.

The functional residual capacity reduces by 10–20% by term, due to the pressure of gravid uterus and a decreased expiratory reserve volume is a definite change.

The minute ventilation increases and the tidal volume increases by 30–35% mainly because of the increased drive exerted on respiratory center by the high levels of circulating progesterone (Fig. 4).

In fact, these changes make the woman prone for hyperventilation, often reported as breathlessness, with higher tendency for respiratory alkalosis.

Pregnant women are at risk of rapid hypoxemia due to decreased functional residual capacity, increased oxygen consumption and intrapulmonary shunting.

Critical Care Issues in Monitoring and Support of the Pregnant Patient due to Physiological Changes[1,2]

The team should be preferably multidisciplinary with obstetrician, anesthesiologist, intensivist, physician, neonatologist and cardiothoracic surgeon. The following special differences in managing a pregnant woman to be noted:
- It should be assumed that the patient has a difficult airway.
- If the uterus is at or above the umbilicus, left uterine displacement is essential during resuscitation.
- The chest compressions are done using standard hand placement for chest compression.
- The usual measures such as defibrillation and administration of medications should not be delayed.

- Intravenous access should be placed above the diaphragm.
- A dedicated timer at 4 minutes should prompt for a perimortem delivery by cesarean section (also called resuscitative hysterotomy) if return of spontaneous circulation (ROSC) is not achieved by then.
- Oxygenation should be 100% O_2 through face mask at rate of 15 L/minute.
- In case she needs intubation and mechanical ventilation, smaller endotracheal tube diameter 0.5–1 mm to be used.
- Low pressure and low volume ventilation to be used.
- Ephedrine, which has both beta-2 properties and alpha-1 agonist properties, is known to increase uterine blood flow and maternal BP and is the vasoactive drug of choice to treat hypotension in pregnant patients.

Let us come back to Mrs A. It is clear that she suffered from PPH from atonic uterus due to hypertension, operative delivery, effect of medication and tissue hypoxia. She developed pulmonary edema due to inadvertent use of crystalloids as packed RBCs were not available in time. The other significant reason is violation of all three Starling's laws of homeostasis in pre-eclampsia. The endothelial integrity of pulmonary capillaries is damaged allowing leak into extravascular space, further aggravated by increase in intracapillary pressure due to hypertension and fall in osmotic pressure of blood due to proteinuria. Thus, such women easily develop pulmonary edema, which is refractory to treatment and improves only after delivery.

The pregnant woman undergoes several important alterations in her physiology, which protect her from blood loss, hypoxia, organ dysfunction, etc. Paradoxically the same changes can take her to the edge of disaster in complicated pregnancies and if poorly understood by care providers, she will be at risk of inappropriate care and inadequate management of pregnancy complications.

■ CHANGED ANATOMY IN PREGNANCY

The anatomical changes that occur during pregnancy have an important role to play in the understanding of why obstetric hemorrhage occurs and an insight into this aspect can help in prevention and timely management.

Case Scenario

Case 2

Mrs B, 32-year-old multigravida delivers vaginally with low forceps application for fetal distress. After placental expulsion, bleeding continues. Uterus is well contracted. After exploration, a high vaginal tear is seen on the right side as an extension of episiotomy, suturing done under good light and local analgesia. Patient continues to bleed. Estimated blood loss is more than 1.5 L, develops hypotension. Patient is taken to OT and explored. There is intractable bleeding from above the apex not controlled by suturing. Packing proves to be ineffective. A decision is made to perform uterine artery embolization. The pelvic angiogram shows up bleeders low in the pelvis, embolized with Gelfoam. After procedure bleeding is controlled.

Why was there intractable hemorrhage?

Why did we not decide on laparotomy and internal iliac artery ligation?

Let us try and answer these questions posed in the case.

Maternal Anatomy

Obstetric hemorrhage has a varied etiopathology but uterine atony causing PPH, placental abruption and placenta previa are the major

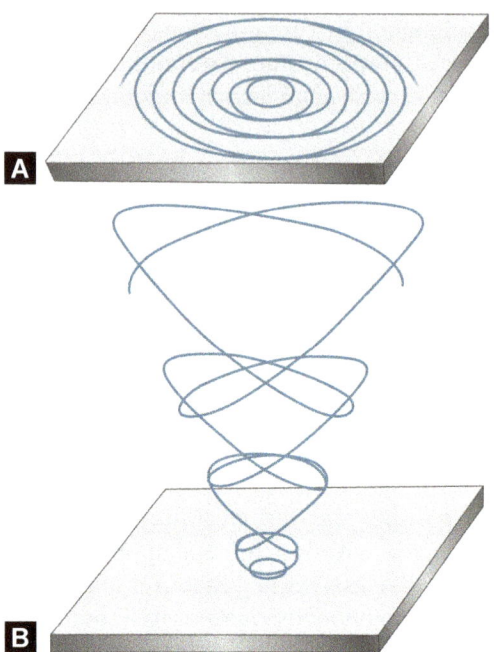

Figs. 5A and B: (A) Circular uterine muscle at rest: two sets of crossing spirals; (B) At term: stretching of the spirals.

causes. The applied anatomy of these will be explored here.

Changes in Pregnancy and Labor

Myometrium

Myometrial anatomy is very important to achieve hemostasis at the placental site during third stage of labor. The myometrium and decidua arrangement is such that powerful muscular contractions after delivery favor hemostasis.[3-5]

Spiral arteries "fan out" to create a low resistance vascular bed in the intervillous space, which facilitates placental blood flow. This flow decreases with muscular activity (Figs. 5A and B).[6]

Third-stage contractions are powerful and prolonged: they act to stop placental blood flow and to separate the placenta and membranes:

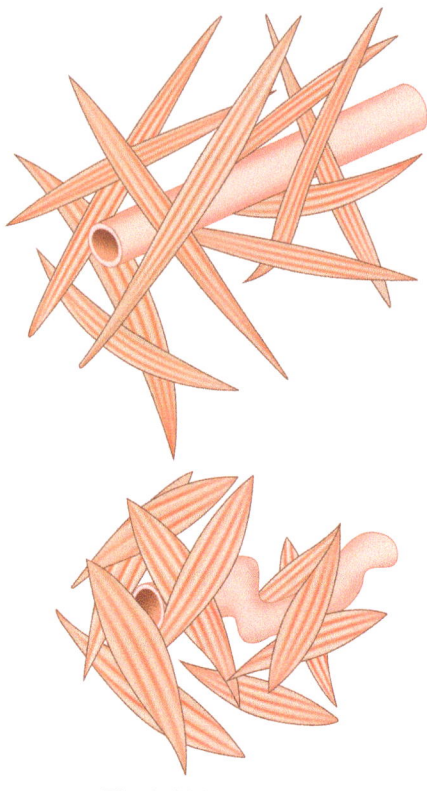

Fig. 6: Living ligatures.

- The innermost part of the muscular layer has been described as superficially "circular" musculature, which is in fact two sets of crossing spirals
- An alternative description is of muscle fibers traveling in all directions
- Both descriptions suggest that blood vessels are compressed during contraction of muscle cells (Fig. 6).

Uterine Atony

The most common cause of PPH is uterine atony, i.e. failure of the uterus to contract. Uterine atony is responsible for 75–90% of primary PPH, but, failure of the uterus to contract may be associated with retained tissue.

The retained material acts as a deterrent against strong uterine contractions needed

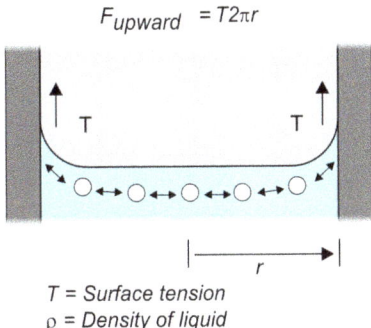

Fig. 7: The Young-Laplace equation. F equals the compressive force acting on the blood vessels, T is the wall tension (generated by the uterine contraction), and r is the radius of the uterus.

to constrict placental bed vessels. Primary hemostasis from the placental bed is due to compression of the uterine vessels as they pass through the myometrium. The degree of compression of these vessels depends on the force acting on the vessels.

This can be explained by the Young-Laplace equation (Fig. 7).

According to the law, the force compressing the vessels cannot be very high if r is large. Therefore, it is essential that the radius of the uterus be made small by emptying the uterus from any blood or placental tissue and increasing the wall tension of the uterus (T) by giving ecbolics.[7]

This is the scientific basis of the initial treatment and the prevention of primary PPH with uterotonics, bimanual compression and surgical compression sutures (like B-Lynch Brace suture) can help to prevent and treat PPH (Figs. 8A and B).

Blood Supply

In pregnancy, there is marked hypertrophy of the uterine vasculature in preparation for establishing and maintaining the uteroplacental circulation. The main blood supply comes from the uterine and ovarian arteries (Fig. 9). The uterine artery is the main branch of the internal iliac artery.

The ovarian artery is a direct branch of the aorta.

The rich cross anastomosis of the four vessels, their branches and tributaries makes it clear that any effort at hemostasis by arterial ligation will require bilateral approach.

It is also evident that bleeding from the cervical and upper vaginal area may not get controlled by uterine or internal iliac artery ligation.

As defined in the writings of Palacios-Jaraquemada, who first used this terminology in 2005, the S1 segment comprises the body of the uterus.[8,9] In Figure 10, the S2 segment corresponds to the lower uterine segment, cervix, upper part of the vagina and the respective parametria. The S1 segment is supplied by ascending branches of the uterine artery and, to a lesser extent, by the descending branches of the ovarian artery. Rarely, the round ligament artery contributes to the collateral blood supply of the uterus. In contrast, the S2 segment is supplied by branches of the uterine, cervical, upper vesical, vaginal and pudendal arteries. All of these blood vessels are located subperitoneally. The blood vessels form a collateral system, which in turn creates a vascular reserve.

A clear understanding of the differences in the blood supply to both uterine segments (S1 and S2) is the basis for the proper selection of a therapeutic intervention, be it surgical or radiological, for the treatment of PPH.

Anatomic evidence: Figure 11 shows a fetal angiographic preparation (representative of adult circulation) illustrating the concept of the rich arterial anastomotic system between the left uterine artery and the corresponding left lower and middle vaginal arteries. These arteries also anastomose with the descending branches of the uterine artery on the ipsilateral

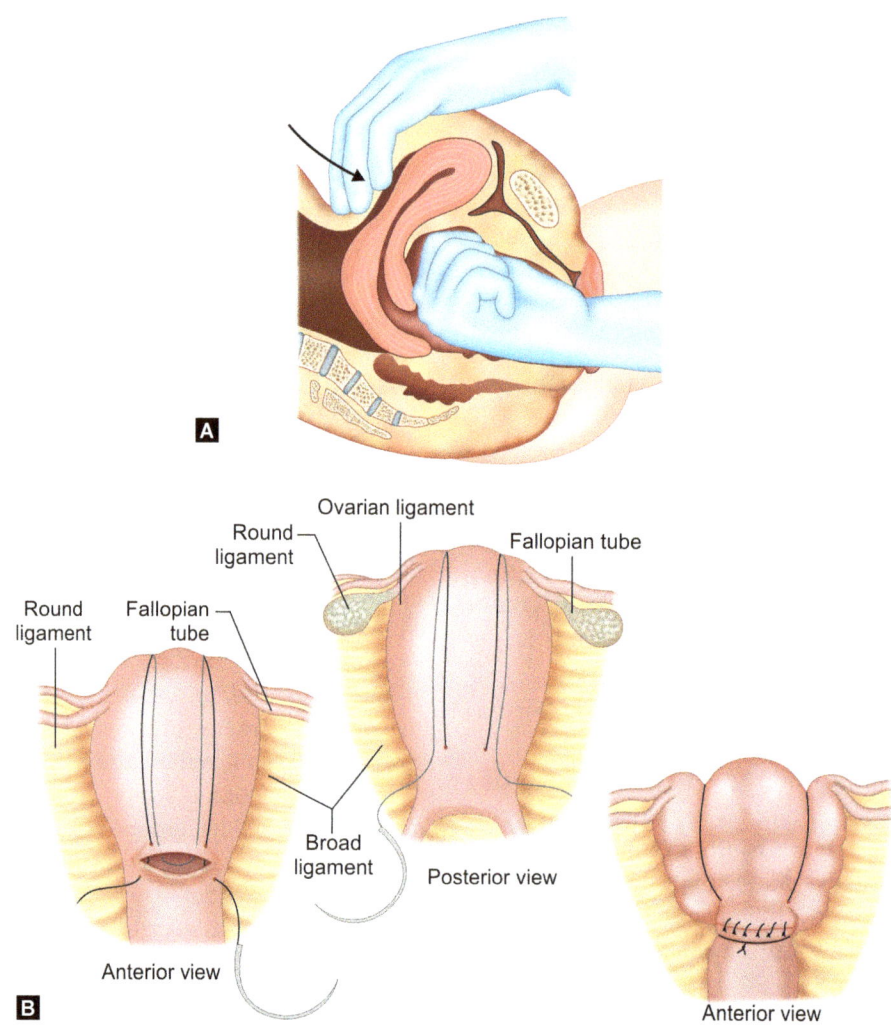

Figs. 8A and B: (A) Bimanual compression; (B) Surgical compression sutures.

side. In other words, this means that the whole of one-half of the lower part of the uterus and the upper part of the vagina receives blood from an interconnected system. The uterine artery and the middle left vaginal artery are branches of the anterior division of the internal iliac artery, whereas the lower left vaginal artery is a branch of the posterior division of the internal iliac artery or it could arise from the internal pudendal artery, which in turn is a branch of the posterior division of internal iliac. This interconnected circulation is responsible for continuation of uterine blood supply when the uterine arteries are embolized and yet future fertility is possible. This is the basis for interventional radiology as a treatment modality in cases of massive blood loss, not responding to uterotonics and when first aid measures have failed. At times, however, when there is neoangiogenesis, as in

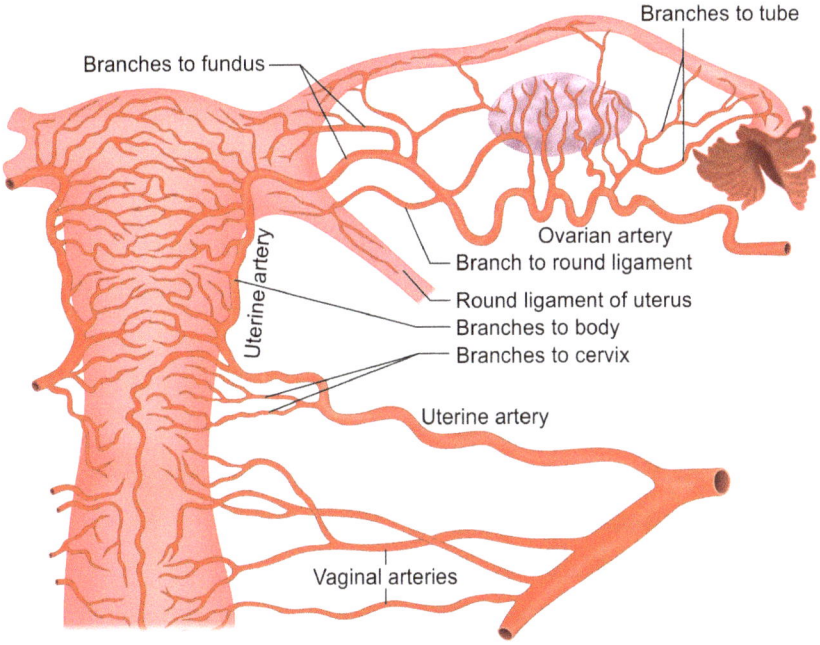

Fig. 9: Blood supply of uterus, vagina, tubes and ovary.

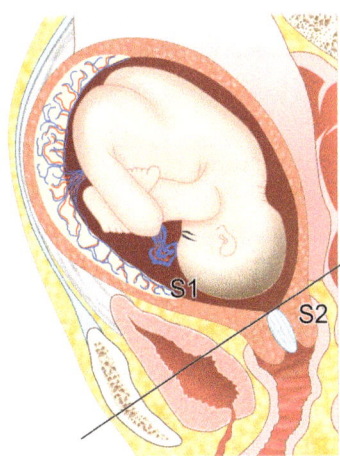

Fig. 10: Uterine segments (S1 and S2).

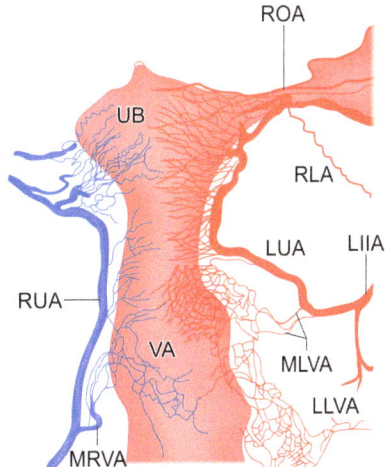

Fig. 11: Arteriography of uterus, ovaries, fallopian tubes, and upper vaginal segment.
(LIIA: left internal iliac artery; LLVA: lower left vaginal artery; LUA: left uterine artery; MLVA: middle left vaginal artery; MRVA: middle right vaginal artery; RLA: round ligament artery; ROA: right ovarian artery; RUA: right uterine artery; UB: uterine body; VA: vagina)
Source: Palacios-Jaraquemada JM, García Mónaco R, Barbosa NE, et al. Lower uterine blood supply: extrauterine anastomotic system and its application in surgical devascularization techniques. Acta Obstet Gynecol Scand. 2007;86:228-34.

adherent placenta, this technique may fail as described later (Fig. 12).

Reasons for failure of some interventional radiological procedures: Figure 13 demonstrates the anatomic basis of why there is failure of some uterine embolization procedure

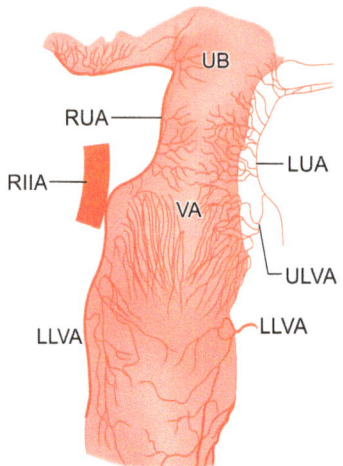

Fig. 12: Arteriography of ovaries, fallopian tubes, uterus, and upper vaginal segment. Demonstrating cross anastomoses between the right and the left uterine arteries over the uterine surface.
(ULVA: upper left vaginal artery; LLVA: lower left vaginal artery; LUA: left uterine artery; RIIA: right internal iliac artery; RUA: right uterine artery; UB: uterine body; VA: vagina)
Source: Palacios-Jaraquemada JM, García Mónaco R, Barbosa NE, et al. Lower uterine blood supply: extrauterine anastomotic system and its application in surgical devascularization techniques. Acta Obstet Gynecol Scand. 2007;86:228-34.

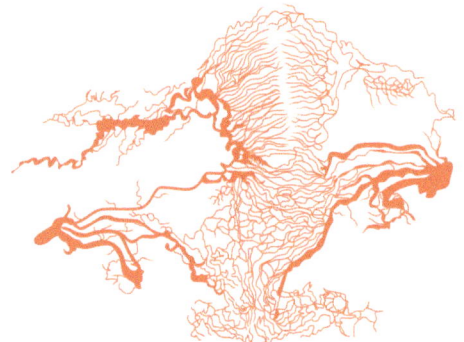

Fig. 13: Failure of some uterine embolization procedure.

in cases of abnormal placentation. It also provides an explanation of why nontarget embolizations occur, especially in the bladder where they may cause necrosis. The interventional radiologists cannot explain these occurrences, because the embolization material has been injected into the uterine artery and the damage is in the area supplied by the vesical artery. Under normal circumstances, the connection between the uterine artery and the vesical artery is microscopic; however, in the presence of *abnormal placentation* and the associated vascular growth factors, these vessels enlarge and represent neovascularization as they lack a tunica media, which in turn allows them to become high flow low resistance systems. When patients undergo interventional radiological procedures in situations involving abnormal placentation, it is important to be aware of the potential for abnormal connections between uterine and vesical arteries. If the embolization material is injected under pressure and if the particle size is small (usually <700 μm), then it is possible to have nontarget embolization to the bladder which occasionally becomes necrotic.

Special Situations

Postpartum hemorrhage following an antepartum hemorrhage.

A rare but catastrophic complication of abruption is extravasation of blood into the myometrium, known as a Couvelaire uterus (Fig. 14), which interferes the physiological uterine contraction/retraction hemostatic process.

Lower Segment as an Implantation Site

Placenta previa: In placenta previa, the placental site is located in an abnormally low position (Fig. 15). Atonic PPH is a recognized complication and, even if cesarean section is performed, severe intraoperative bleeding is a significant risk.[10]

The lower segment is inadequate to maintain hemostasis after delivery as the

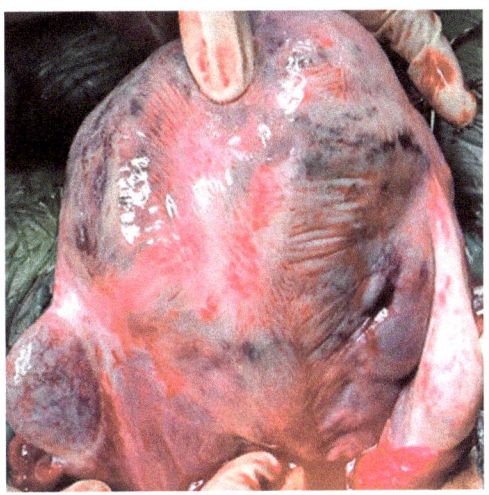

Fig. 14: Couvelaire uterus.

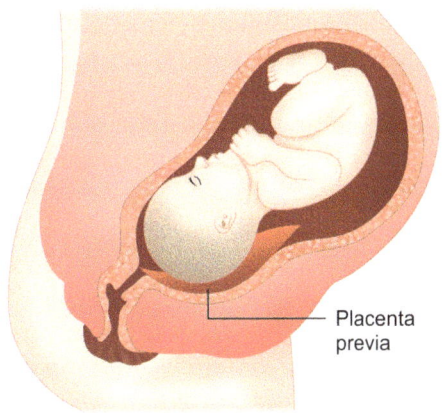

Fig. 15: Placenta previa.

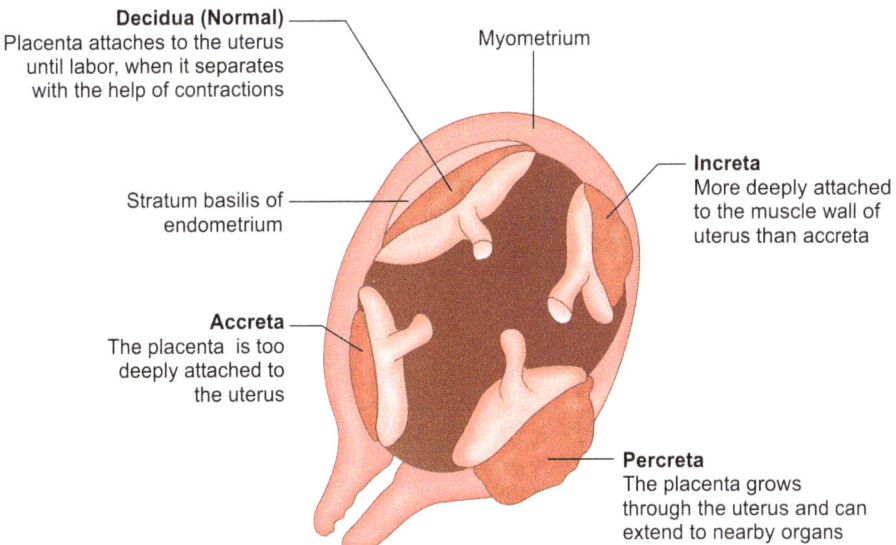

Fig. 16: Types of placenta accreta.
Source: March of Dimes.

muscle layer is thin. Biswas et al.[11] have compared placental bed biopsy changes in placenta previa and normally implanted placenta, showing that previa is associated with significantly higher trophoblastic giant cell infiltration and physiological changes of the myometrial spiral arterioles.

Placenta accreta: The term placenta accreta refers to abnormal adherence, with absence of decidua basalis (Fig. 16).

Placental adherence is also associated with a deficiency of decidua in the lower segment, the most common cause of which is endometrial scarring secondary to previous history of cesarean section. The deficiency of decidua basalis is also the reason why adherent placenta in the lower segment has worse prognosis.

Coming back to Mrs B, there was intractable hemorrhage due to shearing of deep-seated branches of pudendal vessels which bleed through the anastomotic vessels, and so suturing will be of limited value especially when veins are also torn as they may not hold the sutures. Packing is effective for venous bleeds but embolization is necessary for the terminal bleeders from the S2 segment vessels of pelvic vasculature. It is evident that internal iliac artery ligation may not serve the purpose and once performed the option of radiographic uterine artery embolization is lost as the access is blocked.

Therefore, a clear understanding of the anatomical changes helps us to decide the best course of treatment in obstetric hemorrhage.

REFERENCES

1. Roberts SW, Horsager R, Rogers VL, et al. Williams Obstetrics, 24th edition. New York, NY: McGraw-Hill; 2014.
2. American Heart Association. 2015 American Heart Association Guidelines Update for Cardiopulmonary Resuscitation and Emergency Cardiovascular Care. 2015.
3. Goerttler K. Die Architektur der Muskelwand des menschlichen Uterus ind ihre funktionelle Bedeutung. [The architecture of the muscle bonds of the human uterus and their functional behavior.] Gegenbaurs morphologisches Jahrbuch. 1931;45-128.
4. Fuchs A, Fuchs F. Physiology of parturition. In: Gabbe S, Niebyl J, Simpson J (Eds). Obstetrics: Normal and Problem Pregnancies, 2nd edition. New York: Churchill Livingstone; 1991. pp. 147-74.
5. Renn K. Untersuchungen ueber die raeumliche Anordnung der Muskelbuendel im Corpus bereich des menschilichen Uterus. Z Anat Entwicklungsgesch. 1970;132:75-106.
6. Lees MH, Hill JD, Ochsner AJ 3rd, et al. Maternal placental and myometrial blood flow of the rhesus monkey during uterine contractions. Am J Obstet Gynecol. 1971;110:68-81.
7. Drife J. Management of primary postpartum haemorrhage. Br J Obstet Gynaecol. 1997;104: 275-7.
8. Palacios-Jaraquemada JM, Bruno CH. Magnetic resonance imaging in 300 cases of placenta accreta: surgical correlation of new findings. Acta Obstet Gynecol Scand. 2005;84:716-24.
9. Palacios-Jaraquemada JM, García Mónaco R, Barbosa NE, et al. Lower uterine blood supply: extrauterine anastomotic system and its application in surgical devascularization techniques. Acta Obstet Gynecol Scand. 2007; 86:228-34.
10. Konje J, Whalley R. Bleeding in late pregnancy. In: James D, Steer P, Weiner C, Gonik B (Eds). High Risk Pregnancy: Management Options. London: Saunders; 1994. pp. 119-36.
11. Biswas R, Sawhney H, Dass R, et al. Histopathological study of placental bed biopsy in placenta previa. Acta Obstet Gynecol Scand. 1999;78:173-9.

10A

Preventing Hemorrhage in Ectopic Pregnancy

Vidya V Bhat, Bhavana Girish

INTRODUCTION

Ectopic pregnancy (EP) is defined as implantation of a fertilized embryo anywhere outside the endometrial cavity. It is a significant cause of maternal mortality and morbidity and has an estimated prevalence of around 1–2% of pregnancies worldwide.[1] With an increasing number of women conceiving through assisted reproduction, there has been a gradual rise in the incidence of EPs worldwide over the past decade. Most common site of EP is the fallopian tube, which accounts for more than 95% of cases. Other sites of EP include ovarian, abdominal, and cervical pregnancy and cesarean scar pregnancy.[2] Occasionally, pregnancy may be located in both intrauterine and extrauterine sites, termed as a heterotopic pregnancy (HP).

Management of EP should take into consideration both reproductive potential and preferences of the woman as well as minimizing disease- and treatment-related morbidity. The management depends on the clinical condition of the patient, site of EP, and the woman's future reproductive concerns.

TUBAL ECTOPIC PREGNANCY

The most common site of EP is the ampullary portion of the fallopian tube, seen in over 98% of cases.[3] The management options are outlined here.

Expectant Management

Expectant management of an EP involves serial measurement of serum β-human chorionic gonadotropin (β-hCG) and ultrasonography (USG) and waiting for spontaneous resolution of the EP.[4] As per the recommendations of the American College of Obstetricians and Gynecologists, the criteria for expectant management of a suspected EP includes a patient with positive pregnancy test ultrasound does not show a gestational sac or an extrauterine mass and the β-hCG concentration is less than 1,500 IU/mL and declining.[5] However, it is prudent to note that declining levels of serum hCG may still be followed by tubal rupture. Therefore, proper counseling is necessary in case of expectant management, the woman must be kept admitted and monitored for the signs and symptoms of tubal rupture. Furthermore, she should be informed that complete resolution usually occurs between 2 weeks and 3 weeks but may take up to 6–8 weeks, especially with a high pretreatment β-hCG level and this may require prolonged follow-up.

Medical Management

Medical management of EP involves systemic administration of the folate antagonist drug methotrexate (Mtx). There are numerous dosing regimens described in literature such as single dose, two doses or multiple doses regimen. The dosing regimens have

TABLE 1: Methotrexate dosing schedules for ectopic pregnancy.

Protocol	Dosage	Timing of administration	hCG measurement	Additional administration
Single dose	Mtx 50 mg/m² BSA IM	Day 1	Before treatment: Day 1, Day 4, Day 7	Mtx 50 mg/m² BSA, IM on day 7 if hCG drops by <15% from day 4 to day 7
Multiple doses	Mtx 1 mg/kg IM Leucovorin 0.1 mg/kg IM	Mtx: Day 1, 3, 5, 7 Leucovorin: Day 2, 4, 6, 8	Before treatment: Day 1, Day 3, Day 5, Day 7	2nd, 3rd, 4th dose of Mtx 1 mg/kg IM followed by leucovorin 0.1 mg/kg IM if hCG drops by <15% of previous value

(BSA: body surface area; hCG: human chorionic gonadotropin; IM: intramuscular; Mtx: methotrexate)

been presented in Table 1. The single dose regimen is most commonly used due to the convenience of fewer visits to the hospital and lesser adverse effects; however, it may be associated with a higher failure rate as compared to the multiple dose regimen [88%; 95% confidence interval (CI): 86–90% for a single dose vs 93%; 95% CI: 89–96% for multiple doses].[6] Factors predictive of failure of Mtx treatment include initial serum β-hCG greater than 5,000 IU/L, a pretreatment increase in serum β-hCG level of more than 50% over a 48-hour period, presence of moderate-to-large amounts of free fluid in the peritoneal cavity and the presence of fetal cardiac activity on ultrasound.

Prerequisites before administration of Mtx should include assessment of hematologic, hepatic and renal function. Rho(D) immune globulin therapy is recommended in cases of Rh-negative women who are not sensitized. Absolute contraindications to Mtx treatment include breastfeeding mothers; known case of immunodeficiency disorder; alcoholism; chronic liver disease; pre-existing blood dyscrasias; known sensitivity to Mtx; active pulmonary disease; peptic ulcer disease; and hepatic, renal, or hematologic abnormalities. Among the relative, contraindications are high initial hCG levels (>5,000 IU/L),[5] ectopic mass of more than 3.5–4 cm in diameter, presence of fetal cardiac activity detected by transvaginal ultrasound, patients declining blood transfusion or those who are unable to attend follow-up visits. Women under medical management should be explained that they are at risk of tubal rupture after the administration of Mtx, hence, the need to be kept under surveillance as 10% will require intervention due to this.[7] Up to 40% may also suffer from "separation pain", due to separation of the gestational sac from the tubal endothelium after Mtx administration, which may present with abdominal pain and symptoms similar to ruptured EP.[7] Women should be advised to avoid conception for at least 3 months after medical treatment owing to teratogenic effects of Mtx on subsequent pregnancy.

Severe adverse effects are rarely encountered after single dose Mtx treatment for EP, however, unexpected toxicity with Mtx should be kept in mind during its use. The potential severe adverse effects of Mtx treatment are profound and severe myelosuppression, hepatotoxicity, nephrotoxicity, pulmonary toxicity, and risk of infection. Development of myelosuppression and mucositis are more likely in women receiving multiple doses of the drug.

Patients with Mtx toxicity are best managed in intensive care setting with multidisciplinary team management. Folinic acid must be given to counteract the dihydrofolate reductase inhibitory effect of Mtx. Recently, there has been synthesis of a bacterial enzyme called glucarpidase, which hydrolyses Mtx to its inactive metabolites and rapidly causes decline of plasma Mtx levels. In case of failure of these therapies, plasmapheresis may be required.

Surgical Management

Surgical management is indicated in patients who have ruptured EP, hemodynamic instability, completed family, contraindications to medical management or those unwilling for medical management. Laparoscopic approach to EP was first performed in 1973 by Shapiro and Adler and is now the accepted standard of treatment.

There is conclusive evidence from three prospective randomized trials that demonstrate the superiority of laparoscopic approach over laparotomy in terms of lower blood loss, pain medication requirement, cost, and length of hospital stay.[8-10] There are no significant differences in reproductive outcomes, including rates of recurrent EP and subsequent intrauterine pregnancy, between laparotomy and a laparoscopic approach.

Type of Surgery

There are mainly two accepted methods of clearance of the ectopic gestation sac: (1) salpingectomy, which is defined as partial or complete removal of the fallopian tube and (2) salpingostomy (also called salpingotomy) wherein the ectopic gestation sac is removed through an incision over the fallopian tube while leaving the tube in situ.

Salpingectomy: It is recommended in cases of extensive tubal damage and/or rupture, uncontrolled bleeding, prior tubal sterilization, or a large tubal EP (5 cm or more in diameter).[8] The surgical approach should be determined by the status of the patient's contralateral fallopian tube, the patient's plans for future fertility, and surgeon comfort or preference.

Salpingostomy: Linear salpingostomy may be performed in women with contralateral tubal damage, those with history of contralateral salpingectomy, or those who wish to preserve their tube after appropriate counseling regarding risks of subsequent repeat EP and persistent EP (15% incidence of recurrent EP and 4–15% risk of persistent EP).[9] The procedure includes injection of dilute vasopressin into the mesosalpinx at the site of planned incision following which a 1–2 cm linear incision is made using monopolar or bipolar electrocautery, laser or scissors over the bulge in the tube. The products of conception are removed using forceps or high-pressure irrigation, also called hydrodissection. The use of hydrodissection to flush out gestational products may be preferable to piecemeal removal with forceps, as the latter can lead to incomplete removal of trophoblastic tissue. The tubal incision can be left open to heal by secondary intention or sutured closed; a Cochrane review reported an insignificant difference.[10] Women managed by salpingostomy may need follow-up with serial β-hCG levels to ensure complete resolution of the EP.

Laparoscopy in the presence of hemoperitoneum: Hemoperitoneum is no longer a contraindication to performance of laparoscopy. The main goal of surgery would be to enter the peritoneal cavity and secure hemostasis as quickly as possible. In any event, a patient who is hemodynamically unstable must be stabilized first, blood transfusion might be needed. The use of an intrauterine manipulator allows the quick identification of the bleeding site by lifting the uterus away from the pool of blood in the abdominal cavity. The laparoscope should be inserted gradually without touching the blood in the peritoneal cavity to ensure that the tip of the scope will remain clean, allowing optimal visualization of the pelvic organs. Hemostasis should be performed as quickly as possible, most often by salpingectomy.

NONTUBAL ECTOPIC PREGNANCY

Nontubal EPs, though still rare, are being increasingly encountered in the era of assisted reproductive technology (ART). However, there is a lack of consensus and definitive guidelines on its management due to paucity of large-scale data. Expectant and medical management may be attempted in hemodynamically stable patients, but due to the potential of major complications of these EPs, surgical treatment may be preferable.

CERVICAL PREGNANCY

Cervical EP is defined as implantation of the gestation sac in the endocervix, below the level of the internal os. These are extremely dangerous due to high risk of early rupture and risk of trophoblast penetration through the cervical wall into the uterine vessels leading to massive hemorrhage. Management of cervical pregnancies may be medical, surgical or a combination of these. Previously, the safest approach was to perform a hysterectomy in all cases, either pre-emptively or as an emergency due to uncontrolled bleeding.

Medical management may be attempted in an early cervical pregnancy if the patient is hemodynamically stable. Reported success rates for local or systemic Mtx administration range between 60% and 90%.[11] Mtx offers a potential for fertility-sparing treatment, which is extremely important in this patient population, who are often infertile or nulliparous. Recently, Krissi et al. also reported 96% success rate using a combined approach of uterine artery Mtx infusion with systemic Mtx administration.[12]

Options for surgical management include dilatation and curettage, hysteroscopic resection, and hysterectomy. Dilatation and curettage is rarely used in isolation or as a first-line treatment due to the risk of hemorrhage. Measures to reduce blood loss during surgery include uterine artery embolization, uterine balloon tamponade, cervical encerclage, cervical stay sutures, and injection of prostaglandin F2α.

INTERSTITIAL PREGNANCY

Interstitial pregnancy is defined as implantation of the gestational sac at the junction of the interstitial part of the fallopian tube and the uterine myometrium.[13] Interstitial pregnancies are considered a separate entity from tubal EP due to higher risk of early rupture and hemorrhage owing to their location within the highly vascular myometrium, which has vascular supplies from both the uterine and ovarian vessels.

Medical management options include local (intra-amniotic) or systemic injection of Mtx or local injection of potassium chloride. Horne et al. have also reported success with use of systemic Mtx in combination with gefitinib (oral epidermal growth factor receptor inhibitor), with an average time to resolution of hCG levels between 65 days and 68 days (range 25–1,196 days).[14]

Surgical management includes resection of the ectopic sac by laparoscopic approach or laparotomy. Surgical approaches include injection of dilute vasopressin into the myometrium at the cornua to minimize blood loss followed by cornual resection or cornuostomy. Interstitial EPs measuring more than 3-4 cm require cornual resection with removal of the adjacent fallopian tube to prevent recurrence and layered closure as for a myomectomy. Katz et al. have reported successful hysteroscopic clearance of interstitial EP under laparoscopic guidance.[15] During subsequent pregnancies, these women are at increased risk of uterine rupture and patients must be counseled accordingly, although vaginal deliveries have been reported after cornual resection.

CORNUAL PREGNANCY

Implantation of gestational sac in the rudimentary horn of a bicornuate uterus is termed as a cornual EP; it is seen to occur in 0.2-2% of cases.

Management of a cornual EP involves resection of the rudimentary uterine horn by laparotomy or laparoscopic approach.[13] Laparotomy may be preferable due to hemorrhage or large cornual ectopics of advanced gestation and difficulty in retrieval of the specimen necessitating tissue morcellation techniques. In view of the resultant defect in the uterine myometrium, significant concerns remain regarding the risk of uterine rupture in subsequent pregnancies and elective cesarean section is widely recommended.

OVARIAN PREGNANCY

Ovarian pregnancies are quite rare, accounting for 1-6% of EPs. They are highly vascular and up to one-third of patients present with ruptured ectopic and circulatory collapse.[16] An important differential diagnosis to be considered in these women is rupture of corpus luteum of pregnancy. Medical management is usually unsuccessful and surgical management is the mainstay, options include laparoscopic clearance of the gestational sac or ovarian wedge resection. Partial or total oophorectomy must be reserved for cases with uncontrolled hemorrhage. Conservative resection (wedge resection) with ovarian reconstruction can be performed in patients wishing to preserve their fertility and case reports have revealed that these patients successfully conceive following surgery.[17]

ABDOMINAL PREGNANCY

Abdominal EPs are the rarest form of EPs, accounting for 0.9-1.4% of EPs. The gestational sac may be implanted anywhere in the abdominal cavity and derive its vascular supply from various sites including the omentum; organs such as liver, spleen, and bowel; large vessels; pouch of Douglas; broad ligament; and pelvic side wall. Diagnosis requires a high degree of suspicion and is often delayed.

Surgical management is the mainstay of treatment and laparotomy is the conventional method. Laparoscopy may be attempted in an early abdominal EP; however, availability of surgical expertise is crucial. Maternal complications increase with advancing gestation as the implantation site frequently involves large vessels and vital organs. There is no robust data on the conservative management of abdominal pregnancies, although isolated case reports have described leaving placental tissue behind with subsequent Mtx treatment, and ultrasound-guided injection of potassium chloride (KCl)[13] or uterine artery embolization to minimize blood loss.[18]

CESAREAN SCAR PREGNANCY

The number of cesarean scar pregnancies is on a steady rise with the increasing number of cesarean deliveries. It is defined as implantation of the gestation sac over the defective uterine myometrium at the site of previous cesarean scar. The treatment approach depends on various factors like hemodynamic stability, gestational age, availability of endoscopic expertise, feasibility of serial follow-up, and desire for future fertility.

Conservative management options include systemic Mtx, local injection of embryocide, or a combination of both.[19] However, caution must be exercised with Mtx administration as it may lead to separation of the sac leading to life-threatening hemorrhage, necessitating emergency hysterectomy. Apart from Mtx, local injections of potassium chloride, etoposide, and hyperosmolar glucose have been reported with limited success. Medical treatment may also be combined with surgical aspiration of sac, but long-term follow-up with serum β-hCG and imaging is necessary. If β-hCG levels plateau on follow-up or scan shows increasing vascularity on Doppler, then these women are at high risk of internal bleeding or uterine rupture and hence may require surgical procedure.[20]

Several surgical approaches have also been reported, including dilatation and curettage, hysteroscopic and laparoscopic approach. Measures to reduce blood loss include balloon tamponade with a transcervical catheter and application of hemostatic cervical cerclage sutures. Uterine artery embolization has been used as both hemorrhage prophylaxis and salvage therapy in the event of hemorrhage but is not recommended in women desirous of future fertility. Hysteroscopic resection of cesarean scar EPs may be performed using monopolar or bipolar electrocautery, however, it is not recommended when the residual myometrium is less than 3 mm, given the risk of anterior wall perforation and bladder injury.[21] Transabdominal excision by laparoscopy or laparotomy may be preferable when scar pregnancy is deeply implanted and grows towards abdominal cavity and bladder,[20] in such cases as it also allows for revision of the lower uterine segment, which theoretically may reduce risk for recurrence.[21] Principles of laparoscopic approach are excision of the scar pregnancy, removal in endobag, and closure of the uterine defect by endoscopic suturing. Bleeding may be minimized by local injection of vasopressin and hemostasis is achieved by bipolar diathermy.

HETEROTOPIC PREGNANCY

Treatment of an HP is to be individualized depending on the viability of intrauterine pregnancy, specific location of EP, patient's clinical presentation, and clinical stability. Medical management with Mtx is not suitable as it is a known teratogen, treatment options available are local injections of KCl or hyperosmolar glucose solution into the gestational sac under USG guidance. Success rate of medical treatment is variable, over half of tubal HPs managed with local KCl and may require subsequent salpingectomy.[22]

Surgical management has been described more frequently, as patients with tubal HPs present more often with rupture and hemodynamic compromise than those with tubal EPs alone. Mainstay of surgery is salpingectomy by laparotomy or laparoscopic approach, salpingostomy is generally avoided as persistent trophoblastic tissue cannot be monitored in the setting of ongoing intrauterine pregnancy. The viable intrauterine pregnancy must be left undisturbed, uterine manipulation during surgery should be kept to a minimum; however, these women have miscarriage rates up to 30% due to stress of surgery and anesthesia.[23]

FUTURE FERTILITY CONCERNS

Fertility after an EP depends on how that pregnancy was managed, and on the presence or absence of known risk factors for recurrence. Data from observational studies show that women with history of EP have 80–88% chances of subsequent intrauterine pregnancy, although they are at increased rates of recurrent EP of up to 4.2–5%, which is double the risk in the general population.[24,25]

CONCLUSION

With increasing and widespread usage of ART, EP is a relatively common clinical scenario with which all general gynecologist and reproductive medicine specialists must be familiar. While tubal pregnancies are the most common, EPs may occur throughout the abdomen and pelvis. The advances in laparoscopy have done away with the inconvenience of open surgery for many women. Fertility preserving conservative tubal surgery has also become possible with good outcome in subsequent pregnancies.

KEY MESSAGES

- A high degree of suspicion is necessary for diagnosis of EP; in any women with risk factors, one must "think ectopic".
- Treatment in stable patients is often medical, though patients must meet the strict clinical criteria and consent to rigorous follow-up.
- Nontubal EPs may require differing and/or more invasive treatment, the intervention and opinion of a senior gynecologist may be sought.
- Nontubal EPs may be associated with catastrophic life-threatening hemorrhage. Surgeons must be well-versed with techniques to reduce hemorrhage.
- Laparotomy is rarely needed even in women with intraperitoneal hemorrhage, most surgical treatment can be performed by laparoscopy and in some cases by hysteroscopy.

CASE SCENARIOS

Case 1

A 25-year-old primiparous lady married for 8 months with a history of abdominal tuberculosis presented to the emergency department with history of amenorrhea for 1 month and complaints of pain abdomen, vomiting, and dizziness. Urine pregnancy test was positive, and a transvaginal sonography showed a right adnexal mass of 4 × 3 cm with free fluid in the pouch of Douglas. As she was tachycardic and hypotensive on admission, she was planned for emergency laparoscopy. Peroperative findings are shown in Figure 1. This patient was managed with right salpingectomy due to presence of hemoperitoneum and active bleeding from the ruptured tube.

Case 2

A 32-year-old second gravida presented with history of amenorrhea for 1 month and a positive urine pregnancy test done at home. She had a history of infertility and had undergone intrauterine insemination. A transvaginal scan showed empty uterine cavity and a right adnexal mass with gestational sac seen within it. She initially opted for medical management with Mtx, however, after 2 days of administration of Mtx she developed severe abdominal pain.

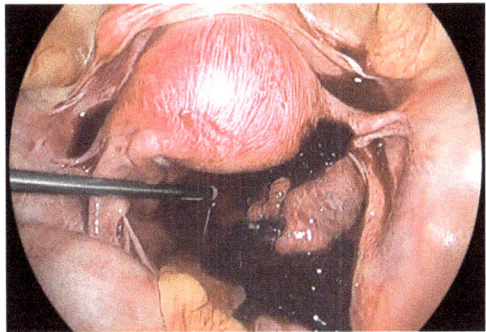

Fig. 1: Laparoscopic image showing ruptured right tubal ectopic pregnancy with hemoperitoneum.

A diagnostic laparoscopy was done showing the findings in Figure 2. Conservative surgery with right salpingostomy was performed as she refused a salpingectomy.

Case 3

A 23-year-old primigravid woman presented to the emergency department with complaints of abdominal pain and bleeding per vagina. Her USG showed a right adnexal mass of 5 × 6 cm with gestational sac within it, both ovaries were seen separate from the mass. On laparoscopy, a ruptured right rudimentary horn pregnancy was seen (Fig. 3), and a right rudimentary horn excision was performed.

Case 4

A 36-year-old multiparous woman presented with history of amenorrhea with positive urine pregnancy test, she had been using an intrauterine device as contraception. A transvaginal USG showed a left adnexal mass which was not seen separate from the ovary, 2 × 3 cm in size with the IUD in situ in the uterine cavity (Fig. 4). She underwent a laparoscopy which showed enlarged left ovary with an area of increased vascularity over it, right ovary and bilateral tubes appeared normal. An incision was given over the left ovary through which the gestational sac extruded out and ovarian reconstruction was performed.

Case 5

A 27-year-old woman presented with amenorrhea of 2 months duration with history of pain abdomen and vaginal spotting on and off. A transvaginal scan showed normal uterine cavity with thick endometrium and

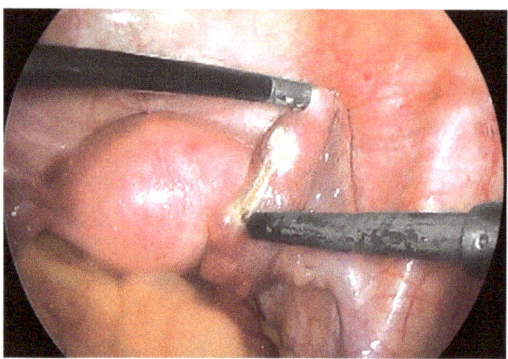 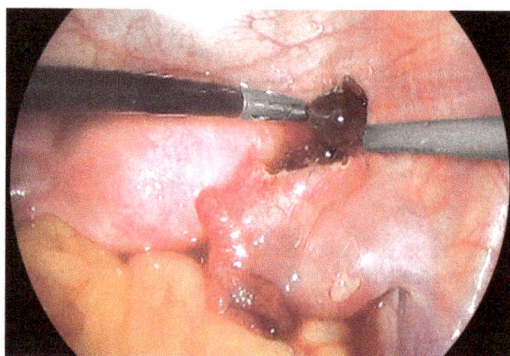

Fig. 2: Laparoscopic image showing unruptured right tubal ectopic pregnancy with salpingostomy incision.

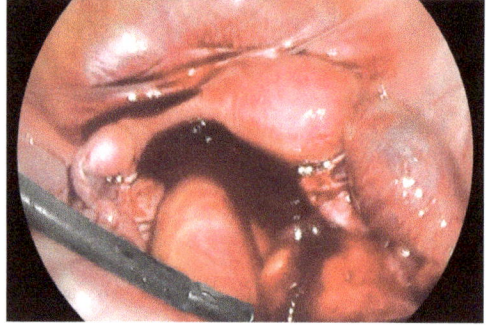 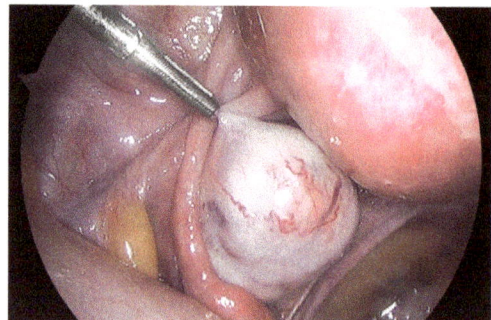

Fig. 3: Laparoscopic image showing ectopic pregnancy in right uterine rudimentary horn.

Fig. 4: Laparoscopic view of left ovarian ectopic pregnancy.

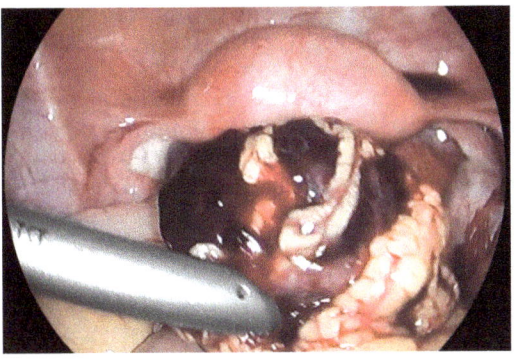 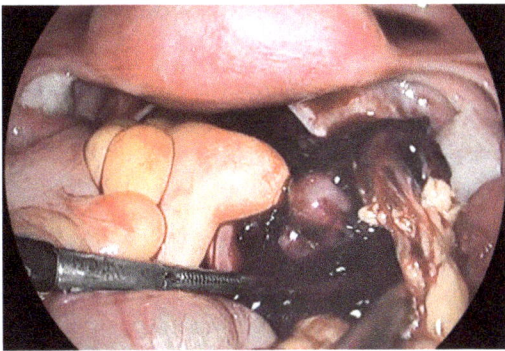

Fig. 5: Laparoscopic view of secondary abdominal pregnancy.

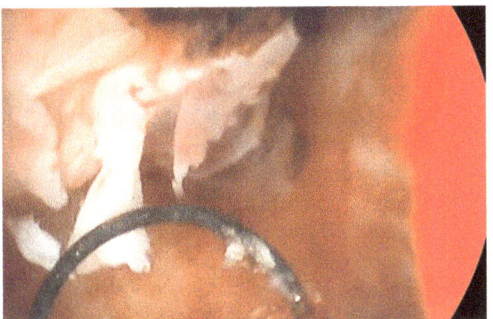

Fig. 6: Hysteroscopic resection of cesarean scar ectopic pregnancy.

bilateral normal appearing tubes and ovaries, there was a mass seen in the pouch of Douglas. A diagnostic laparoscopy showed the findings, an edematous right tube with a 3 × 3 cm heterogeneous mass adherent to the omentum (Fig. 5). A diagnosis of secondary abdominal pregnancy with vascular supply from the omentum was made and omentectomy performed.

Case 6

A 28-year-old second gravida with previous cesarean section presented for an early pregnancy assessment. Her ultrasound showed a low-lying gestational sac with increased myometrial vascularity which was confirmed on magnetic resonance imaging (MRI). With the provisional diagnosis of a scar EP, a diagnostic hysteroscopy was performed as shown in Figure 6. Using a monopolar loop, the gestational sac was excised with minimal damage to the underlying myometrium. Follow-up β-hCG measurements showed resolution of the pregnancy.

REFERENCES

1. Murray H, Baakdah H, Bardell T, et al. Diagnosis and treatment of ectopic pregnancy CMAJ. 2005;173:905-12.
2. Coste J, Bouyer J, Job-Spira N. Epidemiology of ectopic pregnancy: incidence and risk factors. Contracep Fertil Sex. 1996;24:135-9.
3. Bouyer J, Coste J, Shojaei T, et al. Risk factors for ectopic pregnancy: a comprehensive analysis based on a large case–control, population-based study in France. Am J Epidemiol. 2003;157:185-94.
4. Kelly AJ, Sowter MC, Trinder J. The management of tubal pregnancy. RCOG Green-top Guideline No. 21. London: RCOG; 2004.
5. American College of Obstetricians and Gynecologists. ACOG Practice Bulletin No. 94: medical management of ectopic pregnancy. Obstet Gynecol. 2008;111:1479-85.
6. Barmhart KT, Gosman G, Ashby R, et al. The medical management of ectopic pregnancy: a meta-analysis comparing 'single dose and multi-dose' regimes. Obstet Gynecol. 2003;101:778-84.
7. Hajenius PJ, Engelsbel S, Mol BW, et al. Randomised trial of systemic methotrexate versus laparoscopic salpingostomy in tubal pregnancy. Lancet. 1997;350:774-79.

8. Vermesh M, Silva PD, Rosen GF, et al. Management of unruptured ectopic gestation by linear salpingostomy: a prospective randomized clinical trial of laparoscopy versus laparotomy. Obstet Gynecol. 1989;73:400-4.
9. Murphy AA, Nager CW, Wujek JJ, et al. Operative laparoscopy versus laparotomy for the management of ectopic pregnancy: a prospective trial. Fertil Steril. 1992;57:1180-5.
10. Hajenius PJ, Mol F, Bossuyt PMM, et al. Interventions for tubal ectopic pregnancy. Cochrane Database Syst Rev. 2007;24(1):CD000324.
11. Panelli D, Phillips CH, Brady PC. Incidence, diagnosis and management of tubal and nontubal ectopic pregnancies: a review. Fertil Res Pract. 2015;1:15.
12. Krissi H, Hiersch L, Stolovitch N, et al. Outcome, complications and future fertility in women treated with uterine artery embolization and methotrexate for non-tubal ectopic pregnancy. Eur J Obstet Gynecol Reprod Biol 2014;184:172-6.
13. Shen L, Fu J, Huang W, et al. Interventions for non-tubal ectopic pregnancy. Cochrane Database Syst Rev. 2014;7:CD011174.
14. Horne AW, Skubisz MM, Tong S, et al. Combination gefitinib and methotrexate treatment for non-tubal ectopic pregnancies: a case series. Hum Reprod. 2014;29(7):1375-9.
15. Katz DL, Barrett JP, Sanfilippo JS, et al. Combined hysteroscopy and laparoscopy in the treatment of interstitial pregnancy. Am J Obstet Gynecol. 2003;188:1113-4.
16. Casikar I, Condous G. How to effectively diagnose ectopic pregnancy on ultrasound. Expert Rev Obstet Gynecol. 2013;8(6):493-5.
17. Alalade A, Mayers K, Abdulrahman G, et al. A 12-year analysis of non-tubal ectopic pregnancies: do the clinical manifestations and risk factor for these rare pregnancies differ from those of tubal pregnancies? Gynecol Surg. 2017;13:1-7.
18. Rahaman J, Berkowitz R, Mitty H, et al. Minimally invasive management of an advanced abdominal pregnancy. Obstet Gynecol. 2004;103:1064-8.
19. Seow KM, Huang LW, Lin YH, et al. Caesarean scar pregnancy: issues in management. Ultrasound Obstet Gynecol. 2004;23:247-53.
20. Patel MA. Scar ectopic pregnancy. J Obstet Gynaecol India. 2015;65(6):372-5.
21. Wang G, Liu X, Bi F, et al. Evaluation of the efficacy of laparoscopic resection for the management of exogenous cesarean scar pregnancy. Fertil Steril. 2014;101:1501-7.
22. Goldstein JS, Ratts VS, Philpott T, et al. Risk of surgery after use of potassium chloride for treatment of tubal heterotopic pregnancy. Obstet Gynecol. 2006;107(2 Pt 2):506-8.
23. Clayton HB, Schieve LA, Peterson HB, et al. Ectopic pregnancy risk with assisted reproductive technology procedures. Obset Gynecol. 2006;107:595-604.
24. Pisarska MD, Carson SA, Buster JE. Ectopic pregnancy. Lancet. 1998;351:1115-20.
25. Yao M, Tulandi T. Current status of surgical and nonsurgical management of ectopic pregnancy. Fertil Steril. 1997;67:421-32.

10B Chapter
The Dreaded Miscarriages: Incomplete and Septic Abortions

Vidya A Thobbi

INTRODUCTION

Miscarriage is the loss of pregnancy before the period of fetal viability. It is one of the most common complications of pregnancy. The term therefore includes all pregnancy losses from conception up to 20 weeks in North America and 24 weeks in Europe.[1] WHO defines abortion as the expulsion or extraction from its mother of an embryo or fetus weighing 500 g or less when it is not capable of independent survival.[2] This 500 g of fetal development is attained approximately at 22 weeks (154 days) of gestation.

Be that as it may, whatever the reason, there is a common pathway, which includes uterine contractions, placental detachment, and expulsion of uterine contents. Fetal demise may precede expulsion, in a "missed miscarriage", varying degrees of bleeding, is accompanied by expulsion of the embryo and placenta which, may vary from a few drops of blood to torrential hemorrhage.

Different types of abortion are shown in Flowchart 1.

INCOMPLETE ABORTION

Definition

Incomplete expulsion of the products of conception is known as incomplete miscarriage. This is the most frequently encountered type met amongst women.

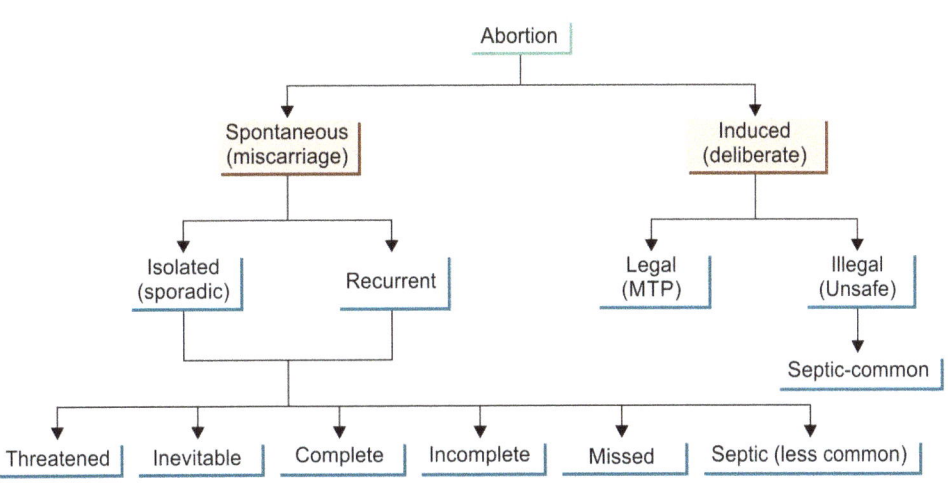

Flowchart 1: Classification or varieties of abortion.[3]

(MTP: medical termination of pregnancy)

Clinical Features

History of expulsion of a fleshy mass per vaginam followed by:
- Lower abdominal pain
- Persistent bleeding per vaginam
- On pelvic examination:
  - Uterus does not correspond with the period of gestation
  - Patulous cervical os usually admits tip of the finger.
- Varying amount of per vaginam bleeding
- Incomplete products of conception
- *Ultrasonography (USG)*: Reveals echogenic material (products of conception) within the cavity.

Complications

The retained products may cause:
- Profuse bleeding
- Sepsis or
- Placental polyp.

The above complications may lead to compromise of mother's well-being and future fertility.

Complications due to Medical Termination of Pregnancy

Abortion-related mortality and morbidity have declined as abortion has been legalized in 1971 in India. Safe and effective method cannot be guaranteed in all cases. However, there are lesser complications (5%) if termination is done before 8 weeks by manual vacuum aspiration (MVA) or suction evacuation/curette. It has been observed that complications are fivefold higher in midtrimester abortions. Safety profile of midtrimester abortions has improved due to use of prostaglandins (PGs) and mifepristone.

Specific Issues of Hemorrhage in Case of Medical Abortion

- Bleeding as a complication is more often seen with medical abortions. It is observed that there is increased risk of hemorrhage in cases of patients with anemia.
- Hence, an important step prior to medical abortion is to counsel women regarding excessive bleeding.

The complications can occur due to:
- Methods used for abortion
- Abortion process.

Immediate

- Traumatic cervical injuries, lacerations, and uterine perforations
- Hemorrhage and shock due to trauma, incomplete evacuation of products of conception, and atonic uterus
- Thrombosis or embolism
- Sepsis pain, bleeding, and low-grade fever due to retained clots or products.

Related to the methods employed:
- *Prostaglandins*: Excessive vomiting, diarrhea, fever, and trauma to cervix and uterus.
- *Oxytocin*: Water intoxication and convulsions.

The incidence of hemorrhage after abortion occurs in <1%, but there is significant associated morbidity. Postabortion hemorrhage blood loss is defined as "more than 250 mL blood loss," more than 500 mL blood loss", "or which require hospitalization" and transfusion.

Incidence

- After vacuum aspiration in the first trimester: 0–3 per 1,000 cases[4-6]
- Bleeding immediately after first trimester abortion is rare

- Delayed bleeding is more commonly seen in first trimester abortions.

On the basis of two recent, large, and registry-based cohort studies found that 1–2% of patients who had first trimester surgical abortion had bleeding that needed a visit or secondary surgical intervention.[8,9] The drawback of these studies was that there is no consistent definition of bleeding and represent overestimates of excessive bleeding after first trimester abortion.

Bleeding following surgical abortion is more common in the second trimester than the first, with estimates ranging from 0.9 to 10 per 1,000 cases.[10,11]

Hemorrhage can be due to:
- Atony of uterus
- Coagulopathy, and
- Abnormal placentation.

Cause of hemorrhage and risk factors:
- *Atony*: Prior lower segment cesarean section (LSCS), gestational age, increasing maternal age, and use of halogenated agents
- *Perforation*: Insufficient cervical dilation and increased gestational age
- *Abnormal placental location*: Uterine scar
- *Cervical laceration*: Nulliparity and incomplete cervical dilatation
- *Retained tissue*: Intraoperative ultrasound
- *Coagulopathy*: Family/personal history of bleeding.

Management

Evacuation and complete removal of product of conception is done. Resuscitation is important before any active treatment is undertaken (Table 1).

Hemorrhage is caused by the abortion process and also by the injury inflicted during the interference.
- Hemorrhage following abortion occurs in less than 1% of abortions, but associated with significant morbidity.
- There is limited evidence on which to make recommendations regarding risk factors and treatment for postabortion hemorrhage.
- Prior cesarean sections women are at higher risk of overall complications from second trimester abortion. Complications are seven times higher among women with two or more cesarean sections.
- According to current standard in the United States, blood grouping should be obtained for all patients undergoing abortion, since it is essential to give anti-D immune globulin for all Rh D-negative patients, including for those in early gestations.
- An organized approach goes a long way in effectively evaluation and treatment of postabortion hemorrhage.

Algorithm for management of postabortion hemorrhage:
- *Assessment and examination*:
  - "Cannula test" is helpful to differentiate lower uterine segment or high cervical bleeding (e.g. site of a previous scar or cervical laceration) from that of atony at the fundus. The cannula test is performed by inserting an 8–10 mm cannula into the fundus and withdrawing it slowly to identify when bleeding through the cannula is more.
- Medical therapy
- Laboratory evaluation
- Resuscitation and evacuation or tamponade for atony massage
- Radiological interventions: Embolization
- Surgery.

Management of Hemorrhage following Abortions[7]

The cause of hemorrhage has to be evaluated first:
- *Cervical injuries and laceration*: Complete inspection of cervix

TABLE 1: Algorithm for classifying women as being at low, moderate or high risk for hemorrhage after abortion.[7]

Hemorrhage risk group	Prevention and preparation measures

Low risk:
• No operative lower segment cesarean section (LSCS) prior
• Lesser than two prior cesarean sections and no previa or accreta
• No history of bleeding disorder
• No history prior obstetric hemorrhage
	Measures for all estimation of:
	• Preoperative hemoglobin or hematocrit values
	• Ultrasound
	• Ripen cervix:
	  – Dilators if gestational age more than 20 weeks
	  – Misoprostol or dilators if more than 13 weeks
	• In cases of Paracervical block, vasopressin can be considered

Moderate risk: • Cesarean sections • Previous cesarean section and low placenta • Bleeding disorder • Obstetrical hemorrhage • Advanced maternal age • Gestational age more than 20 weeks • Fibroids • Obesity	Above factors: • Consent for transfusion • Oxytocics available • Intraoperative ultrasound: – Prepare cervix • Dilators for cervical preparation if > 20 weeks
High risk: • Placenta accreta • History obstetrical hemorrhage requiring transfusion • Any of the "moderate risk" categories may be considered "high risk"	Above factors and then: • Patient should be referred to higher center with blood and blood products availability, anesthesia, and interventional radiology • Consents for transfusion and hysterectomy • Renal function tests, coagulation profile • Blood typing and cross-matching of more than 2 units of blood and blood products

- Uterine atony examination
- *Hematometra*: Seen on ultrasound.

Treatment is divided into primary, secondary, and tertiary treatment (Table 2).

Uterotonics:
- Urgent administration of oxytocics if there is failure of uterine massage. Frequently used are methylergometrine maleate and misoprostol; oxytocin and carboprost are used less often. Repeat doses of oxytocics can be considered if severe bleeding does not reduce with a single agent.

Methylergometrine maleate:
- Onset < 5 minutes
- *Route*: Intramuscularly (most common) or intravenously 0.2 mg dose.

Misoprostol:
- Unknown routes and frequency of dosing.
- *Dose in case of hemorrhage*: 800–1,000 μg are recommended.

Oxytocin:
- Due to lesser oxytocin receptors in midtrimester uterus, effect of oxytocin is unknown and probably less effective than other agents.
- *Dose and route*: 10 U intramuscularly or 10–40 U intravascularly.

Indications of tertiary treatment:
- Confirmed bowel injury
- Unstable patient
- Suspected perforation
- Failure of primary and secondary treatment.

TABLE 2: Treatment of hemorrhage in postabortion.

Primary	Secondary	Tertiary
• Cervical laceration repair • Uterine massage • Oxytocics	• Resuscitation • Laboratory evaluation • Reaspiration • Balloon tamponade	• Embolization • Laparotomy • Laparoscopy • Hysterectomy

Uterine artery embolization:
- Indicated when primary and secondary treatment methods have failed. In a study of 42 patients who underwent uterine artery embolization (UAE) it was observed that there is 100% success in managing hemorrhage which is unresponsive to other treatment methods.
- The UAE shows a success rate of 43% in patients of placenta accreta (hysterectomy was done in four out of seven women).
- Complications:
  - *Contrast reaction*: Diphenhydramine was used for the treatment, and
  - Femoral embolus which required embolectomy.[12]

Uterine injury and to the surrounding structures, e.g. bowels may also occur.
- Infection: Spread leads to:
  - Generalized peritonitis—further spreads to:
    - The fallopian tubes
    - Uterine perforation
    - Endometritis which leads to abscess formation
    - Gut injury
  - Acute renal failure
  - *Lungs*: Atelectasis and acute respiratory distress syndrome (ARDS)
  - Endotoxic shock (Box 1)
  - Thrombophlebitis.

Remote complications:
- Abnormal uterine bleeding
- Chronic pelvic pain
- Recurrent abortions
- Asherman syndrome

Box 1: Endotoxic shock management.

- Shift to obstetric high-dependency unit (HDU) or intensive care unit (ICU)
- Resuscitation with intravenous (IV) fluids and maintenance of electrolyte balance
- Appropriate broad spectrum antibiotics (as mentioned above) and according to reports of blood culture
- Evacuation after the patient stabilizes

- Ectopic pregnancy
- Dyspareunia
- Secondary infertility
- Psychological disturbances.

Method to Decrease Hemorrhage Risk in the Second Trimester Termination of Pregnancy by Surgical Methods: Cervical Preparation

- Decreased risk is seen when cervix is prepared, especially for surgical abortion up to 20 weeks, by way of reducing the incidence of cervical laceration and hemorrhage.[7,13,14]
- Some studies suggest the best method of cervical ripening for abortions up to 20 weeks are osmotic dilators.
- Some regimens used for first trimester abortions are:
  - Cervical ripening done on the same day with misoprostol or Dilapan-S
  - Dilators used overnight
  - Combination of the above two methods.
- A study reviewed recently wherein 6,000 surgical abortions at 12–16 weeks' gestation observed lesser complications with same-day misoprostol cervical

preparation [three perforations (0.04%) and one case of hemorrhage (0.02%)].[15]

Management of Fetal Death

The various strategies used to reduce hemorrhage:
- Increased hemorrhage does not usually occur as a complication in first trimester embryonic demise or early pregnancy failure as there is no evidence to prove it.
- Lesser than 1% of patients (4 of 563) required a blood transfusion in a large trial where comparison of bleeding patterns following surgical versus medical treatment was done.
- Due to the ultrasound, there are fewer and fewer cases of prolonged retained products after fetal death.

Even though there is no proof to suggest any preoperative investigations in instances of fetal death, some suggest acquiring a coagulation board preceding methodology if the fetus has been retained for many weeks.

SEPTIC ABORTION

Definition

An abortion associated with clinical evidences of uterine infection and its contents is called septic abortion. Abortion is considered septic when there are:
- Ascent of temperature of at any rate 100.4°F (38°C) for 24 hours or more,
- Hostile/offensive or purulent discharge per vagina, and
- Different confirmations of pelvic disease, for example, pain in abdomen and tenderness.

Incidence: 10%

Septic abortions are most commonly associated with incomplete/illegal induced abortion, but are seen even after spontaneous abortion. Decidual cast expelled following missed miscarriage abortion.

Mode of Infection

Endogenous organisms are the main cause of sepsis. The microorganisms are:
- *Aerobic*: *Staphylococcus*, *Pseudomonas*, *Escherichia coli*, *Klebsiella*, and group A beta-hemolytic *Streptococcus* (usually exogenous), methicillin-resistant *Staphylococcus aureus* (MRSA). Mixed infection is more common.
- *Anaerobic*: *Clostridium welchii*, *Bacteroides fragilis*, anaerobic *Streptococci*, and tetanus bacillus.

Main cause of sepsis in unsafe induced abortion is due to the following reasons:
- Insufficient antiseptic and aseptic precautions,
- Evacuation which is incomplete, and
- Injury to the genital organs and adjacent structures, e.g. bowels.

Pathology

Endogenous origin organisms are seen in majority (80%) and the infection is limited to the conceptus. The rest 15%, the infection leads to involvement of endometrium and myometrium (endomyometritis), or can spread to the parametrium, fallopian tubes, ovaries, peritoneum, etc. 5% of patients land up in life-threatening conditions such as peritonitis and/or endotoxic shock (Fig. 1).

Clinical Features

Clinical feature varies depending on extent of infection and severity. History of unsafe termination is mostly concealed:
- Sick and anxious
- Temperature: > 38°C
- Chills and rigors (suggest bacteremia)

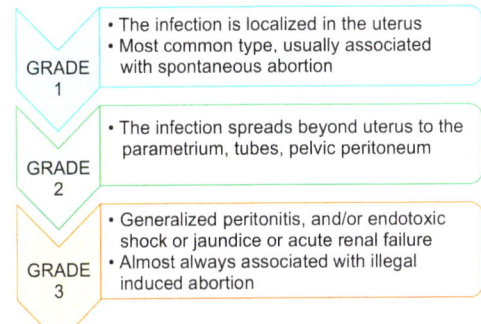

Fig. 1: Different phases of septic abortion.

- Persistent tachycardia ≥ 90 bpm (spreading infection)
- Hypothermia (endotoxic shock) < 36°C
- Abdominal or chest pain
- Tachypnea (RR) > 20 beats/min
- Impaired mental state
- Diarrhea and/or vomiting
- Renal angle tenderness
- *Pelvic examination*: Offensive, purulent vaginal discharge, uterine tenderness, boggy feel in the pouch of Douglas (POD) (pelvic abscess).

Investigations

Routine Investigations

- High vaginal swab is taken for:
  - Isolation of dominant microorganisms by culture
  - Antibiotic sensitivity and resistance
  - Gram staining
- Complete blood count (CBC) and blood group
- Urine routine including culture.

Special Investigations

- *Blood*:
  - Culture
  - Serum electrolytes, C-reactive protein (CRP), serum lactate—as an adjuvant to the management protocol of endotoxic shock. Serum lactate greater than or equal to 4 mmol/L indicates tissue hypoperfusion
  - Coagulation profile
- Ultrasonography to rule out retained products of conception, presence of any foreign body—intrauterine or intra-abdominal, free fluid in the peritoneal cavity or in the POD (pelvic abscess).
- *Plain X-ray*:
  - Abdomen—in suspected cases of bowel injury
  - Chest—for cases with pulmonary complications (atelectasis).

Complications

Immediate Complications

Most of the fatal complications are associated with illegally induced abortions of grade III type.

Prevention

- To boost up family planning acceptance in order to curb the unwanted pregnancies.
- Rigid enforcement of legalized abortion in practice and to curb the prevalence of unsafe abortions. Education, motivation, and extension of the facilities are sine qua non to get the real benefit out of it.
- Taking effective antiseptic and aseptic precautions during examination and during operation.

Management

General Management

- Admission to the hospital
- High vaginal or cervical swab and Gram stain
- Per vaginal examination.

Management Principles

- Sepsis control
- Eradicate the source of infection

- Supportive measures
- Assessment of treatment response.

Grade I Drugs

- Broad-spectrum antibiotics
- Prophylactic antigas gangrene serum and intramuscular dose of antitetanus serum
- Pain relief and analgesia. Blood transfusion is given to improve anemia
- Evacuation of the uterus should be as soon as possible following antibiotic therapy as abortion is often incomplete. Urgent evacuation is needed when there is excessive bleeding per vaginam. Advantage of early evacuation reduces the chances of hemorrhage but also removes the focus of infection. The procedure should be gentle to avoid injury to the uterus.

Grade II Drugs

- *Antibiotics*: Mixed infections are common. Broad-spectrum antibiotics are ideal.
- *Antimicrobial therapy*: A combination of either piperacillin-tazobactam or carbapenem plus clindamycin (IV) gives broadest range of microbial coverage. Empirical therapy is started first and is changed when culture sensitivity report is available:
  - *Piperacillin-tazobactam and carbapenem:* Cover most organisms except MRSA and are not nephrotoxic.
  - Vancomycin or teicoplanin may be added for MRSA resistant to clindamycin.
  - *Clindamycin*: Covers most streptococci, staphylococci including MRSA and is not nephrotoxic.
  - Gentamicin (3–5 mg/kg—single dose) can be given when renal function is normal.
  - *Metronidazole*: Covers anaerobes.
- *Surgery*:
  - When the infection is controlled as well as localized, except if the patient is excessively bleeding.
  - Localized infection in the POD, leads to formation of pelvic abscess for which posterior colpotomy is done. It manifests by spiky rise of temperature, frequent loose stool mixed with mucus called as rectal tenesmus and boggy mass felt through the posterior fornix. Posterior colpotomy and drainage of the pus is effective.

Grade III Drugs

- Antibiotics
- Monitoring clinically
- Supportive management by Ryle's tube aspiration and intravenous crystalloids infusion for treatment of generalized peritonitis.
- *Surgery*: Indications are:
  - Uterine injury
  - Bowel injury
  - Foreign body presents in the abdomen detected by the sonography or X-ray or felt on examination
  - Peritonitis which is unresponsive to treatment most likely suggestive of pus collection
  - Septic shock unresponsive to treatment
  - Enlarged size of the uterus for which safe evacuation per vaginam is difficult.

CONCLUSION AND RECOMMENDATIONS

Based on Good and Consistent Scientific Evidence

- Strong recommendation for evaluation of placenta accreta is of utmost importance in women with a uterine scar and a placenta previa at 16 or more weeks' gestation. Evaluation is to be done by a professional

radiologist or provider experienced in ultrasound. Ultrasound is the first step in evaluating for placenta accreta. MRI is considered if diagnosis is still uncertain.
- Medical abortion is more often associated with bleeding than surgical abortion, though overall hemorrhage incidence is low.

Based on Limited or Inconsistent Scientific Evidence

- Hemoglobin or hematocrit evaluation primarily is done in women undergoing second trimester abortion and those with first trimester medical abortion with anemia.
- Decrease in the risk of incomplete abortion with first trimester surgical abortion and decrease the risk of perforation with standard dilation and evacuation (D and E) with the use of intraoperative ultrasound.
- To decrease blood loss from abortion, vasopressin can be used in a paracervical block.
- In controlling excess bleeding unresponsive to treatment, balloon tamponade is effective.
- Uterine artery embolization can be done before hysterectomy for treatment of bleeding following abortion, a prerequisite being, in patients where perfusion can be maintained during the procedure.
- To control bleeding due to uterine atony, oxytocics are used. For patients bleeding actively, few of the first-line drugs are misoprostol, vasopressin, and methylergonovine maleate.
- There is limited proof that methylergometrine maleate has any use with respect to prophylaxis (for reducing need of reaspiration) before first trimester abortion.

Based Primarily Expert Opinion

- An increased risk of disseminated intravascular coagulation (DIC) is seen when fetal demise with fetus retained for four or more weeks. Though there is no evidence, a preoperative coagulation profile can be done.
- Referral to a hospital service of those patients at a higher risk of bleeding is associated with lesser morbidity.
- After second trimester abortion, oxytocin is a good uterotonic to be used.

REFERENCES

1. Malvasi A, Tinelli A, Di Renzo GC. Management and Therapy of Early Pregnancy Complications: First and Second Trimesters. Berlin, Germany: Springer; 2016.
2. Cunningham FG, Leveno KJ, Bloom SL. Williams Obstetrics, 25th edition. New York, United States: McGraw-Hill; 2018.
3. Konar H. DC Dutta's Textbook of Obstetrics, 8th edition. New Delhi: Jaypee Brothers Medical Publishers (P) Ltd.; 2015.
4. Hakim-Elahi E, Tovell HM, Burnhill MS. Complications of first trimester abortion: a report of 170,000 cases. Obstet Gynecol. 1990;76:129-35.
5. National Abortion Federation. (2011). Clinical Policy Guidelines 2011. [online] Available from: http://prochoice.org/pubs_research/publications/downloads/professional_education/2011%20CPGs.pdf [Last accessed July, 2019].
6. Choudhary N, Saha SC, Gopalan S. Abortion procedures in a tertiary care institution in India. Int J Gynaecol Obstet. 2005;91:81-6.
7. Frick AC, Drey EA, Diedrich JT, et al. Effect of prior cesarean delivery on risk of second-trimester surgical abortion complications. Obstet Gynecol. 2010;115:760-4 [Evidence Grade: III].
8. Engbaek J, Bartholdy J, Hjortso NC. Return hospital visits and morbidity within 60 days after day surgery: a retrospective study of 18,736 day surgical procedures. Acta Anaesthesiol Scand. 2006;50:911-9.

9. Niinimaki M, Pouta A, Bloigu A, et al. Immediate complications after medical compared with surgical termination of pregnancy. Obstet Gynecol. 2009;114:795-804.
10. Altman AM, Stubblefield PG, Schlam JF, et al. Midtrimester abortion with laminaria and vacuum evacuation on a teaching service. J Reprod Med. 1985;30:601-6.
11. Peterson WF, Berry FN, Grace MR, et al. Second-trimester abortion by dilatation and evacuation: an analysis of 11,747 cases. Obstet Gynecol. 1983;62:185-90.
12. Norman WV, Bergunder J, Eccles L. Accuracy of gestational age estimated by menstrual dating in women seeking abortion beyond nine weeks. J Obstet Gynaecol Can. 2011;33:252-7.
13. Kerns J, Steinauer J. Management of post abortion hemorrhage. Contraception. 2013; 87(3):331-42.
14. ACOG practice bulletin. Prevention of Rh D alloimmunization. Number 4, may 1999 (replaces educational bulletin Number 147, October 1990). Clinical management guidelines for obstetrician-gynecologists. American College of Obstetrics and Gynecology. Int J Gynaecol Obstet. 1999;66:63-70.
15. Newmann S, Dalve-Endres A, Drey EA. Clinical guidelines. Cervical preparation for surgical abortion from 20 to 24 weeks' gestation. Contraception 2008;77:308-14 [Evidence Grade: III].

10C

Abnormal Placentation in Early Pregnancy

Mala Arora, Isha Wadhawan

INTRODUCTION

Abnormal placentation leads to hemorrhage and fetal demise. First trimester complications of abnormal placentation could compromise maternal health as well as future fertility. Hence, it is imperative that we handle it efficiently. Transvaginal ultrasound scan and serum beta-human chorionic gonadotropin (beta-hCG) levels are important tools for diagnosis and assessment of the efficacy of a treatment modality. Abnormal placentation may present as:

- Cesarean scar pregnancy (CSP)
- Interstitial pregnancy
- Angular pregnancy
- Subchorionic hematoma
- Morbidly adherent placenta (MAP).

CESAREAN SCAR PREGNANCY

Cesarean scar pregnancy is a rare type of ectopic pregnancy where the fertilized egg implants into the muscle or fibrous tissue of the previous cesarean scar. The *frequency* of CSP is between 1:1,800 and 1:2,226 (0.05–0.04%) of all pregnancies.[1] Interestingly, over half of all CSP cases (52%) have been noted in women after a single cesarean section.[2] With the dramatic increase in cesarean section rate and development of transvaginal ultrasound the incidence and diagnosis of CSP is on the rise. There were only 19 reported cases of CSP up till 2001. Since then, over a 1,000 cases have been added.[1] Promotion of single layer closure of the cesarean scar may be responsible for the sudden rise in the occurrence of CSP.

The etiological factors are not well understood; however, the most likely mechanism is thought to be migration of the implanting embryo through a microscopic tract that forms after prior cesarean.[3]

Recurrence risk has been reported to be up to 5% in women with a previous CSP managed with dilation and curettage.[1,3] Recurrence has also been reported after surgical excision of ectopic and repair of the defect.[1]

Clinical Presentation and Diagnosis

Cesarean scar pregnancy is most often asymptomatic in the initial few weeks. Signs and symptoms, if present, are largely nonspecific. According to one study, the mean gestational age of diagnosis was 7 weeks, and vaginal bleeding was the presenting complaint in most, though some patients also complained of abdominal or pelvic pain.[2] Ouyang et al. reported that the incidence of CSP was higher in women with history of prior cesarean who underwent in vitro fertilization and embryo transfer (IVF-ET).[4] CSP may be diagnosed incidentally on a routine early pregnancy scan or may present with abdominal pain, vaginal bleeding, and rarely hemodynamic instability and collapse due to uterine rupture.[5] Because of this life-threatening potential it is imperative to develop accurate and reliable diagnostic strategies and criteria.

To make a diagnosis of CSP, as with all ectopic pregnancies, one needs to have a high index of suspicion coupled with a good ultrasonographic evaluation. A combined transabdominal and transvaginal approach is superior to either alone.[1] The abdominal scan should be performed first with a full bladder followed by a transvaginal scan after emptying the bladder to have a closer assessment of the lower uterine segment and cervix.[1]

There are two types of CSP based on ultrasound scan:[1,6]
1. *Endogenic or type I CSP* is where the pregnancy grows inwards towards the uterus, this is more difficult to diagnose as CSP.
2. *Exogenic or type II* occurs where the pregnancy grows towards the urinary bladder.

As would be expected, exogenic type has a higher risk of early rupture.

Ultrasound is the main stay for diagnosis of CSP.[7] The characteristic features are listed in Box 1. Three-dimensional ultrasound and MRI are not routinely used, but may be considered as adjunct for diagnosis in cases where diagnosis is unclear; for instance, at later gestational ages or in cases with large fibroids.[6,8]

The two main differential diagnoses for CSP include inevitable miscarriage and cervical ectopic pregnancy. As many as 13.6% of CSP may be misdiagnosed initially.[9] However, surgical evacuation for such misdiagnosed cases may result major hemorrhage which may end in hysterectomy. Therefore, careful radiologic assessment is important. *Ultrasonic "sliding sign"* is a key feature that is noted in cases of inevitable miscarriage; where in gentle pressure on internal cervical os with the probe may displace the gestational sac.[1] Additionally, there is minimal or absent flow noted using color Doppler in such cases. A sliding sign is not seen in a CSP or a cervical ectopic pregnancy. Also, a careful sonographic evaluation would demonstrate a cervical ectopic pregnancy inside the cervical canal. Probe tenderness on touching the cervix as well as ballooning of the cervix may be present. MRI may be used at later gestations or when reliable diagnosis cannot be made sonographically (often in cases of late endogenic CSP).

Management

Cesarean scar pregnancy may be managed in different ways. The choice of treatment depends on certain patient factors, pregnancy characteristics, and the facilities available in the area. The key to therapy is to remove the CSP as soon as possible, which will retain future fertility for the patient.[1] Various modalities have been used for treatment. Their success rates as first-line treatment modality are shown in Table 1.[10]

More often than not, multiple treatment modalities are used together or in a multistep fashion.[11] The medical treatment modality usually precedes the surgical procedures. The interval between the two methods varies from 24 hours to 7 days. Various considerations, advantages, and disadvantages of each of these methods are discussed in Table 2 that follows.

Expectant management is rarely used given the high risks of hemorrhage and

Box 1: Ultrasound features of cesarean scar pregnancy.[1]

- Empty uterine cavity
- Closed cervical canal
- Gestational sac embedded in the cesarean scar
- Absent "sliding organ" sign
- Sac may or may not contain a yolk sac/embryo
- Absent myometrium between the gestational sac and the bladder
- Color Doppler: Typical features of trophoblastic circulation (low impedance blood flow)

TABLE 1: Success rate of therapeutic modalities in cesarean scar pregnancy (CSP).[10]

	Treatment modality	Success rate (as first-line treatment modality)
1	Systemic methotrexate	8.7%
2.	Local therapies, aspiration, embryocidal agents	NA
3.	Uterine artery embolization (UAE)	18.3%
4.	Hysteroscopic excision	39.1%
5.	Dilatation and curettage under ultrasound (US) guidance	39.1%
6.	Laparoscopic excision	NA
7.	Hysterectomy	92.1%

TABLE 2: Factors influencing choice of treatment modalities for cesarean scar pregnancy (CSP).[1]

Patient factors	Symptoms
	Fertility wishes
	Acceptability of prolonged follow-up (surgical methods usually requiring shorter follow-ups then medical methods)
	Associated lesions
	Surgical risk factors
	Response to initial treatment
Pregnancy	Gestational age
	Human chorionic gonadotropin (hCG) levels
	Size of CSP mass
	Type of CSP
	Myometrial thickness
	Viability
Facilities	Interventional radiology
	Surgical expertise/facilities
	Monitoring/intensive care facilities

hysterectomy (29% risk according to one review).[12] An expectantly managed CSP proceeding to the third trimester will most likely have a MAP best managed by a cesarean hysterectomy. A few reports of successful expectant management have been reported in nonviable CSP with declining hCG levels.[13] Systemic methotrexate is the preferred drug for *medical management* as with other ectopic pregnancies. The principles of selecting an appropriate candidate, dosing, and follow-up are similar to that of tubal ectopic pregnancy. Hemodynamically stable patient with an unruptured CSP is the most suitable candidate. She should be explained the need for prolonged follow-up, possible need for additional therapy and/or surgical intervention. Systemic methotrexate is more likely to be successful for patients with beta-hCG < 5,000 IU/L and earlier gestational age (<8 weeks). Full diagnostic workup with complete blood count, liver, and renal function tests are done and all contraindications for methotrexate ruled out before administering the drug.[1] Despite initial belief of effectiveness, more recent data has revealed significantly low efficacy (8.7%) for systemic methotrexate alone, though, interestingly the rate of successful pregnancy is reported to be highest after this therapy.[9] It often requires very long-term follow-up (2 months to up to a year) and may result in multiple complications (nausea, stomatitis, vaginal bleeding, pneumonia, and alopecia) as a result of repeated doses of methotrexate.[2] The remnant tissue may become infected or develop an arteriovenous malformation resulting in further morbidity. Therefore, it is no longer recommended as the first-line therapy. Rotas et al. reported that systemic and local methotrexate, in combination, may be a very effective and complete treatment for CSP with beta-hCG above 10,000 IU/mL.[14] In such cases, the gestational sac is aspirated and most often half the calculated methotrexate dose injected locally under ultrasound guidance and the remaining administered intramuscularly.

Local Therapies

Local embryocidal agents, most commonly, methotrexate or at times potassium chloride (KCl), have been used for administration into the sac under ultrasound guidance.[15] The time required for complete resolution of pregnancy depends on initial sac size and hCG levels. In a small series of 11 cases treated with sac aspiration where the entire dose of methotrexate was given locally, 54% of women required additional systemic methotrexate for complete resolution.[16]

Uterine Artery Embolization

This may be used as a first-line therapy but it is seldom used alone. Close to 80% of cases that undergo a uterine artery embolization (UAE) need additional therapy which may be in form of a dilation and curettage or local methotrexate administration under ultrasound guidance or hysteroscopy in combination with systemic methotrexate administration (in order of effectiveness). UAE may also be used prior to/after surgical removal of the CSP to prevent profuse bleeding.[17,18] However, there are some issues against preference of UAE as first line therapy, firstly it is not freely available in smaller centers and secondly there have been some reports raising concern about future pregnancy following the procedure. Other immediate side effects of UAE are fever, abdominal pain, and pelvic infection. Long-term side effects are infertility, amenorrhea from endometrial atrophy, and premature ovarian aging. Rarely rupture at the site of residual tissue left after embolization and formation of bladder fistula have been reported.

Surgical Methods

A commonly used method for treatment of CSP is *cervical dilation and curettage* under ultrasound guidance. It is appropriate for endogenic CSP, when myometrial thickness surrounding the sac is at least 2 mm. For management and control of bleeding following the procedure, it is advisable to use of Foley's catheter compression or use systemic methotrexate or else to perform UAE.[1]

Abdominal/laparoscopic resection may be performed for removal of the gestation sac and repair of the myometrial defect, if present. It is performed as a primary method or after local or systemic methotrexate injection. Laparoscopic method may be used if appropriate expertise is available.[1] Some report uterine artery ligation to reduce bleeding prior to excision of gestational sac to decrease bleeding.[19]

Another method of surgical resection of CSP under direct visualization and closure of myometrial defect is through *transvaginal route,* which is often combined with transcervical suction curettage.[19] This method may be easier to perform for well-selected patients when expertise is available and may decrease risk of adhesion formation compared to abdominal routes.

Vascular coagulation of the trophoblastic bed under direct visualization under *hysteroscopic guidance* is another option for treatment of CSP. This may be a better method for type I CSP where the sac is growing inwards. There are fewer hemorrhagic complications; however, 61% of patients managed hysteroscopically required additional therapy often in the form of systemic methotrexate and/or dilatation and curettage.[19] Other modalities to reduce hemorrhage are UAE or laparoscopic uterine artery ligation, which are done immediately before the hysteroscopy.[20] In cases of exogenous type of CSP, combined laparoscopic/hysteroscopic excision is preferable.[1,19] Hysteroscopy may also be used to remove remnants of CSP mass after medical management of incomplete surgical management.[17]

There have been case reports of *heterotopic pregnancies* with one CSP and one intrauterine pregnancy. These cases are difficult from a diagnostic and management stand point. Patients have been successfully managed with local KCl injection into the ectopic pregnancy, with continuation of the intrauterine pregnancy.[21] Surgical management with laparoscopy or laparotomy involving removal of the CSP, especially if it is exogenous, is also an option followed by closure of the uterine defect. Though, it does carry the risk of hemorrhage and miscarriage of the normal intrauterine pregnancy.[22]

Patients are ideally followed till the hCG levels decline to zero and/or the CSP mass resolves completely on ultrasound scan, especially when medical or local methods are used. This depends on various factors including gestational age, prior pregnancy size, hCG level, and methods used for treatment. The importance of counseling the patient on the importance of timely and complete follow-up cannot be stressed enough.

Successful pregnancies have occurred after successful treatment of CSP though medical or surgical treatments. Future pregnancies should be screened by early ultrasound to rule out recurrence.[1] There is also an increased risk of MAP in subsequent pregnancies. All future deliveries reported in the literature after CSP have been by a repeat cesarean section, as it is believed to reduce the risk of uterine rupture and allow for proper closure of the uterine defect.[1]

Given the increasing number of CSP and MAP postcesarean deliveries, it is imperative to inform patients about these long-term risk factors especially if the cesarean delivery is performed on maternal request.[1]

INTERSTITIAL PREGNANCY

An interstitial pregnancy is one that implants in the interstitial part of the fallopian tube. It may remain asymptomatic for 7–16 weeks at which point it may rupture spontaneously leading to sudden hemorrhage.[23,24] However, it may be diagnosed prior to rupture with a positive beta-hCG assay and transvaginal ultrasound. In some cases, the diagnosis may not be clear until laparoscopy is performed.[25] The symptoms and signs of presentation are similar to tubal ectopic pregnancy.[25,26]

Cucinella et al., in a systematic review,[26] suggested an algorithm for the treatment of interstitial pregnancy (Flowchart 1). Conservative expectant approach or *medical management* methods may be utilized when:
- Patient is asymptomatic
- Beta-hCG levels are low and declining spontaneously
- Gestational age of > 7 weeks
- Ectopic mass measures less than 35 mm in diameter.[23,26]

These include systemic methotrexate, local injections with embryocidal agents, and/or uterine artery embolization.[23]

If a patient is not a candidate for medical management, she may undergo a conservative or radical *surgical procedure* via laparoscopy or laparotomy depending on the clinical presentation including:
- Size and location of pregnancy,
- Presence of cardiac activity,
- Desire for future fertility,
- Status of contralateral tube and cornua, and
- Skill level of the provider.[26]

Laparoscopic surgery is becoming the mainstay for therapy given its numerous advantages over open surgery.

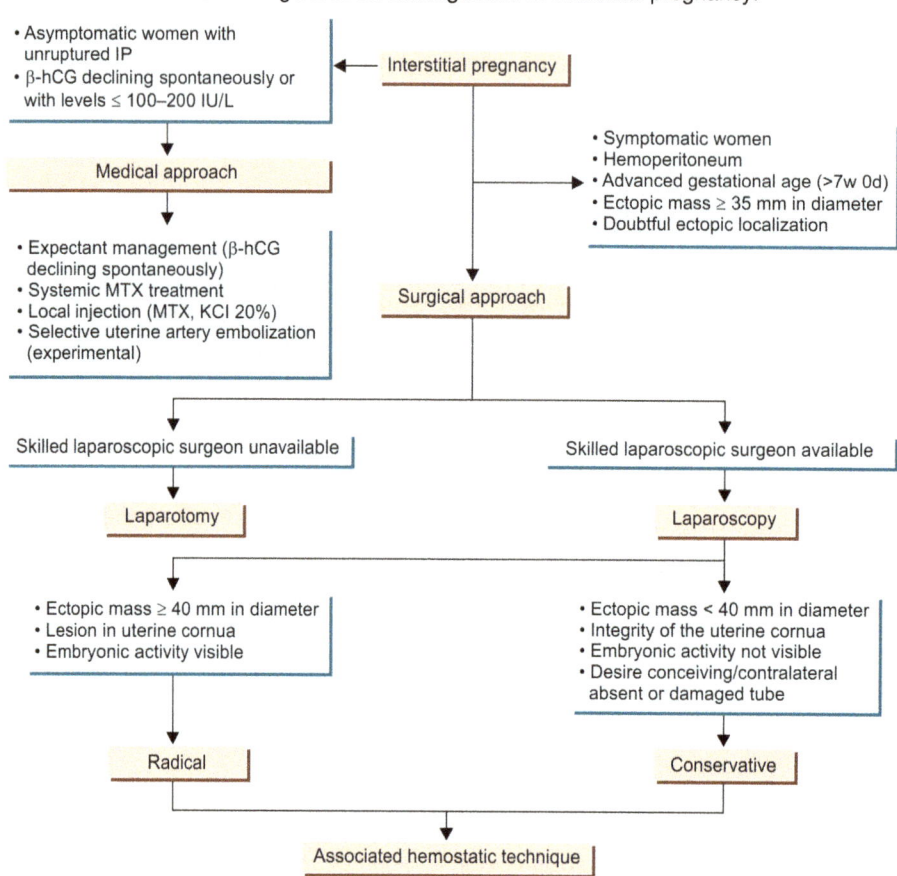

Flowchart 1: Algorithm for management of interstitial pregnancy.[26]

(β-hCG: β-human chorionic gonadotropin; IP: interstitial pregnancy; KCl: potassium chloride; MTX: methotrexate)

The *conservative surgical approach* includes:
- Cornuostomy is a linear incision on the cornua to evacuate the products of pregnancy
- Extended salpingostomy
- Salpingotomy and/or minicornual excision.[24,27]

Radical procedures are cornual (wedge) resection with or without salpingectomy.[24,26,27] *Cornual wedge resection* involves removal of entire cornua, which contains the pregnancy and its surrounding interstitial component of the fallopian tube and the myometrium. This is often performed with a salpingectomy of the ipsilateral side. The defect created in the uterine myometrium after the excision is closed akin to after a myomectomy. The major risk with the surgical approach is that of hemorrhage due to high vascularity of the interstitial and cornual regions. There is also a risk of spontaneous rupture of uterus during a subsequent pregnancy.

Massive hemorrhage due to rupture of the interstitial pregnancy or during its surgical excision may require blood transfusion (4%), conversion of laparoscopic surgery to a laparotomy or conversion from a conservative to a radical procedure.[26] In rare situations, these surgeries may result in major complications like a hysterectomy or may require return to theater for management of hemorrhage (2.6%, only reported in conservative surgeries).[26]

Special hemostatic measures have been used in majority of the cases of interstitial pregnancies reported in the literature. The methods used include:
- Local vasopressin injections below the ectopic mass
- Suturing or endoloop ligation of uterine or ovarian vessels
- Use of special devices, e.g. Surgicel, endostapler, etc.[26]

These were noted to reduce surgical time as well as blood loss compared to cases where only bipolar electrocautery was used.[26]

Adjuvant medical therapy for persistent ectopic pregnancy may also be needed after both conservative and radical procedures in 7–8% cases.[26,28]

Interestingly, even after accounting for these complications the success rate for conservative and radical surgeries are similar and around 86%.[26] Radical surgeries on an average require the patient to stay in the hospital a day longer (3.8 days) than conservative methods (2.7 days).[26] Reported pregnancy rates of 62–72% and live birth rates of 48–62% were comparable for both conservative and radical surgeries amongst the few reported cases in literature.[26] The key to successful management in the first attempt is to select appropriate candidates for the particular treatment approach.

ANGULAR PREGNANCY (TABLE 3)

The terms *"cornual", "interstitial",* and *"angular"* pregnancy need to be clarified.[25]

Interstitial pregnancy actually refers to a pregnancy implanted in the 1–2 cm long

TABLE 3: Differences between an interstitial and an angular pregnancy.[25]

	Interstitial	Angular
Implantation location	Fallopian tube (interstitial segment)	Endometrial cavity (superior lateral aspect, just medial to the uterotubal junction)
Relationship to the round ligament	Lateral	Medial
Relationship to the endometrium	Extraendometrial	Intraendometrial
Is it an ectopic?	Yes	No
Prognosis of fetus	Non viable	Uncertain viability
Prognosis of mother	Significant morbidity and mortality if progresses to rupture	Increased risk of uterine rupture
Imaging findings	• Interstitial line sign = thin echogenic line extending directly up to the center of ectopic pregnancy • Gestational sac seen separately from the most lateral edge of the uterine cavity, with myometrium between sac and endometrium • Thinning of myometrial mantle to < 5 mm thick	Gestational sac primarily surrounded by endometrium with adjacent thicker myometrial layer

interstitial/intramural portion of the fallopian tube. It is *not* a uterine pregnancy. 2–4% of tubal ectopic pregnancies belong to this category which equals 1/2, 500–5,000 live births.[26] The incidence has increased recently due to increased use of assisted reproductive technologies.[29]

Cornual pregnancy was initially described by Johnston as a pregnancy in one horn of uterus with a müllerian anomaly (e.g. bicornuate or unicornuate uterus, didelphys or septate uterus); however, it is also used by many gynecologists for a pregnancy implanted in the cornual region of a normal uterus.[25] Some experts strongly advocate avoiding this term or limiting its use to only cases with müllerian anomalies.

Finally, an *angular pregnancy* was described by an American obstetrician Kelly in 1898 as "implantation of the embryo just medial to the uterotubal junction, in the lateral angle of the uterine cavity". Prior to the frequent use of ultrasound and transvaginal assessment the distinction between an interstitial and angular pregnancy would only be made on surgical evaluation, wherein the former would demonstrate a swelling *lateral* to the round ligament, while later resulted in a *medial* swelling and displacement of the round ligament upwards and outwards.[25] Similarly, previously müllerian anomalies were also only diagnosed surgically. This diagnostic dilemma may have been the reason for the confusion in nomenclature. Now, more often than not the same can be determined sonographically.

Clinical Presentation Diagnosis

Angular pregnancies are difficult to diagnose and may often go undiagnosed. Such a pregnancy may present and act as a completely normal intrauterine pregnancy for majority or part of the gestation, especially when the gestational sac is growing towards the uterine cavity.[30] It may even result in a full-term normal delivery.[31] However, it may also result in life-threatening complications. As such there is no clear point of delineation in the uterine cavity lateral to which an implanted embryo may result in an angular pregnancy.[25] However, the more lateral the implantation, greater the chances of uterine asymmetry, symptoms, and complications. An angular pregnancy should be suspected in cases with asymmetrical appearance of the uterus, abnormal fetal presentation, thickened placenta which is limited to the uterine angle in second or third trimester, and thinning of the angular myometrium from placental growth in a restricted space.[30-32] Angular pregnancy may result in a miscarriage in up to 38.5% of cases, which may be complicated by retained products of conception.[30] Other morbidities during pregnancy include:
- Persistent pelvic pain
- Preterm labor and delivery
- Bleeding and abruption
- Uterine rupture (13.6%)
- Retained placenta
- Postpartum hemorrhage
- Postpartum endometritis
- Placenta accreta
- Severe bleeding leading to hysterectomy.[30]

Transvaginal ultrasound is an excellent diagnostic modality for angular pregnancy, especially in the early gestational weeks. Three-dimensional ultrasound and MRI may help facilitate diagnosis, but when unavailable, some experts strongly support use of serial two-dimensional transvaginal sonography to see if the gestational sac is growing towards to uterine cavity.[25]

Therapeutic Management

Angular pregnancies can be managed conservatively by keeping the complications in mind. There are not clear cut prognostic factors; however, greater the asymmetry of the uterus, higher is the risk of catastrophic complications. If these pregnancies are terminated systemic methotrexate along with a hysteroscopic or laparoscopic-guided uterine curettage may be considered to ensure that all uterine contents are evacuated.[30] When pregnancies progress to viable gestational ages, delivery may be performed as per obstetric indications.[25,30] Often malpresentation may necessitate cesarean delivery. Delivery may be complicated by atonic postpartum hemorrhage as well as due to minimal myometrium in the placenta bed that does not contract well.[30] Uterotonics may be used. Alanbay et al. have applied square sutures with absorbable material, from anterior to posterior wall of uterus in order to obliterate the asymmetrical uterine sacculation. In cases of abnormal or MAP, an obstetric hysterectomy may be needed.

SUBCHORIONIC HEMATOMA

Epidemiology

It is not an uncommon finding on routine or indicated ultrasound in the first or second trimester. The incidence is reported between 1.3% and 3.1% in two large studies.[33] It is seen as hypoechoic area behind the gestational sac and is believed to result from partial detachment of the chorionic membranes from the decidua.[34] At present, the etiology and predisposing factors are poorly understood.

Clinical Presentation and Diagnosis

It may be seen incidentally on routine ultrasound or noted in pregnant woman reporting pelvic pain and/or vaginal bleeding. A subchorionic hematoma may be associated with adverse pregnancy outcomes. This has been noted to be dependent on the:

- Size of the hematoma (>25% of sac volume is associated with worse outcomes),[34]
- Location of the hematoma (worse outcomes are for retroplacental hematomas compared to marginal hematomas),[34] and
- Symptoms (presence of pain and bleeding is associated with worse outcomes then incidental hematomas).[33]

Subchorionic hematoma doubles the risk of spontaneous miscarriage [18 vs 9%; OR; 2.18, confidence interval (CI) 1.29–3.68] and stillbirth (1.9 vs 9%, OR 2.09, CI 1.2–3.67) as reported by a meta-analysis of seven comparative studies; the number needed to harm was 11 and 103, respectively.[34] These women were also at a higher risk for abruption (0.7 vs 3.6%, OR 5.71, CI 3.91–8.33), preterm delivery, preterm premature rupture of membranes (PPROM), but not for fetal growth restriction, or pre-eclampsia. The risk of preterm delivery and stillbirth were dependent on the presence of vaginal bleeding in this meta-analysis.[34] Another large retrospective review of 63,966 women with 1,081 cases of subchorionic hemorrhage noted that after adjusting for confounders it was associated with an increased risk of abruption and preterm delivery and *not for* intrauterine fetal demise, growth restriction, PPROM or pre-eclampsia.[33]

Management

The only management option is expectant with close follow-up. Some providers prefer to repeat ultrasound scan in 2–3 weeks to assess for cardiac activity and change in size of hematoma. This helps to provide reassurance to patients. A recent Cochrane review published in August 2018 reported based on moderate quality evidence that oral progesterone therapy may decrease the risk of miscarriage in patients with first trimester bleeding, which includes patients with symptomatic subchorionic hemorrhage.[35] The evidence on risk of congenital abnormalities from progesterone therapy is low, but there are only a few very poor quality studies available.[35]

Bed rest is not supported by evidence and therefore is not indicated.[35] However, restricted activity and avoiding sexual trauma to the gestational tract is often advised and makes women feel comfortable.

The presence of a subchorionic hematoma is not an indication for an acquired or inherited thrombophilia profile or coagulation profile.[35]

PLACENTA PREVIA AND ACCRETA

Many experts argue that the diagnosis of placenta previa should not be explicitly made prior to 20 weeks of gestation, i.e. the level II or anomaly ultrasound scan which is performed around 18-22 weeks of gestation.[36] This is because as demonstrated by obstetrics as well as radiology literature a placenta covering the internal os or reaching within 2 cm of the internal os can be seen in as many as 42% of the pregnancies till 14 weeks of gestation, while at around 20 weeks it is limited to only about 4% cases and at term between 1.5% and 2 % cases continue to have a placenta previa.[36] As is often explained to the anxious patients this is simply because of the small size of the uterus in early gestation.[37]

No data supports the idea that such a placenta is by itself associated with increased risk of subchorionic hemorrhage or threatened miscarriage. However, most providers recommend pelvic rest (no intercourse and avoiding heavy work outs) to these women.

Evidence-based recommendations for management for low lying placenta diagnosed in the first trimester are lacking. As reported in studies, almost 90% of these issues resolved by 20 weeks of gestation because as the uterus grows the site of implantation and therefore the placenta moves away from the internal os.[36] Therefore, asymptomatic women with such a finding in the first trimester should simply undergo routine level II ultrasound where the placenta may be evaluated again. If a placenta previa is noted at this time, they should have appropriate follow-up and given precautions. If other complications of first trimester pregnancy like threatened abortion or a subchorionic hemorrhage are noted they may be managed accordingly.

A special case scenario of placenta previa with at least one prior uterine surgery and/or cesarean section is increasingly seen. These patients need to be carefully evaluated for MAP or placenta accreta.[37,38] Cali et al. recently reported that MAP may be detected with high sensitivity and specificity in these high-risk women by ultrasound performed as early as 11-14 weeks' gestation.[39] A prospective study carried out at the Harris Birthright Research Center UK screened 22,604 pregnancies and suspected MAP in 1,298 (6%) at 11-13 weeks. All these patients underwent previous uterine surgeries and had low lying anterior placentae. The diagnostic signs were:

- Nonidentifiable cesarean section scar
- Interruption of bladder wall
- Thin myometrium in the retroplacental area
- Intraplacental lacunar spaces
- Identifying arterial blood flow in retro-placental area
- Irregular vascularization of placenta by power Doppler.

However, the diagnostic accuracy improved at a subsequent 12-16 weeks scan, when MAP was suspected in only 14 of these patients, which were confirmed to have MAP at delivery.[40]

Hence, the diagnosis of MAP is more accurate in a two-step screening strategy, first at 11-13 weeks and subsequently at 12-16 weeks.

CONCLUSION

Presentation of abnormal placentation in the first trimester is varied and requires careful assessment with transvaginal ultrasound scan and serial serum beta-hCG before deciding on an appropriate therapeutic option. Surgical procedures are best performed under ultrasound guidance and hysteroscopic vision or laparoscopic guidance. Preservation of future fertility is as important as prevention of maternal morbidity and mortality.

REFERENCES

1. Jayaram PM, Okunoye GO, Konje J. Caesarean ectopic pregnancy: diagnostic challenges and management options. Obstet Gynaecol. 2017;19:13-20.
2. Pedraszewski P, Wlazlak E, Panek W, et al. Caesarean scar pregnancy—a new challenge for obstetricians. J Ultrason. 2018;18(72):56-62.
3. Qian ZD, Guo QY, Huang LL. Identifying risk factors for recurrent cesarean scar pregnancy: a case-control study. Fertil Steril. 2014;102: 129-34.
4. Ouyang Y, Li X, Yi Y, et al. First-trimester diagnosis and management of caesarean scar pregnancies after in vitro fertilization-embryo transfer: a retrospective clinical analysis of 12 cases. Reprod Biol Endocrinol. 2015;13:126.
5. Zhang Y, Gu Y, Wang JM, et al. Analysis of cases with caesarean scar pregnancy. J Obstet Gynaecol Res. 2013;39:195-202.
6. Peng KW, Lei Z, Xiao TH, et al. First trimester caesarean scar ectopic pregnancy evaluation using MRI. Clin Radiol. 2014;69:123-9.
7. Timor-Tritsch IE, Monteagudo A, Santos R, et al. The diagnosis, treatment, and follow-up of cesarean scar pregnancy. Am J Obstet Gynecol. 2012;207(1):44.e1-13.
8. Uysal F, Uysal A, Adam G. Caesarean scar pregnancy: diagnosis, management, and follow-up. J Ultrasound Med. 2013;32:1295-300.
9. Timor-Tritsch IE, Monteagudo A. Unforeseen consequences of the increasing rate of cesarean deliveries: early placenta accreta and caesarean scar pregnancy: a review. Am J Obstet Gynecol. 2012;207:14-29.
10. Kanat-Pektas M, Bodur S, Dundar O, et al. Systematic review: What is the best first-line approach for caesarean section ectopic pregnancy? Taiwan J Obstet Gynecol. 2016;55:263-9.
11. Birch Petersen K, Hoffmann E, Rifbjerg Larsen C, et al. Caesarean scar pregnancy: a systematic review of treatment studies. Fertil Steril. 2016;105:958-67.
12. Smorgick N, Vakin Z, Pansky M, et al. Combined local and systemic methotrexate treatment of viable ectopic pregnancy: outcomes of 31 cases. K Clin Ultrasound. 2008;36:545-50.
13. Al-Hashimi S, Maiti S, Macloy D. Successful conservative management of ectopic pregnancy in caesarean section scar. BMI Case Rep. 2012;1757-90.
14. Rotas MA, Haberman S, Levgur M. Cesarean scar ectopic pregnancies: etiology, diagnosis and management. Obstet Gynecol. 2006;107:1373-81.
15. Ugurlucan FG, Bastu E, Dogan M, et al. Management of caesarean heterotopic pregnancy with transvaginal ultrasound-guided potassium chloride injection and gestational sac aspiration, and review of the literature. J Minim Invasive Gynecol. 2012;19:671-3.
16. Seow KM, Wang PH, Huang LW, et al. Transvaginal sono-guided aspiration of gestational sac concurrent with a local methotrexate injection for the treatment of unruptured caesarean scar pregnancy. Arch Gynecol Obstet. 2013;288:361-6.
17. Jiang T, Liu G, Huang L, et al. Methotrexate therapy followed by suction curettage followed by Foley tamponade for caesarean scar pregnancy. Eur J Obstet Gynecol Reprod Biol. 2011;156:209-11.
18. Zhang B, Jiang ZB, Huang MS, et al. Uterine artery embolization combined with methotrexate in the treatment of caesarean scar pregnancy: results of a case series and review of the literature. J Vasc Intervent Radiol. 2012;23:1582-8.
19. Wang HY, Zhang J, Li YN, et al. Laparoscopic management or laparoscopy combined with transvaginal management of type II caesarean scar pregnancy. JSLS. 2013;17:263-72.

20. Li H, Guo HY, Han JS, et al. Endoscopic treatment of ectopic pregnancy in a caesarean scar. J Min Invasive Gynecol. 2011;18:31-5.
21. Taskin S, Taskin EA, Ciftci TT. Heterotopic caesarean scar pregnancy: how should it be managed? Obstet Gynecol Surv. 2009;64:690-5.
22. Demirel LC, Bodur H, Selam B, et al. Laparoscopic management of heterotopic caesarean scar pregnancy with preservation of intrauterine gestation and delivery at term: case report. Fertil Steril. 2009;91:1293.e5-7.
23. Moawad NS, Mahajan ST, Moniz MH, et al. Current diagnosis and treatment of interstitial pregnancy. Am J Obstet Gynecol. 2010;202(1):15-29.
24. Fylstra DL. Ectopic pregnancy not within the (distal) fallopian tube: etiology, diagnosis, and treatment. Am J Obstet Gynecol. 2012;206: 289-99.
25. Arleo EK, De Filippis EM. Cornual, interstitial, and angular pregnancies: clarifying the terms and a review of the literature. Clin Imaging. 2014;38(6):763-70.
26. Cucinella G, Calagna G, Rotolo S, et al. Interstitial pregnancy: a 'road map' of surgical treatment based on a systematic review of the literature. Gynecol Obstet Invest. 2014;78(3):141-9.
27. Larrain D, Marengo F, Bourdel N, et al. Proximal ectopic pregnancy: a descriptive general population-based study and results of different management options in 86 cases. Fertil Steril. 2011;95:867-71.
28. Siow A, Ng S. Laparoscopic management of 4 cases of recurrent corneal ectopic pregnancy and review of literature. J Minim Invasive Gynecol. 2010;18:296-302.
29. Trabert B, Holt Vl, Yu O, et al. Population-based ectopic pregnancy trends, 1993-2007. Am J Prev Med. 2011;40(5):556-60.
30. Alanbay I, Ozturk M, Karaşahin KE, et al. Angular pregnancy. Turk J Obstet Gynecol. 2016;13(4):218-20.
31. Alves JA, Alves NG, Alencar Júnior CA, et al. Term angular pregnancy: successful expectant management. J Obstet Gynaecol Res. 2011;37:641-4.
32. Kwon JY, Hwang SJ, Shin JE, et al. Two cases of angular pregnancy complicated by preterm labor and placental abruption at mid-pregnancy. J Obstet Gynaecol Res. 2011;37:958-62.
33. Norman SM, Odibo AO, Macones GA, et al. Ultrasound-detected subchorionic hemorrhage and the obstetric implications. Obstet Gynecol. 2010;116(2 Pt 1):311-5.
34. Tuli MG, Norman SM, Odibo AO, et al. Perinatal outcomes in women with subchorionic hematoma: a systematic review and meta-analysis. Obstet Gynecol. 2011;117:1205-12.
35. Wahabi HA, Fayed AA, Esmaeil SA, et al. Progestogen for treating threatened miscarriage. Cochrane Database Syst Rev. 2018;8:CD005943.
36. Mustafá SA, Brizot ML, Carvalho MH, et al. Transvaginal ultrasonography in predicting placenta previa at delivery: a longitudinal study. Ultrasound Obstet Gynecol. 2002;20(4):356-9.
37. Oppenheimer L. Society of Obstetricians and Gynaecologists of Canada. Diagnosis and management of placenta previa. J Obstet Gynaecol Can. 2007;29:261.
38. National Institutes of Health Consensus Development Conference Panel. National Institutes of Health Consensus Development Conference Statement. NIH consensus development conference: Vaginal birth after cesarean: New insights. March 8-10, 2010. Obstet Gynecol. 2010;115(6):1279-95.
39. Cali G, Forlani F, Foti F, et al. Diagnostic accuracy of first-trimester ultrasound in detecting abnormally invasive placenta in high-risk women with placenta previa. Ultrasound Obstet Gynecol. 2018;52(2):258-64.
40. Panaiotova J, Tokunaka M, Krajewska K, et al. Screening for morbidly adherent placenta in early pregnancy. Ultrasound Obstet Gynecol. 2019;53(1):101-6.

Bleeding in Gestational Trophoblastic Disease

PK Sekharan

INTRODUCTION

Gestational trophoblastic disease is a spectrum of abnormal trophoblastic hyperplasia resulting from an abnormal fertilization—an imbalance in the genetic input from the ovum and sperm. In both complete and partial mole, there is an excess of paternal chromosome. In familial recurrent moles, there is an imprinting defect in maternal chromosomes. These will lead to varying degrees of trophoblastic hyperplasia with excess production of human chorionic gonadotropin (hCG). The risk of malignant transformation to invasive mole and choriocarcinoma is 15-20% following complete mole and 1-5% following partial mole. The rare forms of gestational trophoblastic neoplasia (GTN)—the placental site trophoblastic tumor (PSTT) and epithelioid trophoblastic tumor (ETT) can follow any type of pregnancy. Choriocarcinoma following term delivery is diagnosed in the advanced stage as there is no way to predict the development of it after normal delivery.

Bleeding in early pregnancy is the most common clinical presentation in molar pregnancy, especially when diagnosis is made beyond 12 weeks. In remote areas where obstetric care is not optimum, molar pregnancy may progress beyond 16-18 weeks and may report with very heavy vaginal bleeding. With the availability of routine ultrasound evaluation of early pregnancy, the risk of heavy bleeding before evacuation is comparatively less nowadays.

CONTROL OF BLEEDING DURING EVACUATION OF THE HYDATIDIFORM MOLE

Before evacuation, correct anemia and keep blood and blood products ready. Suction evacuation under general anesthesia with ultrasound guidance is the preferred method of evacuation of hydatidiform mole irrespective of the uterine size. An intravenous infusion of oxytocin is started at the beginning of the suction evacuation. Suction evacuation is done using 12-14 size suction cannula.[1] It is important to start and continue oxytocin infusion for one to two hours after evacuation to reduce the risk of excess bleeding.

TWIN WITH HYDATIDIFORM MOLE AND NORMAL FETUS

Rarely a twin pregnancy with a normal fetus and hydatidiform mole can occur. After confirming the normalcy of the fetus with ultrasonography and karyotyping, the pregnancy may be allowed to continue after counseling the couple of the risk of severe bleeding in the course of pregnancy and labor with need for surgical intervention.[2]

BLEEDING AFTER EVACUATION OF HYDATIDIFORM MOLE

Patients may report with heavy bleeding per vagina following evacuation of the molar pregnancy. This may be due to incomplete evacuation of the mole or due to development of GTN. Perform a clinical examination and ultrasonographic evaluation with Doppler study. If there is evidence of retained products, do repeat evacuation under general anesthesia. In cases where the uterine cavity is empty but Doppler study shows vascular nodule in the myometrium, it could be an invasive mole. Do hCG estimation and if found to be elevated, it is a case of GTN. Do the metastatic workup and risk stratification and start chemotherapy as per the International Federation of Gynaecology and Obstetrics (FIGO) stage and risk score. Single agent chemotherapy if the risk score is <7 either with methotrexate/folinic acid regimen or Actinomycin-D. If the risk score is ≥7, start multiagent chemotherapy, the Etoposide, Methotrexate, Actinomycin-D, Cyclophosphamide, Vincristine (EMA/CO) regimen.

To avoid the problem of incomplete evacuation leading to bleeding later on, use oxytocin during evacuation under ultrasound guidance. Do a gentle curettage at the end to make sure the uterine cavity is empty. Do an ultrasonography 1 week after the primary evacuation to make sure the uterine cavity is empty. If there is evidence of retained products, do a curettage. It is mandatory to perform weekly hCG assay with clinical evaluation to diagnose GTN. The normal regression pattern is a fall by one log (1 in 10) every week and normalizes after 8 weeks in 80% of cases.[3] A plateauing of four values over 3 weeks or rise in titer of three values over 2 weeks is diagnostic of GTN. (Plateauing of the hCG is a fall of less than 10% compared to the previous week and a rise in titer is an increase of 10% hCG compared to the previous week).[4]

■ BLEEDING IN INVASIVE MOLE (FIGS. 1 AND 2)

In patients with invasive mole, there is widespread local invasion of the trophoblasts into the myometrium and blood vessels leading to perforation of uterus resulting in heavy intraperitoneal bleed.[5] An emergency laparotomy and a lifesaving hysterectomy have to be performed with transfusion of multiple units of blood and blood products. These patients have to be started on single agent or combination chemotherapy as per the FIGO staging and risk stratification. In order to prevent such catastrophic bleeding due to perforation of the uterus, Michael Seckel et al. (2013) have recommended to start chemotherapy in patients who have serum β-hCG > 20,000 IU/L > 4 weeks after

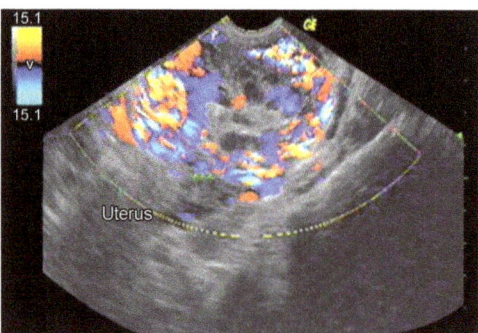

Fig. 1: Doppler appearance of invasive mole with highly vascular myometrial nodules.

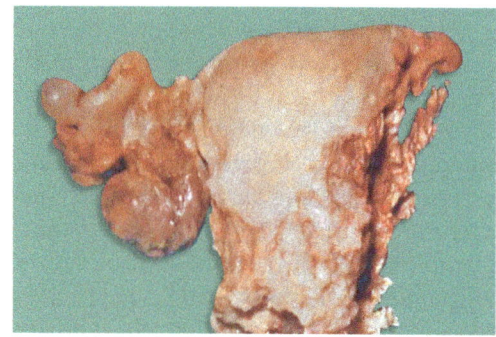

Fig. 2: Specimen of subtotal hysterectomy in perforation of uterus by invasive mole.

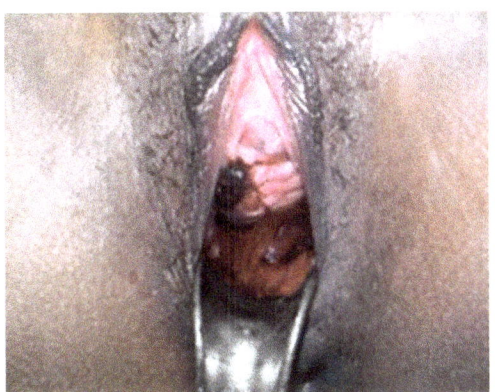

Fig. 3: Suburethral nodule.

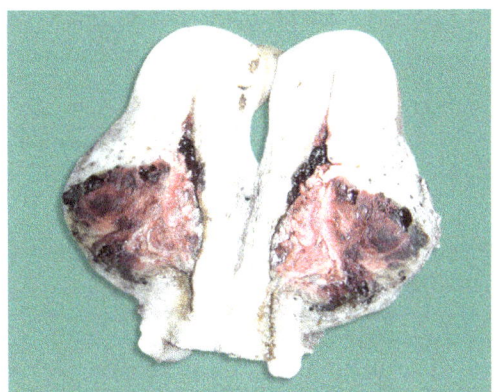

Fig. 4: Hysterectomy to control heavy bleeding in choriocarcinoma.

evacuation.[6] In cases where the perforation is localized to a small area, resection and closure of the perforation is possible and with chemotherapy, reproductive function can be preserved. There were 2 cases of perforation of uterus with intraperitoneal bleed-hysterectomy was the only option for one case, in the other case, resection and closure was possible. This patient subsequently conceived and delivered by cesarean section.

BLEEDING FROM VAGINAL METASTASIS: SUBURETHRAL NODULE (FIG. 3)

Severe bleeding can occur from the vaginal metastasis, typically seen at the suburethral area. Do not try to resect or suture the bleeding point, which will result in severe bleeding. After keeping a Foley's catheter, pack the vagina for 24 hours, which will control the bleeding. If facilities are available, selective embolization could be effective.

BLEEDING IN CHORIOCARCINOMA FOLLOWING NORMAL DELIVERY (FIG. 4)

Choriocarcinoma developing after normal delivery is usually diagnosed at an advanced stage and will present with varying symptoms depending on the metastatic site. One of the ways they may present is with severe vaginal bleeding usually following a period of amenorrhea. Any patient presenting with heavy vaginal bleeding or irregular vaginal bleeding should have a urine pregnancy test done. Emergency hysterectomy will be required to save the life followed by chemotherapy in such cases who present with heavy vaginal bleeding.[7]

CONCLUSION

Life-threatening bleeding during evacuation of hydatidiform mole could be controlled with oxytocin infusion though there is an increased risk of trophoblastic embolization. Perforation of uterus and intraperitoneal bleeding is a real risk in patients with hCG levels of ≥20,000 IU/L after 4 weeks of evacuation and is an indication to start chemotherapy. Hysterectomy is usually required in massive intraperitoneal bleeding in invasive mole leading to perforation of the uterus. In cases with massive vaginal bleeding due to choriocarcinoma, hysterectomy along with chemotherapy can be lifesaving.

REFERENCES

1. Ngan HY, Seckl MJ, Berkowitz RS, Xiang Y, Golfier F, Sekharan PK, Lurain JR and

Massuger L. Update on the diagnosis and management of gestational trophoblastic disease. Int J Gynecol Obstet. 2018;143:79-85.
2. Sebire NJ, Foskett M, Paradinas FJ, et al. Outcome of twin pregnancies with complete hydatidiform mole and healthy co-twin. Lancet. 2002;359:2165-6.
3. Sekharan PK. Gestational trophoblastic disease. J Obstet Gynecol India. 2008;58(4): 299-306.
4. Mangili G, Lorusso D, Brown J, Pfisterer J, Massuger L, Vaughan M, Ngan HY, Golfier F, Sekharan PK, et al. Trophoblastic disease review for diagnosis and management: a joint report from the International Society for the Study of Trophoblastic Disease, European Organisation for the Treatment of Trophoblastic Disease, and the Gynecologic Cancer InterGroup. Int J Gynecol Cancer. 2014; 24(9 Suppl 3):S109-16.
5. Sarwar N, Seckl MJ. Clinical features of molar pregnancies and gestational trophoblastic neoplasia. In: Hancock BW, Seckl MJ, Berkowitz RS (Eds). Gestational Trophoblastic Disease, 4th edition; 2015.
6. Seckl MJ, Sebire NJ, Fisher RA, et al. Gestational trophoblastic disease: ESMO clinical practice guidelines. Ann Oncol. 2013;24 (Suppl 6):vi39-vi50.
7. Tidy J. The role of surgery in the management of gestational trophoblastic disease. In: Hancock BW, Seckl MJ, Berkowitz RS (Eds). Gestational Trophoblastic Disease, 4th edition; 2015.

Ectopic Pregnancy in the Cervix

Chapter 10E

Purnima Kishore Nadkarni, Manisha Singhal

INTRODUCTION

In ectopic pregnancy, fertilized ovum is implanted at any site other than the usual site, i.e. endometrial cavity. Although the majority of the ectopic pregnancies are tubal, other rare sites described are ovary, cervix, and primary abdominal pregnancy. Implantation into cervical canal is known as cervical ectopic pregnancy (CEP). CEP was first described in 1817, and termed/coined in 1860.[1] Cervical pregnancy might land up into torrential hemorrhage requiring massive blood transfusion or many times emergency hysterectomy is required.[2]

INCIDENCE

The incidence of cervical pregnancy as reported in literature varies from 1:1,000 to 1:95,000.[3] However, cervical pregnancy accounts for less than 1% of all ectopic pregnancies.[4-6] The reported cases with cervical ectopic has increased in previous decade with the increasing use of transvaginal sonography in assisted reproductive technology (ART) pregnancies. The incidence of cervical in in-vitro fertilization program ranges from 0.12% to 0.2%.[7,8]

ETIOPATHOGENESIS

The etiology of CEP still remains unknown. Varying hypotheses have been postulated:
- A rapid transport of the blastocyst through an immature endometrium, that is incapable of accepting a fertilized ovum for nidation;
- Delayed fertilization occurring in the endocervix itself with subsequent implantation in the cervical canal. High grade of vascularization of endocervix provide a nidus for implantation of embryo.[9]

Thus, factors that may cause deterioration in the structure of the endometrium, compromising the nidation of the fertilized ovum in the uterine cavity, or those that promote the nidation of the ovum in the endocervical portion of the uterus, can be considered as risk factors that could lead to cervical pregnancy.[10]

RISK FACTORS

Most of the CEPs are iatrogenic in origin. Common risk factors for cervical pregnancy are cesarean section, dilatation and curettage, prior use of the intrauterine contraceptive device (IUCD), prior ectopic pregnancies, pelvic inflammatory disease, Asherman's syndrome, endometriosis, endomyometritis, uterine anomalies or surgery for uterine anamolies.[6,9,11-14] About 70% cases of CEPs had a history of prior curettage.[4,15,16] Majority of women with cervical pregnancy have a low parity.[17] Cigarette smoking is associated with moderate increase in risk for CEPs.[18] These factors cause deterioration in endometrial health making it nonreceptive to implantation of blastocyst.

In recent times, in vitro fertilization and other assisted reproductive technique have been associated with increased risk of cervical pregnancy, reason reported being both presence of endometrial dys-synchrony as well as rapid transit of fertilized ovum into endometrial cavity when the endometrium is nonreceptive.[19,20]

PRESENTATION

The patient with CEPs commonly presents with vaginal bleeding following a period of amenorrhea. Bleeding may be in form of spotting or massive hemorrhage.[6,9] Factors that contribute to high risk of bleeding are:
- Higher vascularity of endocervix
- *Microscopic anatomy of the cervix*: Only 20% of the cervix consists of smooth muscle, the fibrous tissue is noncontractile and also it is difficult to achieve hemostasis with help of uterotonics and mechanical methods.

Torrential bleed may at times require hysterectomy adding to maternal morbidity and might end up in maternal mortality as well. Diagnosis was traditionally made retrospective only.[11] This may be associated with a constant noncramping lower abdominal pain. In advanced cases, urethra may be compressed against the enlarged cervix leading to urinary retention.[6]

Bimanual palpation: Findings may vary, but in general on gentle examination the external os is found open with a soft, globular, and enlarged cervix. Cervical motion tenderness is always present. One must be careful while doing a bimanual examination as massive bleeding can occur while manipulation.

DIAGNOSIS

Pathological diagnosis can be made by examination of excised uterus via Rubin's criteria:[21]

- Presence of cervical glands opposite to the attachment of trophoblastic tissue.
- Trophoblastic tissue is attached below the level of entry of the uterine vessels into the uterus or below the anterior peritoneal reflection.
- Absence of fetal elements from corpus uteri.

Duckman suggested the following diagnostic criteria, in case, in whom, uterus is to be preserved:[22]
- A thinned out enlarged cervix with histologic evidence of products of conceptus.
- External os is patulous.
- Uterus is small and firm and normal sized, resting over the enlarged cervix.

The most widely accepted clinical criteria are those defined by Paalman and McElin.[23] These are:
- Amenorrhea followed by uterine bleeding without cramping pain.
- A softened and disproportionately enlarged cervix equal to or larger than the corporal portion of the uterus (an hour glass-shaped uterus on USG) (Fig. 1).

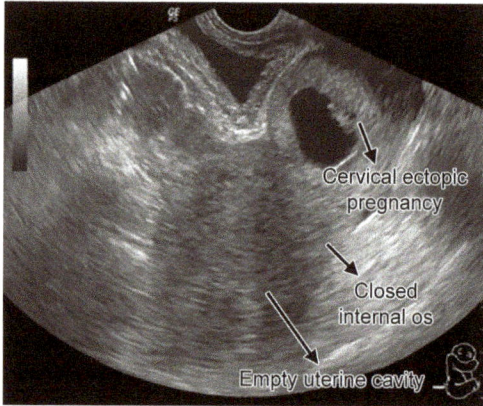

Fig. 1: "Hour glass" appearance of uterus, closed internal os, and gestational sac containing live embryo in intracervical canal.

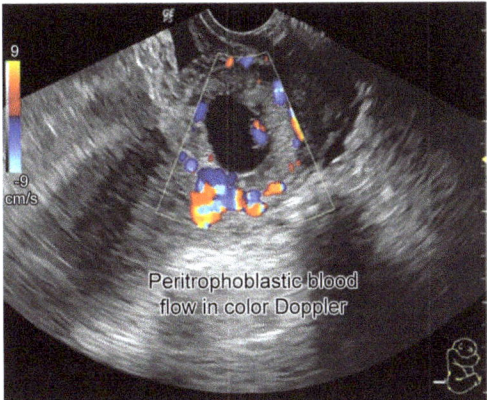

Fig. 2: Color Doppler showing peritrophoblastic blood flow.

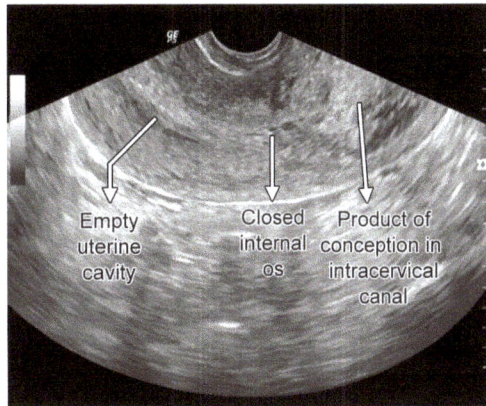

Fig. 3: Empty uterine cavity, closed internal os with product of conception in the intracervical canal.

- Products of conception entirely confined within, and firmly attached to the endocervix (Fig. 2).
- A snug internal os (Fig. 3).
- Partially open external os.

As with the increasing use of transvaginal ultrasound most of the cases of CEPs are detected at an early stage. Ultrasound criteria for cervical pregnancy are summarized in Table 1.[24]

DIFFERENTIAL DIAGNOSIS

Differential diagnosis includes an intrauterine pregnancy in process of abortion. Main differentiating findings are:
- In CEP internal os is closed while it is open in abortion (Fig. 3).
- Presence of "sliding sign" on transvaginal ultrasound.[25]
- Presence of peritrophoblastic blood flow on color Doppler helps to differentiate CEPs from the abortion (Fig. 2).
- The gestational sac of a cervical pregnancy has a regular contour while in an incomplete abortion sac has irregular contour.

Others involve cervical tumor, degenerated uterine polyp, placenta previa, gestational trophoblastic tumor, cervical or prolapsed submucous leiomyoma.

TABLE 1: Sonographic criteria for cervical ectopic pregnancy.

Anatomic structure	Sonographic features
Uterus	Empty
Cervix	Hour-glassed uterus dilated, barrel shaped
Gestational sac	Below the uterine arteries
Sliding sign	Absent (differential diagnosis: miscarriage in progress)
Ostium internum uteri	Closed
Ostium externum uteri	Open
Doppler blood flow	Increased around the gestational sac

CLASSIFICATION

According to site of origin, CEP has been classified into four categories:[26]
1. Isthmicocervical pregnancy
2. Pure cervical pregnancy
3. Cervicoisthmic pregnancy
4. Cervico-isthmic-corporal pregnancy.

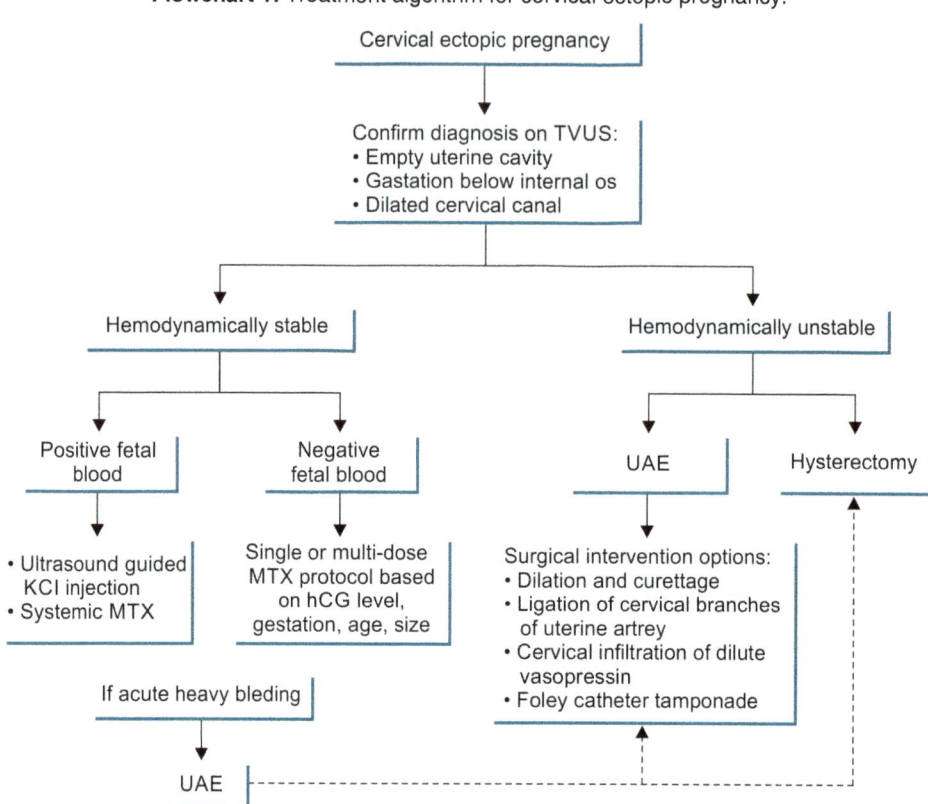

Flowchart 1: Treatment algorithm for cervical ectopic pregnancy.

(hCG: human chorionic gonadotropin; KCl: potassium chloride; MTX: methotrexate; TVUS: transvaginal ultrasound; UAE: uterine artery embolization)

MANAGEMENT

Management of the CEP can be *expectant, medical or surgical* and is dependent on several factors, such as gestational age, fetal cardiac activity, hemodynamic stability of the patient, need for future fertility, and the resources available and expertise of the gynecologists (Flowchart 1). Spontaneous resolution of 69% of cases has been reported.[17] There is a risk of spontaneous torrential hemorrhage in CEPs accounting for maternal death in about 9% of cases.[27]

Expectant Management

An initial human chorionic gonadotropin (hCG) titer less than 1,000 IU/L is recommended and is cutoff for expectant management with successful outcome in 85% of patients.[28]

Medical Management

Systemic therapy with methotrexate (MTX) in single and multiple dose protocols has been adopted for the treatment of CEPs similar to that used for treatment of tubal ectopic pregnancy. Routes of administration can be both systemic as well as local or a combination of both. The dose regimes and contraindication of MTX and side effects have been summarized in Tables 2 to 5. In cases of local administration, any of the following single doses can be used intracervically or intra-amniotically: 4 mg, 5 mg, 10 mg, 12.5 mg,

TABLE 2: MTX treatment protocol.[31]	
Regime	Surveillance
Single dose MTX 50 mg/m² IM	• Measure β-hCG levels on day 4 and day 7 • If difference ≥ 15% repeat weekly till levels are undetectable • If difference ≤ 15% between day 4 and day 7 levels, repeat dose and begin as new day 1 • If fetal cardiac activity present day 7, repeat MTX begin as new day 1 • Surgical management is to be done in cases of failure of fall in β-hCG and persistence of fetal cardiac activity after 3 doses of MTX
Multiple dose MTX 1 mg/kg IM on day 1, 3, 5, 7 Leucovorin rescue 0.1 mg/kg IM on days 2, 4, 6, 8	β-hCG levels to be measured on day 1, 3, 5, 7 prior to MTX dose. Continue alternate day doses of MTX until β-hCG level decreases ≥ 15% in two consecutive samples or up to four doses. Then follow β-hCG weekly till undetectable

(β-hCG: β-human chorionic gonadotropin; IM: intramuscularly; MTX: methotrexate)

TABLE 3: Contraindications to MTX therapy.	
Absolute contraindications	Relative contraindications
• Intrauterine pregnancy • Evidence of immunodeficiency • Moderate to severe anemia, leukopenia, or thrombocytopenia • Sensitivity to MTX • Active pulmonary disease • Active peptic ulcer disease • Clinically important hepatic dysfunction • Clinically important renal dysfunction • Breastfeeding • Ruptured ectopic pregnancy • Hemodynamically unstable patient	• Embryonic cardiac activity detected by transvaginal ultrasonography • High initial hCG concentration (>5,000 mIU/mL) • Ectopic pregnancy > 4 cm in size as imaged by transvaginal ultrasonography • Refusal to accept blood transfusion • Inability to participate in follow-up

(hCG: human chorionic gonadotropin; MTX: methotrexate)

20 mg, 25 mg, 50 mg, or 1 mg/kg. For feticide, in cases with presence of embryonic cardiac activity 2–8 mEq potassium chloride is instilled into amniotic sac.[29,30] After either systemic MTX administration or local MTX administration or both rescue with a 0.1 mg/kg dose of folinic acid to avoid side effects.

Methotrexate is the preferred modality for conservative management of CEPs, with a success rate of 91%. Factors responsible for decreased efficacy of MTX include:
- The gestational age is > 9 weeks
- The β-hCG level is > 10,000 mIU/mL
- Presence of cardiac activity
- Crown-rump length is > 10 mm.[32]

INTERVENTIONS

Other interventions included:
- Bilateral uterine artery embolization[33]

TABLE 4: Treatment and drug side effects associated with MTX.[31]	
Treatment side effects	Drug side effects
• Increase in abdominal girth • Increase in hCG during initial therapy • Vaginal bleeding or spotting • Abdominal pain	• Gastric distress, nausea, and vomiting • Stomatitis • Dizziness • Severe neutropenia (rare) • Reversible alopecia (rare) • Pneumonitis (rare)

(hCG: human chorionic gonadotropin; MTX; methotrexate)

- Vaginal ligation of cervical branches of the uterine arteries
- Dilatation and curettage with or without dilute vasopressin cervical infiltration and Foley catheter tamponade.

TABLE 5: Treatment modalities and respective indications.

Treatment modalities	Indications
Expectant	• Initial serum hCG level < 1,000 (2,000) mIU/mL • Declining serum hCG levels • Absence of severe hemorrhage • Absence of severe abdominal pain
Systemic MTX	• Serum hCG level < 10,000 mIU/mL • Early pregnancy < 9 weeks of gestation • No embryonic cardiac activity • Crown-rump length < 10 mm
Intra-amniotic MTX	Present embryonic cardiac activity
Embryonic intracardiac injection of potassium chloride	Present embryonic cardiac activity
Cervical curettage	• Whenever conservative treatment modalities fail • Precondition: Adequate hemostasis
Cervical cerclage, cervical-stay sutures	Hemostasis before evacuation of the CEP
Ligation/embolization of the descending branches of uterine arteries	• Preoperative hemostasis in cases of expected severe hemorrhage and wish to preserve fertility • Precondition for embolization: Preoperative insertion of an angiographic catheter
Local injection of vasopressin	Noninvasive hemostasis before evacuation of the CEP in cases of expected moderate hemorrhage
Foley balloon tamponade	For noninvasive hemostasis
Hysterectomy	• Terminated family planning • Life-threatening hemorrhage • Second and third trimester CEP

(CEP: cervical ectopic pregnancy; hCG: human chorionic gonadotropin; MTX: methotrexate)

Various treatment modalities and their relative indication have been summarized in Table 5.

Chen et al. reported a case of cervical pregnancy treated with transvaginal ultrasound-guided aspiration and cervical-stay sutures to control hemorrhage.[34]

FERTILITY AFTER TREATMENT

As far as MTX is concerned there is no evidence of impaired fertility after treatment with MTX.[35] Although the shrinkage in size of cervix correlate with falling hCG level, but cervix may still be enlarged if few cases where hCG is undetectable.[36]

CONCLUSION

Cervical ectopic pregnancy is the rarest form of ectopic pregnancy. Often it is misdiagnosis. Mainstay of management is early diagnosis and treatment with systemic or local MTX combined with various conservative measures. Hemostasis is a big challenge; failure to achieve hemostasis might end up into emergency hysterectomy.

REFERENCES

1. Leeman LM, Wendland CL. Cervical ectopic pregnancy. Diagnosis with endovaginal ultrasound examination and successful

treatment with methotrexate. Arch Fam Med. 2000;9:72-7.
2. Kung FT, Chang SY, Tsai YC, et al. Subsequent reproduction and obstetric outcome after methotrexate treatment of cervical pregnancy: a review of original literature and international collaborative follow-up. Hum Reprod. 1997;12:591-5.
3. Celik C, Bala A, Acar A, et al. Methotrexate for cervical pregnancy. A case report. J Reprod Med. 2003;48:130-2.
4. Oliver R, Malik M, Coker A, et al. Management of extra-tubal and rare ectopic pregnancies: case series and review of current literature. Arch Gynecol Obstet. 2007;276(2):125-31.
5. Chetty M, Elson J. Treating non-tubal ectopic pregnancy. Best Pract Res Clin Obstet. Gynaecol. 2009;23(4):529-38.
6. Gun M, Mavrogiorgis M. Cervical ectopic pregnancy: a case report and literature review. Ultrasound Obstet Gynaecol. 2002;19(3): 297-301.
7. Karande VC, Flood JT, Heard N, et al. Analysis of ectopic pregnancies resulting from in vitro fertilization and embryo transfer. Hum Reprod. 1991;6:446-9.
8. Ginsburg ES, Frates MC, Rein MS, et al. Early diagnosis and treatment of cervical pregnancy in an in vitro fertilization program. Fertil Steril. 1994;61:966-9.
9. Kraemer B, Abele H, Hahn M, et al. Cervical ectopic pregnancy on the portio: conservative case management and clinical review. Fertil Steril. 2008;90(5):e1-4.
10. Vitale SG, Rapisarda AM, Laganà AS. Cervical Ectopic Pregnancy: The Role of Hysteroscopy. Cham, Switzerland: Springer; 2018. pp. 171-9.
11. Thomas RL, Gingold BR, Gallagher MW. Cervical pregnancy. A report of two cases. J Reprod. Med. 1991;36(6):459-62.
12. Spitzer D, Steiner H, Graf A, et al. Conservative treatment of cervical pregnancy by curettage and local prostaglandin injection. Hum Reprod. 1997;12(4):860-6.
13. Fylstra DL, Coffey MD. Treatment of cervical pregnancy with cerclage, curettage and balloon tamponade. A report of three cases. J Reprod Med. 2001;46(1):71-4.
14. Cupr Z, Pospisil J, Milickova E. Ectopic pregnancy on the vaginal part of the uterus. Zentralbl Gynakol. 1973;95(39):1385-7.
15. Parente JT, Ou CS, Levy J, et al. Cervical pregnancy analysis: a review and report of five cases. Obstet Gynecol. 1983;62(1):79-82.
16. Pisarska MD, Carson SA. Incidence and risk factors for ectopic pregnancy. Clin Obstet Gynecol. 1999;42(1):2-8.
17. Heer JS, Chao DK, McPheeters RA. Cervical ectopic pregnancy. West J Emerg Med. 2012;13(1):125-6.
18. Agdi M, Tulandi T. Surgical treatment of ectopic pregnancy. Best Pract Res Clin Obstet Gynaecol. 2009;23(4):519-27.
19. Surampudi K. A case of cervical ectopic pregnancy: Successful therapy with methotrexate. J Obstet Gynaecol India. 2012;62(Suppl 1):1-3.
20. Samal SK, Rathod S. Cervical ectopic pregnancy. J Nat Sci Biol Med. 2015;6(1):257-60.
21. Rubin IC. Cervical pregnancy. Surg Gynecol Obstet. 1911;13:625.
22. Duckman, S. Cervical pregnancy. Am J Obstet Gynecol. 1951;62:1381.
23. Varghese U, Fajardo A, Gomathinayagam T. Cervical pregnancy. Oman Med J. 2008;23:53-4.
24. Kung FT, Lin H, Hsu TY, et al. Differential diagnosis of cervical ectopic pregnancy and conservative management with combination of laparoscopic-assisted uterine artery ligation and hysteroscopic endocervical resection. Fertil Steril. 2004;81:1642-9.
25. Jurkovic D, Hacket E, Campbell S. Diagnosis and treatment of early cervical pregnancy: A review and a report of two cases treated conservatively. Ultrasound Obstet Gynecol. 1996;8:373-80.
26. David MP, Bergman A, Delighdish L. Cervico-isthmic pregnancy carried to term. Obstet Gynecol. 1980;56;247-52.
27. Ehrenberg-Buchner S, Sandadi S, Moawad NS, et al. Ectopic pregnancy: role of laparoscopic treatment. Clin Obstet Gynecol. 2009;52(3):372-9.
28. Trio D, Strobelt N, Picciolo C, et al. Prognostic factors for successful expectant management of ectopic pregnancy. Fertil Steril. 1995;63(3):469-72.
29. Cepni I, Ocal P, Erkan S, et al. Conservative treatment of cervical ectopic pregnancy with transvaginal ultrasound-guided aspiration and single-dose methotrexate. Fertil Steril. 2004;81:1130-2.

30. Ushakov FB, Elchalal U, Aceman PJ, et al. Cervical pregnancy: past and future. Obstet Gynecol Surv. 1997;52:45-59.
31. Practice Committee of American Society for Reproductive Medicine. Medical treatment of ectopic pregnancy: a committee opinion. Fertil Steril. 2013;100(3):638-44.
32. Hung TH, Shau WY, Hsieh TT, et al. Prognostic factors for an unsatisfactory primary methotrexate treatment of cervical pregnancy (a quantitative review). Hum Reprod. 1998;13:2636-42.
33. Kaur R, Singh R. Effective management of early cervical pregnancy with bilateral uterine artery embolization followed by immediate evacuation and curettage: A case report. J Obstet Gynaecol India. 2017;67(1):66-9.
34. Chen D, Kligman I, Rosenwaks Z. Heterotopic cervical pregnancy successfully treated with transvaginal ultrasound-guided aspiration and cervical-stay sutures. Fertil Steril. 2001;75:1030-3.
35. Oriol B, Barrio A, Pacheco A, et al. Systemic methotrexate to treat ectopic pregnancy does not affect ovarian reserve. Fertil Steril. 2008;90:1579-82.
36. Yoshida S, Furuhashi M, Itakura A, et al. Conservative handling of the uterus in a 10-week cervical pregnancy case. Nagoya J Med Sci. 1997;60(3-4):139-43.

Chapter 10F

Postabortion Hemorrhage

Nozer Sheriar, Rajneet Bhatia

INTRODUCTION

An estimated 10–20% of pregnancies result in a spontaneous abortion.[1] An estimated 56 million abortions are reported worldwide each year.[2] This makes abortions, both spontaneous and induced, an important fact of women's lives, second only to childbirth and also means that abortion-related complications, particularly postabortion hemorrhage have serious implications for maternal morbidity and mortality. This risk to women's lives and health is further vitiated by unsafe abortion, with an estimated one woman dying every 8 minutes due to complications arising from these abortions in the developing world.

Abortion is permitted for the more liberal indications including social or economic reasons in just 16% of developing countries as compared with 80% of developed countries.[3] This difference is particularly significant, given that countries with restrictive abortion laws have higher rates of abortion-related mortality (34 per 100,000 births) as compared to those with liberal laws (1 or fewer per 100,000 births).[4]

Even after legalization of abortion in many countries, unsafe abortion still remains a major public health issue. In India, the burden of unsafe and illegal abortions still persist despite Medical Termination of Pregnancy (MTP) Act legislated in 1971, with unsafe abortion still reported to cause a third of all maternal deaths.

PREVALENCE

It is estimated that around 47,000 women die due to unsafe abortion and an estimated 5 million women get admitted each year for abortion-related complications.[3] Abortion-related complications cover a wide spectrum of severity and include hemorrhage, sepsis, and cervical and uterine injury. Prevention and management of these complications by the provision of safe and legal abortion care have the potential to avert most of this abortion-related mortality and morbidity, even in developing countries.

Hemorrhage after abortion is rare, occurring in approximately 1% of abortions, numerically substantial given the large number of spontaneous and induced abortions. The associated morbidity is significant and associated with life-threatening events.[5] Although medical abortions bleed more than surgical abortions, the overall bleeding associated with both the procedures is generally minimal and clinically insignificant. A study of 2,055 second trimester abortions reported severe hemorrhage in 1.9%, many of these requiring transfusions.[6]

There is no accepted definition for hemorrhage, but severe hemorrhage is defined as bleeding more than or equivalent to 500 mL which needs hospital admission with or without the need for blood product transfusions. In the first trimester, hemorrhage (14%) is the second common cause of abortion-related mortality following infection (33%).

In the second trimester, hemorrhage is the most common cause of mortality, with 33% following induction terminations and 40% following second trimester dilatation and evacuation.[5]

ETIOPATHOGENESIS

Uterine Atony

The most common cause of postabortion hemorrhage, like most obstetric hemorrhage, is an atonic uterus. The principal mechanism of uterine hemostasis is contraction of the myometrium, which mechanically compresses the blood vessels supplying the placental bed. In addition, local hemostatic factors such as tissue factor type 1 plasminogen activator inhibitor, systemic coagulation factors such as platelets, and circulating clotting factors also contribute in preventing hemorrhage.[7]

An inadequate contraction of the uterine myometrial cells in response to endogenous oxytocin released during abortion leads to hemorrhage. The delivery of the placenta leaves disrupted spiral arteries, which do not have myometrium and are dependent on contractions to mechanically squeeze them for hemostasis. Greater gestational age, advanced maternal age, and previous scar on the uterus are associated risk factors.[8]

Abnormal Placentation

Placental invasion in and beyond the myometrium can be a major risk factor complicating the abortion. The incidence of placenta accreta is rising due to the increased rates of cesarean sections and this complication is also dangerous for the woman undergoing abortion. She will be at risk of hemorrhage though relatively lesser than the third trimester pregnancies.[9]

While the exact pathogenesis is not known, placental adherence can be due to one or combination of factors including primary deficiency of decidua, abnormal maternal vascular remodeling or excessive trophoblastic invasion. Placenta previa is generally not considered to be associated with hemorrhage occurring with abortions. However, whenever there is excessive bleeding during the procedure of midtrimester and late-first trimester medical and surgical abortions and postabortion hemorrhage, complete or marginal previa or placentation low in the uterine cavity should be considered.[5,10]

Retained Tissue

Retained products of conception refer to the partial or complete retention of the parts of the first trimester gestation, placenta or other decidual tissues within the uterus. These are more common after medical abortion, though can also occur after surgical abortion. The incidence is dependent on gestational age and occurs frequently after second trimester abortions. A study of 2,055 second trimester abortions reported the need for evacuation of retained products in 3.6%.[6]

Retained products of conception are cause of both primary or secondary obstetric hemorrhage, most significant cause of maternal morbidity and mortality worldwide. The major cause of retained products is the abnormal adherence of placenta, either whole or in part, to the underlying uterine wall. Patients usually present with abdominal pain, bleeding, and fever. Though these symptoms are not specific but they play a critical role in early diagnosis and management thereby preventing associated consequences.[11]

Cervical Lacerations

Forced dilatation of the cervix always causes microscopic tears of the cervical musculature. Small tears rarely cause major bleeding episodes. High lateral cervical tears in the area of uterine arteries can lead to significant hemorrhage.[5]

The use of injectable 15-methyl PGF2 alpha as practiced earlier had a distinct association with bucket handle tears of the cervix. These were believed to be the result of strong uterine contractions with lagging cervical dilatation and highlight the necessity of priming the cervix and permitting gradual progress with second trimester medical abortion.

Cervical injuries are now uncommon with the contemporary methods. The medical priming of the cervix for surgical abortion and the use of misoprostol with or without mifepristone prepares the cervix and gives it protection from injury.

Perforation

Uterine perforation, although rare, is an extremely dangerous complication of abortion particularly when it goes undiagnosed at the time of the abortion. It can lead to trauma to visceral structures or uncontrollable hemorrhage requiring hysterectomy or even leading to death.

Multiparae have been found to be at least three times at higher risk than primiparae. Uterine anomalies are also associated with higher chances of perforation. Several studies have also found that the risk of uterine perforation is also related to the seniority and experience of the surgeon performing the procedure.

Uterine position is a critical factor in determining the site of the perforation (anterior, posterior, isthmic, fundal or cornual). The posterior wall is more commonly involved in anteverted uterus, while anterior wall is perforated in retroverted uterus. The lateral wall of the uterus and cervix can also be at risk of perforation if the uterine angle is deviated to either direction.[12]

The site of perforation is important as the visceral organs at that anatomical site are at risk of injury.

Perforation is likely to occur whenever there is a discrepancy between the surgeon's estimates and the actual size of uterus.[13] The most common perforating instruments are suction cannula, uterine sound or a uterine dilator, all contributing almost equally.

Perforation is particularly dangerous and life-threatening when associated with unsafe abortions performed by unsafe providers more so because of the delay in diagnosis, accompanying sepsis, and peritonitis.

Bleeding Disorders

Women on anticoagulants and with bleeding disorders are obviously at an increased risk of hemorrhage, if these are not stopped in time. The difficulty in stopping the anticoagulants in time may be because of the urgent need to undertake the completion of a spontaneous abortion or the need to perform the abortion while staying on anticoagulants due to an underlying medical condition.

Postabortion Triad

The triad of pain, bleeding, and low-grade fever are frequently seen in emergency situations and the diagnosis of retained products of conception is usually the cause.

Postabortion Syndrome

This presents as progressively worsening lower abdominal pain and hemodynamic compromise in the absence of postabortal vaginal bleeding. This is due to the collection of blood and/or retained products of conception in the uterus, causing overdistention of the uterine cavity, which is then unable to contract in order to expel its contents. It either results from cervical stenosis or sudden excessive bleeding, which is the uterus is unable to expel.[14]

DIAGNOSIS

The diagnosis and quantification of abortion-related hemorrhage is challenging because of the different techniques, procedures, and gestational ages at which abortions are occur or are performed.

Surgical Methods

Accurate measurement of blood loss is possible both with manual vacuum aspiration (MVA) where the syringe collects all products and estimates blood and electric vacuum aspiration (EVA) where the suction apparatus allows for accurate measurement. Of course, depending on the gestational age, amniotic fluid would have to be subtracted from the collected fluid.

Medical Methods

With medical methods of abortion (MMA) in the first trimester, the assessment of blood loss depends on the woman and hence has an element of subjectivity. The usage and frequency of change of sanitary napkins would be a guide as to the severity of blood loss and must be explained to the woman as a part of counseling. Since late medical abortions occur in healthcare facilities the estimation immediately postprocedure can be made by the provider.

Estimation of Hemorrhage

The vagina has the capacity to hold more than 500 mL of blood in the supine position without significant external bleeding hence a bimanual examination should always be performed for postabortion hemorrhage.

Occasionally, cervical stenosis may result in an intrauterine blood collection with the hematometra, which could reach substantial proportions. The presentation has the absence of any bleeding or discharge associated with severe pelvic pain. Clinically the uterus is enlarged, tense and tender, with the diagnosis being confirmed and the collection quantified by a pelvic ultrasound.

MANAGEMENT

The management of postabortion hemorrhage generally follows the protocols and levels of management described for postpartum hemorrhage (Table 1). While the primary

TABLE 1: Levels of management for postabortion hemorrhage.

Primary	Cervical laceration	Pressure suturing
	Atonic uterus	Bimanual massage Uterotonic agents Oxytocin, methylergometrine maleate, 15-methyl PGF2 alpha, misoprostol
Secondary	Atonic uterus Retained products or blood clots	Fluid resuscitation Blood components transfusion Tamponade effect Uterine pack Foley's catheter/Bakri balloon/condom or glove Suction evacuation or manual vacuum aspiration preferably under ultrasound guidance
Tertiary	Intensive surgical interventions	Uterine artery embolization Compression sutures B-Lynch, Cho sutures Stepwise devascularization Laparoscopy or laparotomy for perforation Hysterectomy

Box 1: Management of atonic uterus.

Stabilization of the patient:
- Monitor vitals
- Trendelenburg position
- Blood investigations
- Fluid resuscitation
- Blood transfusion
- Broad-spectrum antibiotics

Mechanical methods:
- Empty bladder
- Bimanual massage

Uterotonic agents:
- Oxytocin 10U in 500 mL saline
- Methylergometrine maleate 0.2 mg IM/slow IV 5 doses 2–4 hours apart
- 15-methyl PGF2 alpha 250 µg IM 8 doses every 15–20 minutes
- Misoprostol 800 µg orally

Uterine packing:
- Roller gauze
- Foleys catheter
- Condom catheter or glove
- Bakri balloon

Conservative methods:
- Uterine tamponade with condom, BAKRI balloon, RUSCH catheter, etc.
- Uterine artery embolization
- B-Lynch or Cho sutures
- Stepwise devascularization

Last resort:
- Total or subtotal hysterectomy.

management may be medical or surgical depending on the etiology, the severe or intractable hemorrhage requires intensive intervention either by interventional radiology or surgical techniques.

Uterine Atony

Since most of the cases of postabortion hemorrhage are caused by uterine atony, a systematic therapeutic approach is essential. Uterine size and tone should be assessed and a uterine massage should be commenced if the uterus is flaccid and not well contracted (Box 1).

The mechanical methods to initiate uterine contraction and decrease bleeding include emptying bladder and bimanual massage. Simultaneously, uterotonics should be administered. Oxytocin is the recommended first-line agent given intravenously in a bolus of 5 units followed by an infusion of 10 units in 500 mL normal saline.

If the bleeding is not controlled with bimanual massage and oxytocin, the recommended second-line drug is methylergometrine maleate. Intravenous or intramuscular injection of 0.2 mg should be given for maximum of five doses; 2–4 hours apart. Hypertension is a contraindication for ergot derivatives while the Rh negative group constitutes a relative contraindication.

In patients refractory to oxytocin and methylergometrine maleate, 15-methyl PGF2 alpha has been found to be effective in 80–90% of cases. The recommended dose is 250 µg intramuscular or intramyometrial injection, which can be repeated every 15–20 minutes up to a maximum of 2 mg (8 doses). Bronchial asthma is an absolute contradiction whereas a state of hypovolemic shock is a relative contraindication as absorption of the drug would be compromised.

Misoprostol is a valuable and low-cost drug that is now considered an alternative of oxytocin particularly in low-resource settings. International Federation of Gynaecology and Obstetrics (FIGO) recommends a single dose of 800 µg misoprostol sublingually as soon as the hemorrhage is diagnosed if oxytocin is not available. The rectal route is not recommended as it is associated with lower serum concentrations and hence has longer time for onset of action than buccal route. The patient may experience transient shivering, chills, and fever which can be managed with antipyretics or physical cooling. Rarely, they may also experience transient diarrhea, nausea, and vomiting which responds to appropriate symptomatic management.

If the uterus does not contract and bleeding persists despite medical management, uterine tamponade is the logical next step. Packing of the uterus can be therapeutic or an initial option till surgical facilities are prepared or a shift to a tertiary care setting is organized. The uterus and vagina are packed manually under direct vision using a roller gauze. In few cases, uterine packing itself can control bleeding and the pack is removed after 24 hours. Broad-spectrum antibiotics are administered to prevent infection. Intrauterine catheters create a tamponade effect, which can successfully control bleeding. The large bulb Foley's catheter inflated with 30–50cc of saline can be used. An especially designed catheter, the Bakri balloon, has been used to control hemorrhage. In low resource centers, surgical gloves or condoms and even condom catheters may be used.

For cases refractory to tamponade, further management is carried out by uterine artery embolization (UAE) by experienced interventional radiologists. When UAE is not possible or when bleeding still persists, immediate laparotomy should be adopted. Initial step should be compression sutures, B-Lynch or Cho sutures, which hold the anterior and posterior walls together and rapidly control bleeding. These techniques are simple to perform and may be effective rapidly as an alternate to hysterectomy. Stepwise devascularization of the uterus is the safe and effective step to save the uterus, especially in patients who desire to retain fertility. Patients not responding to internal iliac artery ligation have no other option left than hysterectomy. Total hysterectomy is preferred even though subtotal hysterectomy will be faster and effective to control bleeding related to uterine atony but it may not be effective for lower segment, cervix or vagina-related hemorrhages. Bleeding posthysterectomy can be controlled by packing the vagina with a gauze for 24 hours.

Abnormal Placentation

With an increased incidence of adherent placentae due to the increased prevalence of cesarean section, it would be critical to make the diagnosis beforehand, as intraoperative preventive measures can significantly reduce the blood loss thereby avoiding substantial morbidity and mortality. The diagnosis is made by gray-scale ultrasound, which can be confirmed with MRI for better delineation of the extent of placental invasion, though this is rarely possible with abortion. Aggressive use of uterotonics prophylactically is the mainstay of treatment. Conservative management, even placental preservation, can be carried out with subsequent methotrexate therapy or pelvic artery embolization. If hemorrhage still persists despite all prophylactic measures further medical and surgical management should be instituted as described in the previous section.[15]

Cervical Injury

Damage during abortion can occur during dilatation, especially in a rigid and tight cervix. Priming of the cervix using misoprostol 400 mg per vaginally or orally 2–3 hours prior to the procedure is protective as it helps soften the cervix making the dilatation easier and prevent tears. In bleeding episodes, cervix should be inspected visually and digitally. Small lacerations less than 0.5 cm will respond to adequate pressure. Highly vascular or lacerations greater than 1 cm need to be repaired using absorbable sutures. If bleeding is persistent after high cervical tear repairs the possibility of uterine artery laceration should be considered. It is suggested that the patient should be shifted to operating room in case vaginal exploration is required for patients with heavy bleeding.[5]

Retained Tissue

Ultrasound is useful in evaluating intrauterine echogenic tissue, is suggestive of retained products of conception. Sometimes necrotic decidua and blood clots may be very difficult to differentiate from retained tissue, wherein combined gray scale and color Doppler may be of help. Once the diagnosis is confirmed, treatment should be decided as per the symptoms of the patient. If the patient is stable with minimal bleeding, expectant management using uterotonic medications like prostaglandins E1 analogs or oral methylergometrine maleate can be used and patient can be reassessed with ultrasound a week after her next menses.

For persistent retained products after medical management or in cases of delayed bleeding, evacuation of the uterus is advised under hysteroscopic vision. The goal of this procedure is to decrease the thermal damage to the endometrium, preserve the integrity of the uterine cavity minimizing the rates of intrauterine adhesions and fertility issues. Additional advantage includes identification and treatment of uterine cavity anomalies, which may be the underlying cause. However, this technique is not recommended in immediate postpartum period and hence surgical methods like vacuum aspiration or suction evacuation should be considered. It is suggested the above procedures be carried out under ultrasound guidance for complete evacuation, thus preventing the complications of perforation.[11]

Uterine Perforation

Kafrissen et al. studied a cluster of four abortion-related deaths at a single facility, and hemorrhage as a result of perforation was the cause of death in two of the four patients.[16]

Cervical priming before the procedure facilitates dilatation of the cervix, thus minimizing the chance of perforation. It is also recommended that the dilator and cannula should be passed just beyond the internal os and also the products should be sucked from that position only as much as possible.[13] Uterine evacuation should be done only when the uterus is well contracted.

The uterine sound is associated with 20% of perforations and hence avoiding the use of this instrument can reduce the risk to certain extent. Uterine sound may be reserved for cases where determination of the size and position of the uterus is in doubt. The high negative pressure transmitted through the suction cannula can easily traumatize the bowel and other abdominal viscera in case of perforation. MVA is hence the recommended technique of surgical abortion for pregnancies up to 12–14 weeks of gestation as it is associated with fewer complication. Sharp curettage should be avoided.

The experience of the operator is the main determining factor and hence training of the young professionals should concentrate on the safe use of these instruments. Procedures under ultrasound guidance reduce the risk of perforation by many folds. Ultrasound indicates the direction and depth of the uterine cavity and hence evacuation can be done without undue pressure on the uterine walls, especially in the cases of second trimester abortions. Small perforations remain undiagnosed and hence the true incidence of uterine perforations is significantly underestimated. Therefore, patients feeling unwell postabortion should be asked to follow-up to rule out undiagnosed perforations.

Broad-spectrum antibiotic coverage is recommended for all cases of uterine perforation following abortion because of the high incidence of postoperative fever.

Injury by instruments during abortions may occur even in the hands of the most experienced gynecologist. A careful assessment of the uterine size and position, vigilance in the use of the uterine sound and dilators, greater care in the use of suction cannula, and experience in vacuum aspiration will decrease the incidence of uterine perforation during elective abortions. A high degree of suspicion together with early diagnosis and treatment will prevent the potential complications that may arise from uterine perforation.

If a perforation is suspected after completion of evacuation, the patient is observed for 2 hours. Vital parameters monitored, intravenous fluids and oxygen started, and intravenous antibiotics and intravenous or intramuscular methylergometrine maleate administered. If the condition gets worse and the bleeding does not stop, then laparoscopy with a possible laparotomy may be necessary to locate and repair the source of the bleeding.

If a perforation is suspected during the procedure, the procedure is stopped immediately and the instrument responsible left in place. Laparoscopy is performed to assess the damage to the uterus and abdominal organs and the damage repaired by laparoscopy or laparotomy. The intestines are traced, other organs checked and appropriate repair undertaken. Evacuation is completed under direct vision. If the perforation is extensive, hysterectomy may also be necessary. Simultaneously, patient is stabilized with oxygen, intravenous fluids, and blood transfusion, if necessary. Uterotonics should also be administered during and even postprocedure.[3,12]

Bleeding Disorders

Patients with inherited coagulopathies must receive an individualized treatment from multidisciplinary team including hematologists. For the patient on anticoagulants, elective abortion procedures should be carried out 48 hours after the stoppage of medication. Postabortion hemorrhage in these patients is managed with close observation and aggressive use of uterotonics in a tertiary care setting.

CONCLUSION

Although hemorrhage after abortion is rare, it is associated with significant morbidity and mortality. Definitions of hemorrhage across studies are inconsistent and consensus needs to be built towards a consistent definition. Future research is needed regarding the prophylactic use of uterotonics and the use of ultrasound during abortion. Not only will these advances benefit the large number of induced abortions, they will also benefit and make spontaneous abortions safer.

REFERENCES

1. Robinson GE. Pregnancy loss. Best Pract Res Clin Obstet Gynaecol. 2013;28(1):169-78.
2. Sedgh G, Bearak J, Singh S, et al. Special tabulations of updated data from abortion incidence between 1990 and 2014: Global, regional and subregional levels and trends. Lancet. 2016;388:258-67.
3. WHO. (2012). Safe abortion: technical and policy guidance for health systems. [online] Available from: https://www.who.int/reproductivehealth/publications/unsafe_abortion/9789241548434/en/ [Last accessed July, 2019].
4. Bashar MA, Bhattacharya S, Singh A. Unsafe abortions in India: Removing the bottlenecks. Int J Med Public Health. 2018;8(1):42-4.
5. Kerns J, Steinauer J. Management of postabortion hemorrhage. Contraception. 2013;87(3):331-42.
6. Bhathena RK, Sheriar NK, Guillebaud J. Late abortion practice in a teaching hospital in India. J Obstet Gynecol. 1990;10:299-303.
7. Al-Mehaisen L, Al-Kuran O, Amarin ZO, et al. Secondary postpartum hemorrhage following placental site vessel subinvolution: a case report. Arch Gynecol Obstet. 2008;278(6):585-7.

8. Gill P, Van Hook JW. Uterine Atony. USA: StatPearls Publishing; 2018.
9. AbdElfatah EA, Mohamed Awad E, Abd-Eldaym T, et al. Outcome of patients with placenta accreta at El Shatby Maternity University Hospital. Obstet Gynecol Int J. 2017;7(7):725-33.
10. Tantbirojn P, Crum CP, Parast MM. Pathophysiology of placenta accreta: The role of decidua and extravillous trophoblast. Placenta. 2008;29(7):639-45.
11. Guarino A, Di Benedetto L, Assorgi C, et al. Conservative and timely treatment in retained products of conception: A case report of placenta accreta retention. Int J Clin Exp Pathol. 2015;8(10):13625-9.
12. Chen LH, Lai SF, Lee WH, et al. Uterine perforation during elective first trimester abortions: A 13-year review. Singapore Med J. 1995;36:63-7.
13. Mittal S, Misra SL. Uterine perforation following medical termination of pregnancy by vacuum aspiration. Int J Gynecol Obstet. 1985;23(1):45-50.
14. Sajadi-Emarzarova KR, Martinez CL. Abortion Complications. USA: StatPearls Publishing; 2018.
15. Bauer ST, Bonanno C. Abnormal placentation. Semin Perinatol. 2009;33(2):88-96.
16. Kafrissen ME, Grimes DA, Hogue CJ, et al. Cluster of abortion deaths at a single facility. Obstet Gynecol. 1986;68:387-9.

Section 3: Antepartum Hemorrhage

- **Imaging in Antepartum Hemorrhage**
  Narendra Malhotra, Amitha Indersen, Prerna Keshan, Neharika Malhotra Bora, Rishabh Bora, Jaideep Malhotra
- **Surgical Challenges in Placenta Previa**
  Suchitra N Pandit, Swati Bhargava
- **Abruptio Placentae**
  Saswati Sanyal Choudhury
- **Rupture Uterus: The Catastrophe Compendiously Summarized**
  Pratima Mittal, Sheeba Marwah
- **Expectant Management of Placenta Previa**
  Gomathy Narayanan, Narayanan R
- **Morbidly Adherent Placenta (Placenta Accreta Spectrum): Prearm and Perform**
  VP Paily

11A
Chapter

Imaging in Antepartum Hemorrhage

Narendra Malhotra, Amitha Indersen, Prerna Keshan, Neharika Malhotra Bora, Rishabh Bora, Jaideep Malhotra

INTRODUCTION

Antepartum hemorrhage (APH) is defined as bleeding from or into the genital tract occurring after 24 completed weeks of gestation. APH complicates around 3.5–4% of pregnancies. The causes can be:
- Placental:
    - Abruptio placentae (15%)
    - Placenta previa (10%).
- Antepartum hemorrhage of unknown origin
- Extraplacental causes:
    - Rupture uterus
    - Excessive show
    - Trauma
    - Vulvovaginal infections
    - Genital tumor
    - Vasa previa
    - Incidental bleed from cervical polyp, erosion, or malignancy.

Undiagnosed APH can result in significant maternal and fetal compromise. Hence, the key point is that absence of placenta previa should be confirmed by imaging before doing a pervaginal examination of a female presenting with bleeding during the third trimester. Expeditious diagnosis by ultrasonography (USG) becomes the mainstay of management in APH. Only when placenta previa and abruptio placenta are ruled out by imaging, we can think of alternate causes of APH.

Antepartum hemorrhage is invariable always an obstetric emergency and mandates clinical acumen, prompt diagnosis, and efficient management. It can present with overt bleeding or with subtle signs that have to be identified. It is always better to initially suspect the possibility of placenta previa or abruption in cases with bleeding and then proceed to rule them out. APH can present in the antenatal period when the patient is not in labor, at the onset of cervical dilation or in active labor. By definition APH is any bleeding per vaginam presenting between 24 weeks of gestation up to term irrespective of presence of pain or contractions.

RISK FACTOR ASSESSMENT BEFORE SUBJECTING TO IMAGING

- Multifetal gestation
- Hypertension in pregnancy
- Polyhydramnios in any previous scan
- Number of previous cesarean sections if any
- History of APH in previous pregnancy
- History of bleeding diathesis/thrombophilias
- Previous history of abortions
- Assisted reproductive technology (ART) pregnancy
- Smoking
- Extreme of age.

DETAILED HISTORY OF BLEEDING IN THE CURRENT PREGNANCY PRIOR TO IMAGING

- History of trauma
- Amount and nature of hemorrhage

- Color of the blood—dark colored or bright red
- Whether there is any associated pain?
- Whether the bleeding is continuing?
- Whether any previous episode of bleeding has occurred in the current pregnancy?
- History of intercourse
- Any passage of stained liquor for evidence of membrane rupture.

PLACENTAL ABRUPTION

Abruption placenta is defined as the premature separation of a normally implanted placenta, after 20 weeks and before the third stage of labor. Patients typically present with uterine tenderness, contraction, may or may not have overt bleeding and variations of varying degrees in the maternal circulatory system. It is an emergency where the mother can exsanguinate, and the fetus can suffer distress as the placental insertion gets detached. Placental abruption is commonly associated with maternal hypertension, preterm labor/premature rupture of membranes, overdistended uterus, chorioamnionitis, trauma, etc.

Placental abruption can be marginal (most common), retroplacental or preplacental depending on where the rupture of the decidual arteries happens.

It is important that a high index of suspicion is maintained and clinical judgment often overrides imaging modalities.[1]

Ultrasound diagnosis of placental abruption is not very reliable as the appearance of the hemorrhage may be variable. It is usually hyperechoic or isoechoic immediately following the hemorrhage and can be difficult to identify. Another reason is that in presence of abruption and revealed hemorrhage, the bleed could have been passed per vaginam and is not imaged on the ultrasound. When there are associated fetal signs like

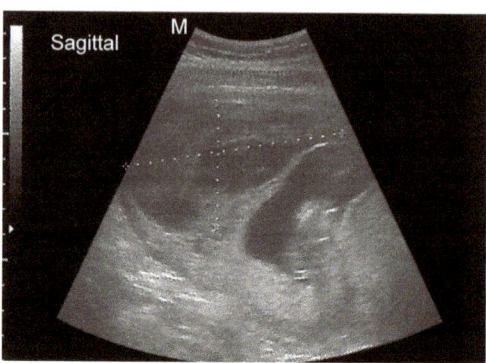

Fig. 1: Ultrasonic image of subchorionic abruption.

bradycardia or signs of fetal hypoxia seen in the Doppler studies, the prognosis is poorer and necessitates emergent intervention.

Magnetic resonance imaging (MRI) can accurately identify abruption and can be considered if the ultrasound examination is normal or noncontributory and if the diagnosis would change the management plan.

The hemorrhage appears as medium to high intensity signals between the uterus and the placenta on T2-weighted images.

Recent advances in imaging have significantly increased the sensitivity of detecting abruption by USG (Fig. 1). Although USG is considered specific for placental abruption but the sensitivity is still questionable. On USG, the following findings can be noted:
- *Early hemorrhage:* Hyperechoic or isoechoic
- *Resolving hemorrhage:* Hypoechoic in 1 week
- Sonolucent in 2 weeks of abruption
- *Acute hemorrhage:* It may be misinterpreted as homogeneous thickened placenta or fibroid

Locations of Placental Abruption (Figs. 2A to C)

- *Retroplacental:* Blood is collected behind the placenta (between the placenta and the myometrium)

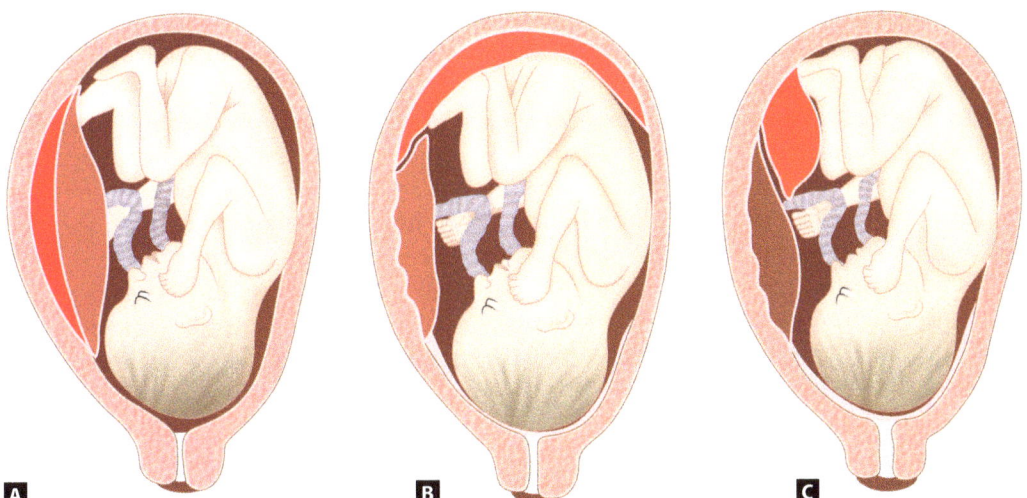

Figs. 2A to C: Types of placental abruption. (A) Retroplacental; (B) Subchorionic; and (C) Preplacental.

- *Subchorionic:* Blood dissects along the chorion (between the placenta and the membranes)
- *Preplacental/subamniotic:* Blood collects anterior to the placenta within the amnion and the chorion (between the placenta and the amniotic fluid)
- Location and extent of hemorrhage is directly related to fetal morbidity. Retroplacental hematomas carry poorer prognosis than subchorionic hemorrhage.
- *Large retroplacental hematomas:* A retroplacental hematoma of volume more than 60 mL is related to increased fetal mortality.

PLACENTA PREVIA

Placenta previa is one of the causes of APH that can be detected prior to the episode of bleeding if a proper ultrasound examination is done. The diagnosis enables adequate counseling of the patient during pregnancy, planning of care options and a prepared and planned delivery. Placenta previa can present with sudden heavy bleeding which needs immediate management, of which conservative management may not be sufficient in cases with excessive bleeding and can warrant termination of the pregnancy irrespective of the gestational age, in the interests of the mother.

It early pregnancy, the area of decidual reaction can be identified clearly from around the 7-8th week of pregnancy. By the 11-12 weeks the placenta is well demarcated. During this period very often, the placenta can be seen extending up to the level of the internal os or sometimes the lower margin may overlap the internal os. This can be a cause for minor bleeding in the first trimester when the marginal sinuses or the capillaries rupture. As the pregnancy advances, the placenta tends to migrate up and away from the cervix except in a few. The diagnosis of placenta previa is ideally made around the time of the target scan at 18–22 weeks. This allows for precautions to be taken, monitoring and patient counseling through pregnancy. The diagnosis of placenta previa is to be revisited at around 34–36 weeks to re-evaluate, if the placenta is low lying or has migrated up. If the placenta lies within 2–2.5 cm from the internal os,[2] the patient runs the risk of bleeding when labor sets in and the cervix dilates.[3] The placenta may be the presenting part in a complete or central placenta previa and can bleed torrentially. If the placenta lies in the lower segment but not covering the os, it can still interfere with the descent of the presenting part, especially if the placental tissue lies over the sacral promontory and in the sacral hollow as in grade I and II posterior placenta previa. The grading of placenta previa helps to assess the risk of bleeding during labor, the need for cesarean section,[4] and also planning outpatient care.

Placenta previa can be graded as placenta previa major or minor as below:
- Grade 1—(minor) the placenta extends up to the lower segment but not up to the internal os.
- Grade 2—(marginal) the placenta reaches up to the internal os but does not cover it.
- Grade 3—(major) the placenta partially covers the cervix.
- Grade 4—(major) the placenta completely covers the cervix.

Another descriptive classification is:
- *Complete placenta previa*—where the major bulk of the placenta is seen covering the cervical os completely.
- *Partial placenta previa*—where the cervical os is partially covered by the placental edge.
- *Marginal placenta previa*—where the placental edge reaches up to the cervical os by does not overlap it and is not seen in front of the presenting part when the cervix dilates.

For the diagnosis of placenta previa, transvaginal ultrasound is preferred[5] and ideally performed with a partially full bladder. Transabdominal ultrasound is not very reliable. On transvaginal ultrasound, it is easy to clearly demarcate the placental edge and measure the distance from the internal os (Figs. 3A and B). When there is a contraction in the lower segment, placenta can easily be mistaken to be low lying. During a transvaginal ultrasound, gentle insertion under visualization does not cause any increased risk of hemorrhage as the probe is in the cervical fornice and does not injure the placental bed even in the presence of bleeding.[1,6] It has the additional advantage being able to pick up vasa previa, especially in low lying placenta and marginal cord insertions.

Presence of any of the risk factors like history of previous placenta previa, cesarean section, uterine cavitary surgical procedures, and previous curettage increases the risks of placenta previa.

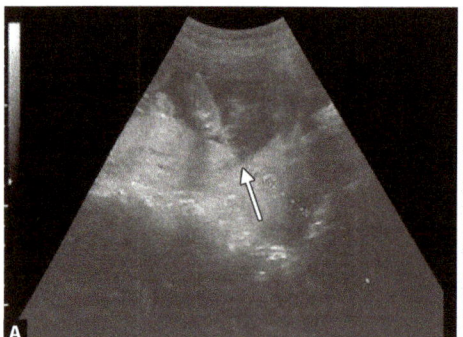 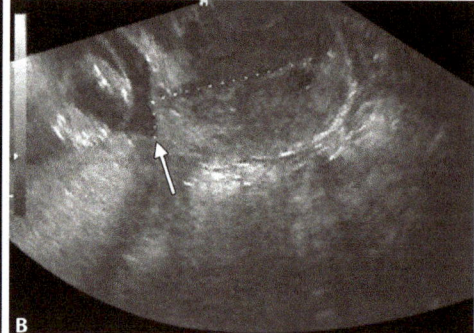

Figs. 3A and B: Transabdominal and transvaginal sonography of low lying placenta--------->edge.

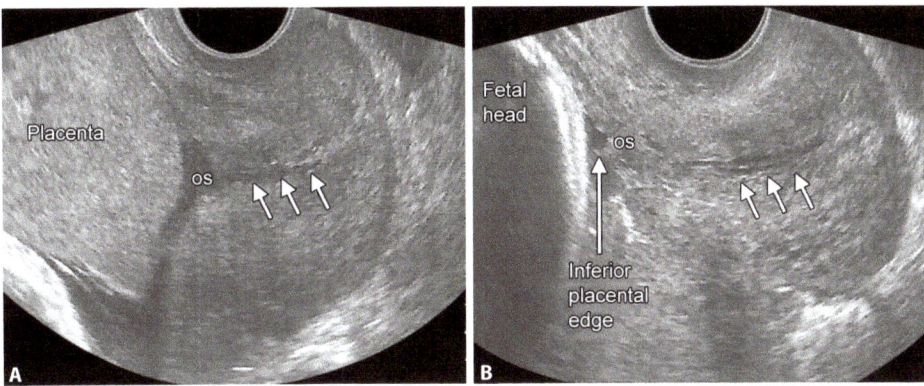

Figs. 4A and B: (A) True placenta previa; (B) Low-lying placenta.

The gold standard in diagnosis of placenta previa is now MRI. This is especially useful in late gestations, where the presenting part is low and obscures the posterior placenta.

Placenta previa is defined as presence and implantation of placenta over or adjacent to the cervical internal os.

Ultrasonography shows two variables:
1. *True placenta previa*: The internal cervical os is completely covered by the placental tissue (Fig. 4A).
2. *Low lying placenta*: Placenta lies within 2 cm of the internal os but does not cover it (Fig. 4B).

Placental migration with the advancement of pregnancy is common. If a placenta previa is diagnosed during the second trimester, a repeat USG must be done in the early third trimester at 32 weeks. Over 90% of placenta previa diagnosed in the second trimester resolves by term pregnancy. The incidence of resolution of placenta previa depends on:
- Timing of the assessment and diagnosis
- Whether there is placental margin extension over the internal cervical os (true placenta previa diagnosed in the second trimester will persist into the third trimester)
- Location of the placenta—anterior placenta previa is less likely to migrate away from the internal cervical os than posteriorly located placenta.

A significant number of placenta previa is now detected antenatally with imaging techniques before the onset of any episode of massive bleeding.

Transabdominal USG can detect almost 95% of placenta previa whereas the reproducibility of transvaginal sonography (TVS) is as high as 100%. A transabdominal sonography (TAS) followed by TVS in doubtful cases is not contraindicated provided the probe does not come in contact with the cervix. In a suspected case of placenta previa, USG is first done in full bladder and then rescanned after emptying bladder.

Imaging helps in differentiating the variants of placenta previa—whether accreta, increta, or percreta variant (Fig. 5).
- *Placenta accreta:* It refers to the abnormal attachment of the placental tissue to the uterine lining because of an absence of deciduas basalis and an incomplete development of the fibrinoid layer.
- *Placenta increta*: Extension of the placenta into the uterine myometrium.
- *Placenta percreta:* Placenta extends through the uterine myometrium toward the bladder mucosa.

Two-dimensional (2D) USG findings in a case of placenta accreta:
- Loss of hypoechoic retroplacental myometrial zone

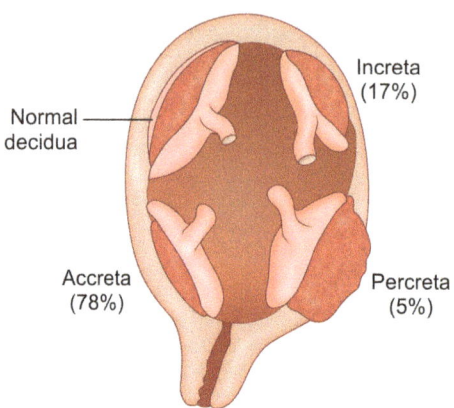

Fig. 5: Variants of placenta previa.

- Thinning and disruption of the uterine serosa—bladder wall interface
- Focal exophytic regions within the placenta
- Numerous intravascular placental lacunae.

Color Doppler Findings in Placenta Accreta

- Diffuse and focal intraplacental lacunar blood flow
- Hypervascularity of the bladder and uterine serosa
- Prominent subplacental venous complexes
- Loss of subplacental Doppler vascular signals
- Myometrial thickness <1 mm with large intraplacental venous lakes is highly predictive of invasive placentation.

MRI for Placenta Previa

Magnetic resonance imaging is used to diagnose and assess the extent of invasion of placental tissue into the surrounding parametrium and bladder. Useful criterion for diagnosis of abnormal placentation using MRI is:
- Uterine bulging
- Heterogeneous signal intensity within the placenta
- T2 dark intraplacental bands.

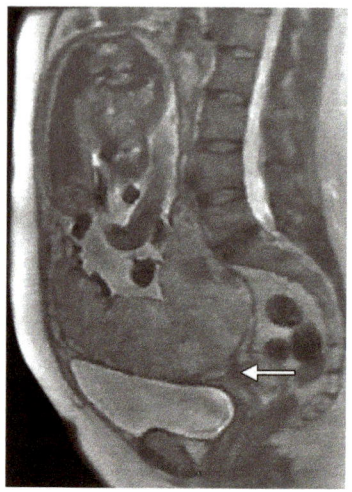

Fig. 6: Sagittal T2-weighted imaging—placenta covering os.

Preoperative MRI evaluation in cases of suspected morbidly adherent placenta significantly reduces maternal mortality rate by delineating topographic extension into the parametrial regions and identifying the cervicotrigonal vascular hyperplasia, thus helping in planned surgical approach and dissection (Figs. 6 to 8).

Placenta Accreta

Placenta accreta indicates abnormally adherent placenta with the placental tissue or the villi encroaching into the myometrium due to a defect in the decidual basalis. The placental myometrial interface is lost as the chorionic tissue invades into the myometrial zone. More severe variations depending on the depth of invasion are placenta increta where the placental villi invades deep into the myometrial layer and placenta percreta where the placental villi grows through the entire thickness of the myometrium and perforates the serosal layer of the uterus.

The risk factors for placenta accreta are presence of placenta previa, previous placenta previa, increasing maternal age,

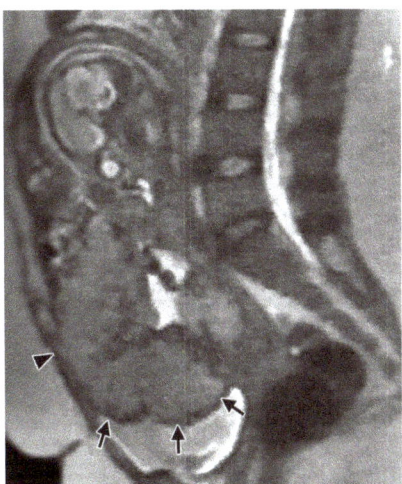

Fig. 7: Sagittal T2-weighted imaging with loss of normal placental myometrial interface and bulging contour.

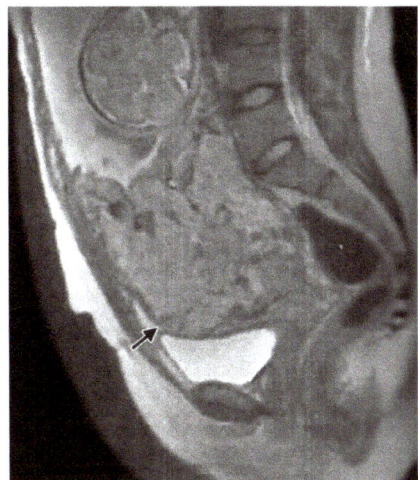

Fig. 8: Sagittal T2-weighted image with thickened heterogeneous placenta and lobulation with loss of myometrial margin.

previous uterine scar like previous cesarean or myomectomy scar, uterine anomalies, previous uterine curettage, or any condition where the decidua basalis is disrupted.

The ultrasound criteria for the diagnosis of placenta accreta are as follows:

- Marked thinning or obliteration of the retroplacental hypoechoic placental myometrial interface.
- Interruption if the vesicouterine interface in placenta percreta with or without a mass with placental echogenicity abutting the bladder serosa or invading into it.
- Presence of placenta lakes or prominent vessels with low velocity flow within the placeta or myometrium. Presence of placental lacunae has the highest sensitivity in the diagnosis of placenta accreta, with a detection rate of 78–93% after 15 weeks of gestation with a specificity of 78.6%.[7] The placental lacunae appear as "moth eaten" hypoechoic areas with turbulent blood flow unlike the placental lakes which have a laminar flow of low velocity.

Overall, the detection of placenta accreta on ultrasound has a sensitivity of 89.5%, positive predictive value of 68%, and negative predictive value of 98%.[8] The detection is better using high frequency transducers and transvaginal scans.

Magnetic resonance imaging is a very useful tool and is the gold standard in the diagnosis of abnormally invasive placentae. It is especially useful to assess posterior placenta and lateral wall placenta, where the visualization of the placental myometrial interface is difficult and suboptimal with ultrasound. On T2-weighted images, the invasive mass appears hyperintense and sometimes heterogeneous. T2-weighted MR images are useful in the assessment of focal thinning of the myometrium and interruption of the junctional zone. A study by Lax et al. found that the most useful findings were uterine bulging, heterogeneous signal intensity within the placenta, and dark intraplacental bands on T2-weighted images. When uterine bulging is present, a focal outward contour bulge can be seen, or there can be disruption of the normal pear shape of the uterus, with the lower uterine segment being wider than the fundus. Heterogeneous signal intensity in the placenta with increased vascularity is also associated with placental invasion, especially when the heterogeneity is marked, and may represent either areas of hemorrhage in the placenta or the lacunae that can be visualized on ultrasound. Dark intraplacental bands can also be seen in patients with PA, appearing as nodular or linear areas of low signal intensity on T2-weighted images. These bands usually extend from the uterine-myometrial interface and have varying thickness and a random distribution, features that help differentiate them from normal placental septa. They are thought to represent areas of fibrin deposition within the placenta. If the placenta is homogeneous and without placental bands, it is unlikely that the patient has invasive placentation.[9]

PLACENTAL INFARCTION

Placental infarction may or may not cause APH, the pathology is not often detectable because in initial phase the echogenicity on a USG scan is isoechoic like placenta. If there is associated hemorrhage, the lesion becomes hypoechoic with a hyperechogenic rim and no blood supply to the area on power Doppler imaging. Normal color flow imaging may not be sensitive enough to demonstrate presence or absence of flows. 3D placental vascular imaging and SMI (superb microvascular imaging) can be used to provide accurate assessment and prediction of perinatal outcome (Figs. 9 to 12).

OTHER CAUSES OF APH

The other causes of APH are much rarer and often do not present with as heavy bleeding as in the above causes which can be life threatening.

Trauma

Following any injury to the abdomen and the gravid uterus there can be bleeding. Following blunt injury there can be a formation of a retroplacental hematoma, which presents and acts as in a case of abruptio placenta depending on the severity. There can be marginal separation of the placenta, chorioamniotic separation, or just bruising of the uterine myometrium. All of these can

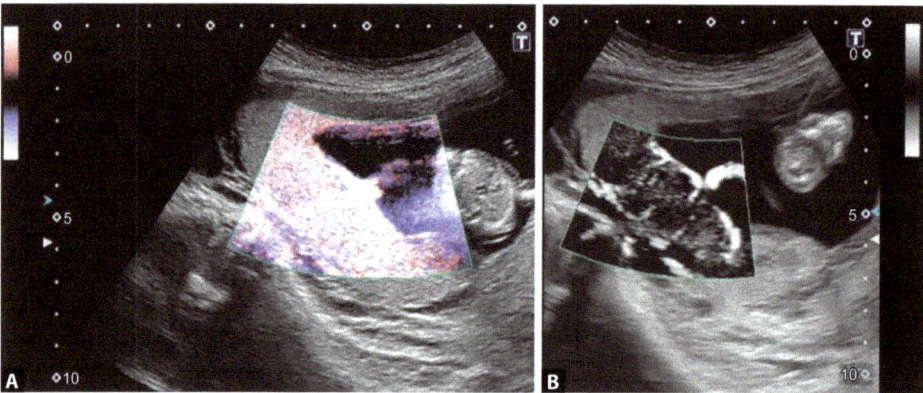

Figs. 9A and B: Comparison between conventional color Doppler (A) and SMI (B) at same pulse repetition frequency in visualizing small vessels in the placenta during mothers' respiratory motion at 14 weeks of gestation.

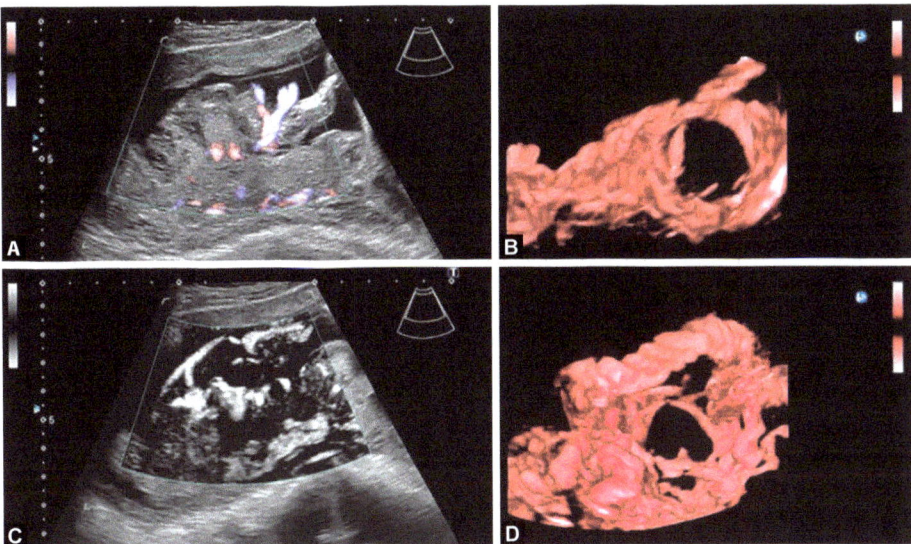

Figs. 10A to D: Doppler ultrasound image showing chorionic vessels in the placenta depicted using conventional color Doppler (A and B) and SMI (C and D). Though, small vessels cannot be detected by conventional Doppler, in the images of SMI, it reveals that the villous trees are not depicted in the placenta and branching vessels become congested. (A and C): 2D; (B and D): 3D image.

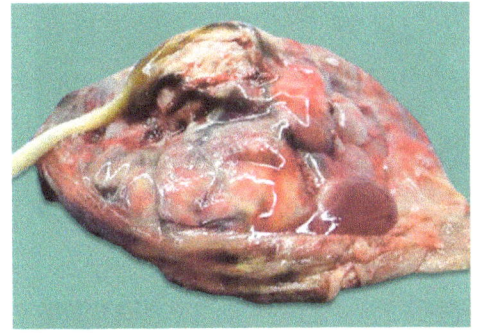

Fig. 11: Image of the placenta. Multiple placental infarctions with fibrin deposition are observed.

be directly visualized on ultrasound.[10] The presence of these with fetal cardiac rate declarations or bradycardia is ominous and patient will then require intensive monitoring or delivery, if the bleed increases or the heart rate deceleration persists. There is also a risk of rupture of fetal vessels like a vasa previa and fetal exsanguination can happen rarely (Figs. 13 and 14).

Vasa Previa

It is the presence of fetal vessels over the cervical os. Velamentous cord insertion may also occur and fetal vessels may run between bilobed or succenturiate lobed placenta.

Ultrasonography Findings in Vasa Previa

Color Doppler and pulse Doppler mapping documents umbilical vessels over the cervical os.

CERVICAL POLYP

This can cause irregular bleeding especially in the first and second trimesters of pregnancy. The bleed is usually of small quantity or spotting in each episode but can be a persistent problem. In pregnancy, the vascularity and size may increase. The presence of polyp is easily diagnosed on ultrasound, where a well-defined often hyperechoic lesion is seen in the cervix with a vascular pedicle or as a sessile mass.

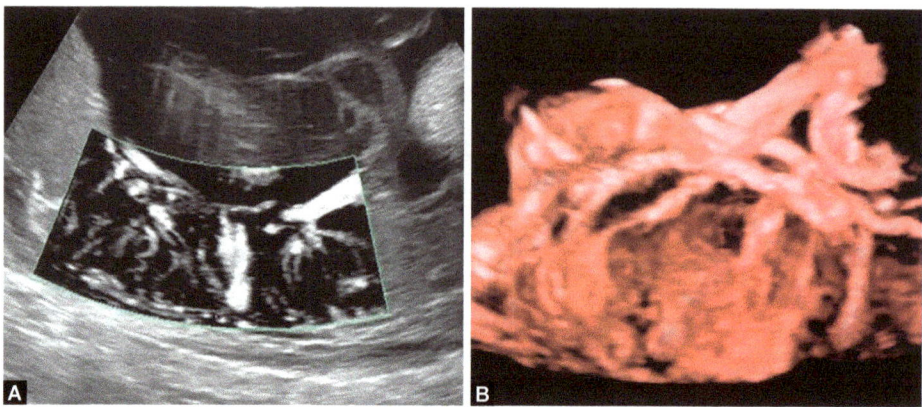

Figs. 12A and B: Doppler ultrasound image of another placenta on the same gestational day obtained using SMI. The branching vessels to the peripheral villous trees in the cotyledons are clearly depicted by 2D (A) and 3D SMI (B).

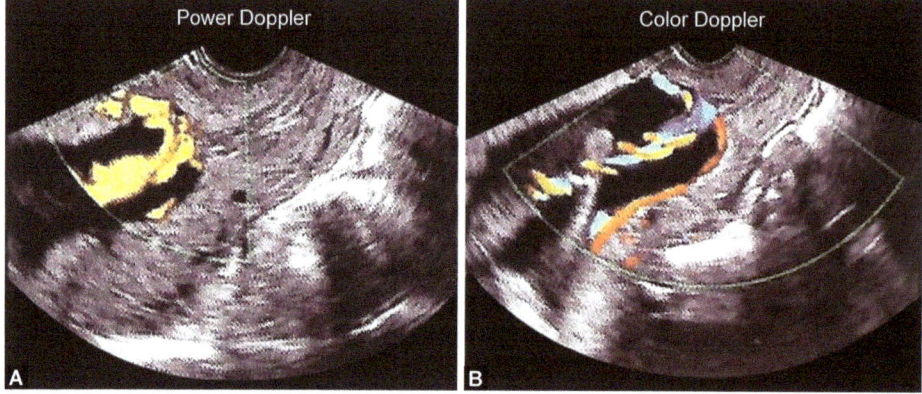

Figs. 13A and B: (A) Vasa previa and (B) Velamentous cord.

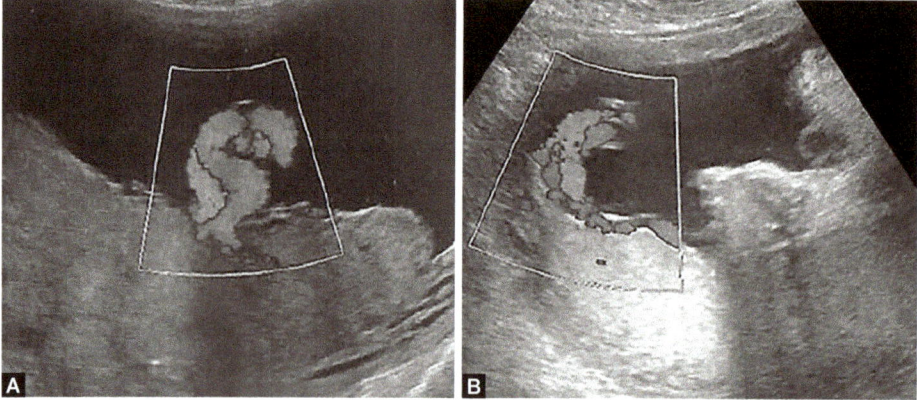

Figs. 14A and B: Placental cord insertion—(A) Central (normal) and (B) Marginal cord insertion.

CERVICAL EROSIONS

During pregnancy, there is an increase in the vascularity of the cervix and the transitional zone of the cervical mucosa can move outward or get everted under the influence of the pregnancy hormones. This can present with occasional spotting or episodes of bleeding which may not be very severe usually. Cervical erosions are easily diagnosed by a speculum examination of the cervical mucosa. Ultrasound examination may not be contributory unless a cervical hypertrophy is present or cervicitis is present which appears as a thickened cervix with congestion.

CONCLUSION

- Antepartum hemorrhage is a life-threatening condition, which complicates pregnancy.
- Timely ultrasound can recognize more than 50% of the causes of APH.
- Meticulous antepartum fetal surveillance with routine use of Doppler USG in all cases of APH is the mainstay of improving perinatal outcome.
- Good maternal-fetal units with trained imaging specialists and obstetricians should take care of these cases in tertiary care centers.

REFERENCES

1. Glantz C, Purnell L. Clinical utility of sonography in the diagnosis and treatment of placental abruption. J Ultrasound Med. 2002;21(8):837-40.
2. Oppenheimer LW, Farine D, Ritchie JW, et al. What is a low-lying placenta? Am J Obstet Gynecol. 1991;165:1036-8.
3. Wortman AC, Twickler DM, McIntire DD, et al. Bleeding complications in pregnancies with low lying placenta. J Matern Fetal Neonatal Med. 2016;29(9):1367-71.
4. Oppenheimer LW, Farine D. A new classification of placenta previa: Measuring progress in obstetrics. Am J Obstet Gynecol. 2009;201(3):227-9.
5. Merz E. Ultrasound in Obstetrics and Gynaecology, 2nd edition. New York, NY: Thieme; 2007.
6. Farine D, Fox HE, Jakobson S, et al. Vaginal ultrasound for diagnosis of placenta previa. Am J Obstet Gynecol. 1988;159:566-9.
7. Baughman WC, Corteville JE, Shah RR. Placenta accreta: Spectrum of US and MR imaging findings. radiographics. 2008;28(7):1905-16.
8. Esakoff TF, Sparks TN, Kaimal AJ, et-al. Diagnosis and morbidity of placenta accreta. Ultrasound Obstet Gynecol. 2011;37(3):324-7.
9. Lax A, Prince MR, Mennitt KW, et al. The value of specific MRI features in the evaluation of suspected placental invasion. Magn Reson Imaging. 2007;25:87-93.
10. Hasegwa J, Suzuki N. SMI for imaging of placental infarction. Placenta. 2016;47:96-8.

11B Chapter
Surgical Challenges in Placenta Previa

Suchitra N Pandit, Swati Bhargava

INTRODUCTION

Placenta previa is a condition where placenta may lie wholly or partially in lower segment, it completely or partially covers the internal os or lies adjacent to internal os. Placenta previa can be either anterior or posterior low lying placenta depending on the location of placenta in relation to uterine wall. Placenta previa is divided into four types.[1] Type I—placental lower edge is in lower uterine segment. Type II—placental lower edge reaching internal os (marginal placenta previa). Type III—incomplete central previa. Type IV—complete central previa. Woman with placenta previa presents with painless unprovoked bleeding and may have resulting neonatal anemia.[2] Prevalence of clinically significant placenta previa is estimated to be 4-5/1,000 pregnancies.[3,4] Placenta previa is a risk factor for postpartum hemorrhage, preterm deliveries, and cesarean hysterectomy. Placenta previa is associated with significant maternal and neonatal mortality and morbidity. Due to increased rates of primary cesarean sections and assisted reproductive technology, incidence of placenta previa is increasing; however, maternal mortality due to placenta previa has decreased due to early diagnosis by advent of ultrasonography, improvements in general condition of patients, availability of blood and blood products and better surgical techniques. Though in comparison to low risk pregnancies, perinatal morbidity (due to preterm deliveries) and maternal morbidity (due to preoperative and postpartum blood loss).[3] It can raise an emergency for surgical intervention at any point of time during the course of pregnancy.

Increased maternal age, history of abortion, previous cesarean delivery, multiparity, assisted reproductive techniques, smoking, and cocaine use during pregnancy are the risk factors for placenta previa.[4-6] Transvaginal sonography is the diagnostic modality of choice, and placenta previa type IIb and above is an indication for cesarean section.

SURGICAL CHALLENGES

Preoperative Decision Making and Preparation

The decision and the goal of management depend on the following points:
- Location of placenta in relation to uterine wall (anterior/posterior)
- Distance from internal os
- Presence or absence morbidly adherent placenta
- Presence of vessels over lower uterine segment
- Optimal time for planned cesarean delivery, if placenta previa persists.

Reduce the Risk of Bleeding

Monitoring placental localization, as the lower uterine segment is formed by 28 weeks, it gradually increases in size and placental edge appears to migrate upward. Serial ultrasonography may aid to determine placental migration, as placental lower edge <2 cm from internal os is an indication for cesarean section. In placenta previa type I, IIa vaginal delivery can be attempted.

Mode of Delivery

A cesarean delivery is always indicated when there is sonographic evidence of placenta previa and a viable fetus. Vaginal delivery may be considered in rare circumstances, such as in the presence of a fetal demise or a previable fetus, as long as the mother remains hemodynamically stable. Cesarean delivery is indicated for— severe and persistent vaginal bleeding such that maternal hemodynamic stability cannot be achieved or maintained. Active labor—a nonreassuring fetal heart rate tracing unresponsive to resuscitative measures. Usually, the first hemorrhage is a warning sign so one must be prepared that this may recur. Conservative management is preferred to help fetus gain more maturity and steroids can be given to enhance lung maturity. There are neonatal benefits from avoiding preterm delivery but maternal risks from persistent or recurrent bleeding probably increase, so it is essential to balance the risks of fetal benefit versus maternal risk. If the subsequent vaginal bleeding is significant, it should warrant urgent delivery of the fetus by cesarean section. The gestational age and amount of bleeding considered significant are matters of clinical judgment and the setup one is operating in. The decision to deliver these pregnancies is made on a case-by-case basis while observing the patient's course on the labor unit. Delivery should not be delayed to administer antenatal corticosteroids, if the bleeding is severe. It is always advisable to deliver such women in a tertiary care center where blood is available as chances of postpartum hemorrhage (PPH) are very high.

Excluding Morbidly Adherent Placenta

Women with documented ultrasonographical diagnosis of placenta previa may need color Doppler or magnetic resonance imaging (MRI), especially in those patients with previous cesarean sections to rule out placenta accreta, increta, or percreta.

Placenta accreta is a rare condition, though last decade has seen a rise in incidence by 10 folds, due to increased rate of primary cesarean sections. Ultrasound can be used for diagnosis in majority of cases, if there is inconclusive finding in ultrasonography, MRI or color Doppler may play a role in diagnosis. They are adjunct imaging techniques. Features of morbidly adherent placenta on MRI are abnormal uterine bulging, disorganized intraplacental vascularity, and dark intraplacental bands.

If present, cesarean delivery is scheduled earlier in gestation than for previa alone and preoperative preparation includes planning for cesarean hysterectomy (which is usually required) and interventions that will reduce the risk of massive hemorrhage (which is more common than with previa alone).

Precautions to be Taken

- Measures to reduce preoperative and intraoperative bleeding.
- Intrauterine growth restriction to be ruled out.
- Decision between inpatients and outpatient monitoring.
- Administration of antenatal corticosteroids.
- Patient should be delivered at a tertiary center where adequate blood bank facilities are available.
- Presence of neonatal care unit.
- Experienced team always helps.

When to Operate

A cesarean delivery is performed after 37 weeks, if there is no further vaginal bleeding in an uncomplicated placenta previa.[7-9]

Preferred anesthesia: Risk of hemorrhage is lower with regional anesthesia than general anesthesia for cesarean delivery and considered to be safe in women with placenta previa. However, patient and attenders to be counseled about the necessity of conversion to general anesthesia, if required.[10]

Royal College of Obstetricians and Gynaecologists (RCOG) Greentop Guidelines [107]:
- Vertical skin and/or uterine incisions when gestational age is below 28 weeks, and fetus is in transverse lie.
- Ultrasonography to determine the location of placenta and to decide site of incision.
- Immediate clamping of umbilical cord postdelivery, if there is transection of placenta to avoid excessive fetal blood loss.
- Intrauterine tamponade and compression sutures to be applied at the earliest if pharmacological measures fail to control bleeding.
- Use of interventional radiological techniques like uterine artery embolization at the earliest, if necessary.
- Early resort to cesarean hysterectomy if conservative measures fail to arrest bleeding.

Site of Incision

Increased maternal bleeding is seen in patients with anterior placenta previa, where placenta is transected. It was found in a retrospective cohort study, that avoiding placenta during uterine incision after 24 weeks of gestational age reduces the necessity for intra- and postoperative blood transfusion.[11]

Another cohort study found that J-shaped intrauterine incision aids to reduce blood loss during cesarean and aids in easier delivery of fetus.[12]

As the fetal blood circulates within the placenta, on incision of placenta there is both maternal and fetal blood loss causing neonatal anemia. In 71–96% of cases, lower segment transverse incision is practiced. To avoid incising placenta during transverse incision in cases of placenta previa, various surgical techniques are used along with ultrasonological localization of placenta before surgery. These are classical cesarean incision, inverted T-shaped incision, J-shaped incision, and medial transverse incision.

However, studies do not show much difference in blood loss with these incisions. Hence after confirming the position of placenta, lower uterine segment is incised without cutting through the placenta, it is separated gently from the uterus by inserting a finger so that bag of membranes is approached, membranes ruptured and fetus can be delivered.

So if USG is available, the lie of the fetus can be confirmed as it facilitates delivery by knowing where the foot of the fetus would be. However, this technique is limited in presence of morbidly adherent placenta. So using lower uterine transverse incision in cases of placenta previa is safe, cost-effective as number of imaging studies for placental localization is reduced, suturing is simple, less blood loss, less hospital stay, and less damage to uterus. Hence, lower uterine transverse incision is preferred.

MANAGEMENT OF PPH IN PATIENTS WITH PLACENTA PREVIA

Conservative management includes pharmacological management, use of balloon tamponade, compression sutures, and uterine artery occlusion, which have less morbidity compared to cesarean hysterectomy and preferred increasingly.

Balloon tamponade includes use of Bakri balloon,[13,14] Sengstaken–Blakemore tube,[15] and condom tamponade. Their use in placenta previa reduces blood loss by 75–88%.[16] Factors associated with failure of balloon tamponade include anterior placenta, previous cesarean, if patient is already in disseminated intravascular coagulation (DIC), and blood loss of > 500 cc within 1 hour of placement.[17]

Selective en masse bilateral uterine artery ligation can be done to reduce the bleeding. For this, the uterus should be exteriorized. Uterovesical peritoneum is separated and bladder is pushed down so uterine artery ligation can be done without damaging the ureter.

Compression sutures like B Lynch, Hayman's, and Cho's sutures aid in reducing blood loss in women with atonic PPH, B Lynch is best technique postcesarean and was described by B lynch in 1997.[18] Combine use of B Lynch suture and balloon tamponade has been proved successful in control of PPH in patients with placenta previa.[19]

Prior to using this suture one must ensure that uterus is firmly grasped and gently massaged while the oxytocics are being given. Using polyglycolic acid (PGA) sutures is advisable. Once the bleeding is arrested and uterus has started to contract there are concerns about hematoma formation between the apposed uterine walls sutures.

Interventional radiology techniques like uterine artery or internal iliac artery embolization,[20] and temporary balloon occlusion have also been used successfully to control PPH in patients with placenta previa.[21]

We have used this internal iliac artery temporary balloon occlusion in two of our patients and found bleeding significantly reduced; follow-up studies have found no impact on menstruation or fertility in these women.[22-24]

Preparation: Anticipation of PPH is important. This will help in planning and ensure availability of oxytocics, blood or blood products, human personnel, or a transfer to a tertiary care can be planned. 2–4 units of packed red blood cells should be available for the cesarean delivery. Appropriate surgical instruments for performance of a cesarean hysterectomy should also be available since these patients are at increased risk of morbidly adherent placenta.

Appropriate written informed consent should be taken. Evaluation for placenta previa-accreta should have been performed antenatally, with appropriate preparations for management, if present.

Placenta previa is frequently accompanied by accreta, and the maternal and perinatal outcome depends on the type of placenta previa, major or minor and the presence or absence of accreta.[25-27] After delivery of the placenta, severe bleeding may occur from the placental bed—in a systematic review, 16–29% of postpartum hemorrhage was documented.[28] The reason for the increased risk of PPH is thought to be that the myometrium of the lower uterine segment does not contract as effectively as the upper uterine segment, and thus may impede physiological hemostasis from a lower segment placental bed. In some cases, hemorrhage is due to focal placenta accreta.

Postpartum hemorrhage is approached in the following ways:
- Administration of oxytocin and tranexamic acid
- *Arrest focal bleeding:* The following options may control bleeding from a small focal area:
  - Hemostatic square sutures (Cho's method).
  - Placement of fibrin glue or patch over area of oozing to promote clotting.

- Application of ferric subsulfate (Monsel's solution) to oozing area.
- Excision, if the area is small and easily accessible, particularly in cases of focal placenta accreta with persistent bleeding.
- Hemostatic square sutures—ligation of myometrial vessels at the placental site will control focal bleeding in patients who have a focal placenta accreta and some patients who responded poorly to intravenous uterotonic therapy.
- The Affronti endouterine hemostatic square suture technique involves making four to six 2 by 2 cm squares in the area of placental bed bleeding.[29] The 1.0 polyglactin 910 sutures should penetrate the decidua and extend into the myometrium but not beyond the uterine serosa. The ends of the sutures are tied down tightly to compress the enclosed vessels.
- Placental site injection of vasopressin may reduce significant blood loss.
- Tying uterine vessels and utero-ovarian vessels (O-leary stitch):
  - It can decrease diffuse uterine bleeding by reducing perfusion pressure in the myometrium.
- Use of intrauterine balloon tamponade or compression sutures:
  - If bleeding persists, the next step is either placing compression sutures or intrauterine balloon tamponade. Compression sutures are more effective for atony and fundal bleeding, whereas the balloon may be more effective for lower segment bleeding. However, an advantage of placing the balloon first is that it is a quick and easy procedure and if it does not work, the balloon can be deflated, compression sutures can be placed, and then the balloon can be reinflated, if needed. If the compression sutures are placed first, then they will have to be removed in order to place a balloon.
  - *Intrauterine balloon tamponade:* The stem of a balloon catheter is passed through cervical os and then vagina, after introducing through uterine incision; an assistant then pulls the end of the catheter out of the introitus. If it is difficult to pass the catheter through the cervical os, an assistant can pass the tip of a small forceps from below.[30] Surgeon then places the stem of the catheter into the open tip so the assistant can pull it into the vagina while the surgeon places the balloon end in an appropriate place within the uterine cavity. The balloon can be left deflated or inflated with 50–100 mL sterile saline to reduce the risk of puncture when the hysterotomy incision is closed. After the uterine incision is closed, the assistant inflates the balloon to its maximum volume with sterile fluid while the surgeon inspects the uterus from above. Uterine compression sutures, if balloon tamponade is ineffective, the balloon can be deflated and a B-Lynch uterine compression suture is applied. The hysterotomy site is then closed, the uterus replaced in the pelvis (if previously exteriorized), and the balloon is reinflated, thereby applying pressure to both the outer and inner surfaces of the myometrium.[30,31] It is important to observe the myometrium and stop instilling fluid before undue blanching occurs at the compression suture sites, which might lead to rupture or uterine necrosis. It is also important to observe for vaginal

bleeding to see if hemorrhage has been controlled.

Arterial Embolization

When the above measures have failed, uterine or hypogastric artery embolization is an option in an appropriate setting.

Cesarean Hysterectomy

Hysterectomy is a definitive treatment of uterine bleeding when fertility preserving procedures have not reduced the bleeding to a manageable level. Ideally, it should be performed before severe hypovolemia, tissue hypoxia, hypothermia, electrolyte abnormalities, and acidosis have developed, which further compromise the patient's status.

Placenta Previa Accreta Spectrum Surgical Approach

In patients with placenta accreta instead of an attempt to separate placenta, cesarean hysterectomy with placenta in situ reduces blood loss. In those patients when depth and surface area of placental implantation can be identified and implantation area is accessible without deep pelvic invasion, uterus preserving surgery like partial myometrial resection may be done; however, it should be attempted by experienced surgeons working as a team, after appropriate counseling and taking informed and written consent. There are little data for placement of ureteral stents in patients undergoing placenta accreta spectrum surgeries; however, it can be used in women with placental invasion of urinary bladder.

Position of placenta, depth of invasion, and extension to parametrium assessed by USG or MRI determine the choice of surgical technique to be adopted.[32]

Intraoperative findings during surgery and clinical presentation also help in decision of surgical technique. ACOG recommends planned cesarean hysterectomy with placenta left in situ, as attempt to remove placenta accreta spectrum may result in severe hemorrhage.[33] In cases of high suspicion of placenta accreta, it is better to proceed with cesarean hysterectomy according to SMFM and FIGO expert panel.[34-38]

Steps for cesarean hysterectomy in women with placenta previa accreta:[39] Eight measures to be opted which are "universally achievable":
- Informed and written consent
- Placement of internal iliac arteries balloon catheter by interventional radiology
- Ureteral stent placement is usually needed if there is an anterior placenta accreta
- "Holding the cervix" for site of transaction
- Baby delivered by incision on uterine fundus
- Avoid uterotonics
- Ovarian ligament ligated by "M-cross double ligation"
- "Filling the bladder" to know the placental separation site, and "opening the bladder" in cases of bladder invasion in morbidly adherent placenta
- Medial side of parametrium or cervix to be clamped and use of "double edge pickup" for ligation.

■ CONCLUSION

Understanding pathophysiology, appropriate surgical skills and team approach play a vital role in management of placenta previa and associated conditions. Time of uterine incision to fetal delivery has to be minimized to prevent excessive blood loss. Prompt decision making and expertise of obstetrician can handle any challenges faced in handling a case of placenta previa.

REFERENCES

1. Oyelese Y, Smulian JC. Placenta previa, placenta accreta, and vasa previa. Obstet Gynecol. 2006;107:927-41.
2. Bizzarro MJ, Colson E, Ehrenkranz RA. Differential diagnosis and management of anemia in the newborn. Pediatr Clin North Am. 2004;51:1087-107.
3. Iyasu S, Saftlas AK, Rowley DL, et al. The epidemiology of placenta previa in the United States, 1979 through 1987. Am J Obstet Gynecol. 1993;168:1424-9.
4. Faiz AS, Ananth CV. Etiology and risk factors for placenta previa: an overview and meta-analysis of observational studies. J Matern Fetal Neonatal. Med 2003;13:175-90.
5. Ananth CV, Smulian JC, Vintzileos AM. The association of placenta previa with history of cesarean delivery and abortion: a metaanalysis. Am J Obstet Gynecol. 1997;177:1071-8.
6. Rosenberg T, Pariente G, Sergienko R, et al. Critical analysis of risk factors and outcome of placenta previa. Arch Gynecol Obstet. 2011;284:47-51.
7. Society for Maternal-Fetal Medicine (SMFM). Electronic address: pubs@smfm.org, Gyamfi-Bannerman C. Society for Maternal-Fetal Medicine (SMFM) Consult Series #44: Management of bleeding in the late preterm period. Am J Obstet Gynecol. 2018;218(1):B2-B8.
8. Spong CY, Mercer BM, D'alton M, et al. Timing of indicated late-preterm and early-term birth. Obstet Gynecol. 2011; 118:323.
9. American College of Obstetricians and Gynecologists. ACOG Committee opinion no. 560: Medically indicated late-preterm and early-term deliveries. Obstet Gynecol. 2013;121:908.
10. RCOG Greentop Guidelines No. 27a. Royal College of Obstetrics and Gynaecologists; 2018. pp. 21-48.
11. Verspyck E, Douysset X, Roman H, et al. Transecting versus avoiding incision of the anterior placenta previa during cesarean delivery. Int J Gynaecol Obstet. 2015;128:44-7.
12. Zou L, Zhong S, Zhao Y, et al. Evaluation of "J"-shaped uterine incision during caesarean section in patients with placenta previa: a retrospective study. J Huazhong Univ Sci Technolog Med Sci. 2010;30:212-6.
13. Maher MA, Abdelaziz A. Comparison between two management protocols for postpartum hemorrhage during cesarean section in placenta previa: Balloon protocol versus non-balloon protocol. J Obstet Gynaecol Res. 2017;43:447-55.
14. Soyama H, Miyamoto M, Sasa H, et al. Effect of routine rapid insertion of Bakri balloon tamponade on reducing hemorrhage from placenta previa during and after cesarean section. Arch Gynecol Obstet. 2017;296:469-74.
15. Uygur D, Altun Ensari T, Ozgu-Erdinc AS, et al. Successful use of BT-Cath balloon tamponade in the management of postpartum haemorrhage due to placenta previa. Eur J Obstet Gynecol Reprod Biol. 2014;181:223-8.
16. Ishii T, Sawada K, Koyama S, et al. Balloon tamponade during cesarean section is useful for severe post-partum hemorrhage due to placenta previa. J Obstet Gynaecol Res. 2012;38:102-7.
17. Cho HY, Park YW, Kim YH, et al. Efficacy of intrauterine Bakri balloon tamponade in cesarean section for placenta previa patients. PLoS One. 2015;10:e0134282.
18. B-Lynch C, Coker A, Lawal AH, et al. The B-Lynch surgical technique for the control of massive postpartum haemorrhage: an alternative to hysterectomy? Five cases reported. Br J Obstet Gynaecol. 1997;104:372-5.
19. Yoong W, Ridout A, Memtsa M, et al. Application of uterine compression suture in association with intrauterine balloon tamponade ('uterine sandwich') for postpartum hemorrhage. Acta Obstet Gynecol Scand. 2012;91:147-51.
20. Inoue S, Masuyama H, Hiramatsu Y; Multi-Institutional Study Group of Transarterial Embolization for Massive Obstetric Haemorrhage in Chugoku & Shikoku Area Society of Obstetrics and Gynecology. Efficacy of transarterial embolisation in the management of post-partum haemorrhage and its impact on subsequent pregnancies. Aust NZJ Obstet Gynaecol. 2014;54:541-5.
21. Broekman EA, Versteeg H, Vos LD, et al. Temporary balloon occlusion of the internal iliac arteries to prevent massive hemorrhage during cesarean delivery among patients with placenta previa. Int J Gynaecol Obstet. 2015;128:118-21.

22. Sentilhes L, Gromez A, Clavier E et al. Fertility and pregnancy following pelvic arterial embolisation for postpartum haemorrhage. BJOG. 2010;117:84-93.
23. Doumouchtsis SK, Nikolopoulos K, Talaulikar V, et al. Menstrual and fertility outcomes following the surgical management of postpartum haemorrhage: a systematic review. BJOG. 2014;121:382-8.
24. Soro MP, Denys A, de Rham M, et al. Short and long term adverse outcomes after arterial embolisation for the treatment of postpartum haemorrhage: a systematic review. Eur Radiol. 2017;27:749-62.
25. Ha JW, Chung IB, Cho HC, et al. The comparison of the pregnancy outcomes according to the types of placenta previa. Korean J Obstet Gynecol. 2005;48:51-7.
26. Won HS, Lee PR, Lee IS, et al. Maternal and perinatal outcomes in pregnancies complicated with placenta previa totalis. Korean J Perinatol. 1998;9:375-80.
27. Kim SP, Lee CH, Kim SJ, et al. A clinical study of placenta previa. Korean J Obstet Gynecol. 1999;42:481-6.
28. Fan D, Xia Q, Liu L, et al. The Incidence of Postpartum Hemorrhage in Pregnant Women with Placenta Previa: A Systematic Review and Meta-Analysis. PLoS One. 2017;12:e0170194.
29. Arduini M, Epicoco G, Clerici G, et al. B-Lynch suture, intrauterine balloon, and endouterine hemostatic suture for the management of postpartum hemorrhage due to placenta previa accreta. Int J Gynaecol Obstet. 2010;108:191.
30. Matsubara S, Kuwata T, Baba Y, et al. A novel 'uterine sandwich' for haemorrhage at caesarean section for placenta praevia. Aust NZJ Obstet Gynaecol. 2014;54:283.
31. Yoong W, Ridout A, Memtsa M, et al. Application of uterine compression suture in association with intrauterine balloon tamponade ('uterine sandwich') for postpartum hemorrhage. Acta Obstet Gynecol Scand. 2012;91:147.
32. Silver RM. Abnormal placentation: Placenta previa, vasa previa and placenta accreta. Obstet Gynecol. 2015;126:654-68.
33. Committee on Obstetric Practice. Committee opinion no. 529: placenta accreta. Obstet Gynecol. 2012;120:207-11.
34. Mehrabadi A, Hutcheon JA, Liu S, et al.; Maternal Health Study Group of Canadian Perinatal Surveillance System (Public Health Agency of Canada). Contribution of placenta accreta to the incidence of postpartum hemorrhage and severe postpartum hemorrhage. Obstet Gynecol. 2015;125:814-21.
35. Jolley JA, Nageotte MP, Wing DA et al. Management of placenta accreta: a survey of Maternal-Fetal Medicine practitioners. J Matern Fetal Neonatal Med. 2012;25:756-60.
36. Esakoff TF, Handler SJ, Granados JM, et al. PAMUS: placenta accreta management across the United States. J Matern Fetal Neonatal Med. 2012;25:761-5.
37. Wright JD, Silver RM, Bonanno C, et al. Practice patterns and knowledge of obstetricians and gynecologists regarding placenta accreta. J Matern Fetal Neonatal Med. 2013;26:1602-9.
38. Cal M, Ayres-de-Campos D, Jauniaux E. International survey of practices used in the diagnosis and management of placenta accreta spectrum disorders. Int J Gynaecol Obstet. 2018;140:307-11.
39. Masturbara S, Kuwata T, Usui R, et al. Important surgical measures and techniques at cesarean hysterectomy for placenta previa accrete. Acta Obstetricia et Gynecologica Scandinavica a 2013 Nordic Federation of Societies of Obstetrics and Gynecology. 2013;92:372-7.

11C Chapter

Abruptio Placentae

Saswati Sanyal Choudhury

INTRODUCTION

Abruptio placentae is defined as premature, partial, or complete separation of normally situated placenta from uterine wall before delivery after 20 weeks of pregnancy. Approximately 10% of all preterm births and 10–20% of all perinatal deaths are caused by placental abruption in developed countries. Maternal mortality although rare but found to be seven times higher than overall maternal mortality rate (Table 1).[1]

INCIDENCE

Incidence varies from 1–4.5% and it is three to five times more common in pre-eclampsia. Incidence in European American and East Asian population is 0.4–1%.[1-3] Recently, a report by Mukherjee et al. from Mumbai reported an incidence of 4.4% in 7,164 cases.[4] One-third of all antepartum hemorrhage (APH) comprises abruptio. Incidence peaks at 24–26 weeks. Recurrence rate is 11% after one and 25% after two episodes in previous pregnancy. This recurrence may occur 1–3 weeks prior than the first abruption. There is a strong relationship of preterm labor and abruptio. Abruptio is present in 12% of preterm labor in comparison 1% in term labor. Histological diagnosis of abruptio is found to be 32% of preterm delivery compared to 2% in term.[5]

ETIOLOGY AND RISK FACTOR[1-4,6-9]

- Trauma—1–6% in minor trauma and 20–25% in major trauma cases[1]
- Heavy smoker—in 40% or more
- Alcohol consumption
- Acute chorioamnionitis (OR 2.5–3.3)[1]
- Previous history of abruptio (OR 3.2–25.8)[1]
- Maternal coagulopathies (OR 1.4–7.7)[1]
- Cocaine abuse (10%).

Risk Factors

- Grand multiparity (OR 1.6 95% CI 1.1–2.4)[10]
- Chronic hypertension (OR 1.8–2.4)[1]
- Elderly gravida[11]
- Sudden decompression in polyhydramnios
- External cephalic version (ECV)
- Hyperhomocysteinemia (OR 1.8–5.3)[1]
- Folic acid deficiency

TABLE 1: Sociodemographic and behavioral risk factors for placental abruption.[1]

Risk factor	Odds ratio
Sociodemographic:	
• Maternal age ≥35 years	• 1.3–2.6
• Maternal age <20 years	• 1.1–1.5
	• 1.1–1.4
• Parity ≥3	• 1.3
• Black race	• 1.2–1.5
• Unmarried or single mother	
Behavioral:	
• Smoking cigarette	• 1.5–2.5
	• 1.6–2.8
• Alcohol use	• 3.9–8.6
• Cocaine use	• 1.2–2.4
• Unexplained infertility	

- Preterm premature rupture of membrane—2–5% (OR 9.5 95% CI 6.9–13.1)[10]
- First trimester bleeding 1–1.4%
- Gestational hypertension (OR 7.4 95% CI 5.1–10.8)[10]
- Pre-eclampsia (OR 2.9 95% CI 1.9–4.6)[10]
- Thrombophilia
- Uterine septum and fibroid
- Circumvallate placenta
- Multiple gestation—2–3 fold risk[1]
- Race—more in Afro-American and Caucasian
- Family history[12]
- Nonvertex presentation
- Short umbilical cord
- Amniocentesis
- Prior fetal demise
- Low body mass index (BMI)
- Diabetes mellitus (OR 2.7).[1]

PPROM and Chorioamnionitis

Preterm premature rupture of membrane (PPROM) before 37 weeks has a good association with abruptio and approximately 4–12% of PPROM may develop abruptio. The less the duration of pregnancy more is the chance of abruption probably due to sudden reduction of uterine volume. Prolonged PPROM delivery interval is also associated with abruptio, if the interval is more than 24 hours.[1]

Ascending uterine infection in PPROM increases the chance of abruptio. 4.8% with infection and 0.8% without infection.[1] In all abruptio, chorioamnionitis is present in 6.7% cases. Severe chorioamnionitis is strongly associated with placental abruption in both term and preterm.

Smoking

It is a preventable risk factor and cessation of smoking reduces many adverse outcome of pregnancy including abruptio. Approximately in 15–25% cases, smoking may be a contributing factor although mechanism involved is usually speculative. Possible mechanism may be higher homocysteine level causing thrombosis of placental vascular bed or nicotine induced vasoconstriction in uterine and umbilical arteries and hypoxia caused by carbon monoxide which may lead to placental infarcts with increased capillary fragility and arterial rupture.[13] Paternal smoking can also be a risk factor due to passive smoking.

Trauma

Trauma is an important factor for abruptio. Mechanism is directly related to the injury. Elastic uterus can change its shape in reaction to forces whereas placenta is not, and therefore it leads to a shearing effect leading to separation of placenta from deciduas. ACOG recommends a minimum monitoring of 4 hours following any trauma and especially with uterine contraction or tenderness, non-reassuring cardiotocography (CTG), vaginal bleeding rupture of membrane, or serious maternal injury.

Alcohol and Cocaine

Alcohol easily crosses placenta and passes to fetus and amniotic fluid. Alcohol disturbs fetomaternal hormonal balance and also causes vasoconstriction in placenta and umbilical cord giving rise to abruption. Cocaine also causes vasoconstriction and its use is independent risk factors although there are associations with use of smoking and other drugs.

PATHOLOGY

Weakening of the wall by pathologic alteration in pre-eclampsia leading to rupture of spiral arteriole may cause the hemorrhage. Venous rupture following thrombosis of the decidual arterioles may also cause this. There is decidual necrosis. There is also venous outflow obstruction. Acute vasospasm of small vessels precedes separation of placenta. Clinical abruptio may not be associated with discernible placental pathology in all cases. In 35% with retroplacental hematoma, abruptio is diagnosed clinically. Separation causes defunctionalization of overlying placenta and then infarction with utero-placental ischemia, if retroplacental hematoma is large. Chronic marginal separation is common in circumvallate placenta as well as abruptio. In Couvelaire uterus, there is continuous bleeding and entire placenta is separated and there is extravasation of blood in myometrium which makes blotchy blue areas. This is diagnosed visually or by biopsy or both. There is no loss in contractility of myometrium due to this as believed before.

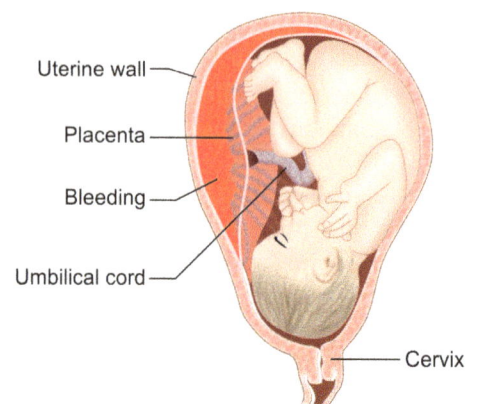

Fig. 1: Concealed abruptio.

PREDICTION OF ABRUPTIO

A recent study of 34,271 women indicated that first trimester low level of pregnancy-associated plasma protein-A (PAPP-A) had an increased risk of placental abruption (FASTER trial).[14] Recent study has shown a complex relationship between placental telomere length, mitochondrial deoxyribonucleic acid (mtDNA) copy number, and placental abruption. Placental telomere shortening and increase mtDNA may be associated with abruptio.[15]

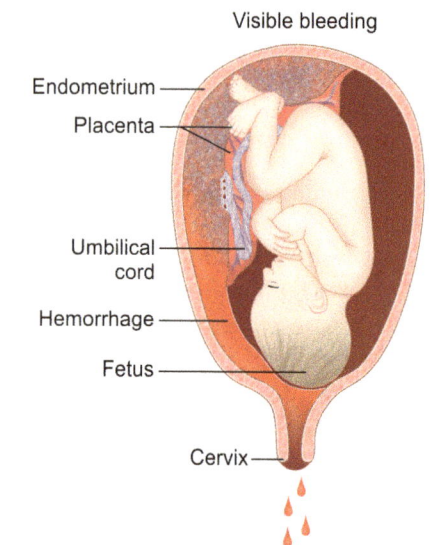

Fig. 2: Revealed abruptio.

VARIETIES OF ABRUPTIO (FIGS. 1 AND 2)

There are three varieties of abruptio:
1. *Revealed*: Most common type where following separation of placenta blood insinuates downward between membrane and deciduas and then comes out through cervical canal.
2. *Concealed:* Blood collects behind the separated placenta or collected between membranes and deciduas and bleeding is not visible outside.
3. *Mixed:* Some parts blood collects inside and some expelled.

GRADES OF ABRUPTIO

Depending on the degree of placental abruption and its clinical effects, there are four grades of abruptio.

Grade 0: Asymptomatic

Diagnosis is usually retrospective when there is a presence of blood clot after delivery of placenta.

Grade 1: Mild (40%)

- Mild vaginal bleeding or no bleeding
- Mild tenderness over uterus
- Maternal pulse and blood pressure within normal limits
- No signs of fetal distress.

Grade 2: Moderate (45%)

- Moderate vaginal bleeding or no vaginal bleeding
- Significant uterine tenderness with titanic contractions
- *Change in vital signs:* Maternal tachycardia and orthostatic changes in blood pressure
- Signs of fetal distress
- Mild clotting profile alteration—hypofibrinogenemia.

Grade 3: Severe (15%)

- Severe vaginal bleeding or no bleeding
- Titanic uterus or board like rigidity on palpation
- Maternal shock
- *Clotting profile alteration:* Hypofibrinogenemia and coagulopathy
- Fetal demise.

CLINICAL PRESENTATION

Classic clinical triad of presentation is uterine bleeding, tetanic uterine activity, and abdominopelvic pain with nonreassuring CTG or poor biophysical profile or fetal demise. Other clinical sign and symptoms include the following:

- Pain—sudden severe sharp pain in abdomen or backache
- Loss of fetal movements
- Preterm labor
- Uterine tetany
- Pre-eclampsia features
- Intrauterine growth restriction (IUGR)
- Raised blood pressure
- Tachycardia
- Pallor
- Shock
- Unduly distressed with pain
- Woody uterus
- Difficulty in palpating fetal parts
- 50% in established labor
- Elevated baseline tone
- Contraction of uterus, high frequency but low amplitude, saw toothed
- Cardiotocography—fetal bradycardia, late deceleration, sinusoidal pattern, and saw toothed uterine contraction
- Increased abdominal girth or raised fundal height suggesting concealed hemorrhage
- Hypotension and anemia may not be an obligatory sign in extreme concealed hemorrhage
- With more than 50% separation of placenta maternal and fetal compromise is likely. Once the placental separation exceeds 50%, there is grave risk of fetal and maternal compromise.

Cause of Pain in Abruptio

Extravasation of blood in myometrium causes pain and spasm of uterus.

Complications of Abruptio

Maternal peripartum risks include obstetric hemorrhage, need for blood transfusion, emergency hysterectomy, DIC, renal failure, and maternal death. Fetal risks are fetal growth restriction (FGR), low birth weight (LBW), preterm delivery, birth asphyxia stillbirth, and perinatal death.

- *Consumptive coagulopathy*: It is found in one-third cases of fetal death and is rare with live fetus. In concealed hemorrhage, higher intrauterine pressure forces more thromboplastin in maternal venous circulation, which is responsible for coagulopathy. There is also activation of intravascular coagulation with varying degrees of defibrination consequently activation of plasminogen leading to plasmin formation, which lyses fibrin microemboli. Later on hypovolemic shock requiring large volume transfusion exacerbate DIC leading to low fibrinogen, high fibrin degradation product (FDP) and high D-dimers.
- *Renal failure*: Ischemic damage to kidney due to hypovolemic shock leads to acute tubular necrosis and bilateral cortical necrosis. Hypoxia also leads to obstruction by focal fibrin deposits in precapillary arterioles from DIC, if treatment of hypovolemia is delayed. According to Lindheimer et al.,[16] acute cortical necrosis in pregnancy is usually due to abruption. Renal failure in abruptio is mostly reversible with prompt and vigorous treatment.

DIAGNOSIS OF ABRUPTIO

Ultrasonography (USG) and clinical signs and symptoms are mainstay of diagnosis. Sensitivity of USG in diagnosing abruptio is low 24% but specificity is 96% with a positive predictive value of 88% and negative predictive value of 53%.

USG Findings

- Preplacental collection under chorionic plate
- Jell-O like movement of chorionic plate with fetal activity
- Retroplacental collection
- Marginal hematoma
- Subchorionic hematoma
- Increased heterogeneous placental thickness of more than 5 cm in perpendicular pain
- Intra-amniotic hematoma.

Timing and severity of the condition can be speculated from the echogenicity, size, and location of hematoma. If the hematoma is hyperechoic than placenta, it suggests duration of 0–48 hours; if isoechoic, it is around 3–7 days old and it becomes hypoechoic in 7 days and anechoic after 2 weeks. Larger size predicts bad prognosis and size more than 60 mL retroplacental then chances of fetal mortality is 50%. The hematoma may be located behind the placenta: retroplacental, between the membranes and myometrium: subchorionic, or between placenta and amniotic cavity: preplacental. Subchorial is the most common location consisting of 67% of placental hemorrhage by USG. Retroplacental hemorrhage on USG is characterized by placental thickening or retroplacental clots and consists of 29% of cases. Preplacental forms occur due to rupture of membrane near the placental detachment and blood reaches amniotic cavity. The volume of hemorrhage is estimated by the measurement of 3 perpendicular diameters.[17]

Other Investigations

- Blood grouping and cross matching
- Complete blood count
- Hematocrit
- Coagulation study—prothrombin time (PT), international normalized ratio (INR), and activated partial thromboplastin time (aPTT)

- Serum fibrinogen
- Urine routine
- Renal function tests blood urea nitrogen (BUN), creatinine, and urea
- Bedside tests—5 mL blood in test tube is taken and to wait for 8 minutes suggest coagulopathy, if no clot retraction after 1 hour, it suggests thrombocytopenia and if clot dissolves within 1 hour, it suggests excessive fibrinolysis.

PREVENTION OF ABRUPTIO

Lifestyle modification in terms of stoppage of smoking, alcohol, and cocaine use may be helpful in prevention. Folic acid supplementation may also help. There is a definitive role of control of blood pressure in pregnancy induced hypertension in prevention of abruptio. Similarly, use of magnesium sulfate in severe PIH also has a role. Needle puncture during amniocentesis should be under USG guidance to avoid placental injury. Avoidance of forceful ECV under anesthesia, avoiding sudden decompression of uterus in hydramnios by doing amniocentesis rather than amniotomy, and routine administration of folic acid are other preventive aspects in abruption.

TREATMENT

Women classified with mild variety and pregnancy below 37 weeks may be managed conservatively. Hospitalization for monitoring of maternal and fetal status is needed. Intravenous access and cross-matched blood should be stored and monitoring continues till fetal maturity is achieved.

Goals of treatment in moderate and severe abruptio are prevention of hypovolemia; prevent anemia by keeping hemoglobin above 10 g/dL preventing DIC hematocrit level maintenance above 30% to keep the oxygen carrying capacity and keeping urinary output at least 30 mL/hour. These goals will prevent most of the severe complications of abruptio.

After diagnosis of abruptio of severe variety two IV cannula of large bore should be given and crystalloids are transfused. Packed call blood to be given in low hematocrit level. Fresh frozen plasma (FFP) transfusion is to be considered, if fibrinogen level is less than 100 mg/dL, and platelet transfusion if platelet count is less than 20,000 or 50,000/dL. Blood pressure and pulse rate may mislead in relation to amount of retroplacental hemorrhage especially in concealed type. 30% of fetal demise will show coagulopathy so one must be vigilant in severe form of abruptio and average intrapartum blood loss in fetal demise is 2,500 mL. So in severe form, aggressive intravascular fluid resuscitation is done to avoid organ damage. Irrespective of patient's general condition at least one liter of blood transfusion is minimum when the diagnosis is concealed accidental hemorrhage. The best guide is to monitor central venous pressure, which is maintained at 10 cm of water. Blood counts may also mislead as intense vasoconstriction may show normal blood counts. In concealed hemorrhage, there is always a chance of underestimation and when vital signs deteriorate there is severe hypovolemia and it becomes difficult to replace fluid adequately. In massive blood loss, the goals are to keep hemoglobin at more than 8 g/dL platelet count more than 75,000/cmm, aPTT less than 1.5x mean control and fibrinogen level to be maintained at more than 150 mg/L.

Continuous electronic fetal heart monitoring for fetal status monitoring is mandatory.

OBSTETRIC MANAGEMENT

Vaginal delivery is the goal in fetal demise. Routine amniotomy is done to release intrauterine pressure, better compression of spiral artery to arrest bleeding, avoiding of intramyometrial extravasation, and reduction in entry of thromboplastin into maternal circulation and possible DIC. Oxytocin drip to be started, if labor does not follow with amniotomy or to expedite delivery. Prostaglandin induction is to be taken with caution in a live fetus as it can have deleterious effect on the compromised fetus and resting intrauterine pressure is as high as 40 mm of Hg. Oxytocics to be used to prevent PPH after delivery in the form of oxytocin 10 IU intramuscularly or methylergometrine.

Operative delivery is to be used judiciously in presence of experienced obstetrician, anesthesiologists and provision of blood. Indications of cesarean section are severe abruption with live fetus, unfavorable cervix where amniotomy could not be done and prospect of immediate vaginal delivery is remote and appearance of adverse features like fetal distress, oliguria falling fibrinogen level, etc. and other obstetric indications. Coagulation factors are to be replaced during surgery. Surgeon should be quick, meticulous hemostasis to ascertain and closed drain at incision may be required in selected cases. For third stage management in case atony, surgical tamponade is useful. Couvelaire uterus is to be managed as normal uterus and it is not an indication of obstetric hysterectomy as thought before.

Expectant Management in Mild Cases

Close monitoring is necessary in the form of weekly nonstress test (NST), biophysical profile, and fetal weight gain by ultrasound. Antenatal glucocorticoids are necessary in preterm fetus. Role of tocolysis is doubtful but there may be some role of magnesium sulfate which may reduce further separation of placenta and as a neuroprotective in premature fetus.[18] Anti-D prophylaxis for Rh negative mothers within 72 hours and regular Kleihauer-Betke test is to be done.

MANAGEMENT OF COAGULOPATHY

If fibrinogen level is normal as in nonpregnant state then also one should suspect hypofibrinogenemia as level of fibrinogen rises in pregnancy. Less than 200 mg/dL is suspicious and clinical bleeding usually occurs when it goes below 100 mg/dL. Coagulation profile to be done every 2 hours and D-dimer and FDP level is most sensitive for diagnosis of DIC. RCOG guideline recommends 4 units of FFP, 10 units of cryoprecipitate while waiting for results of coagulation studies. One unit of FFP raises plasma fibrinogen by 25 mg/dL.

POSTNATAL CARE

Early ambulation is advised in postnatal period. One should be vigilant for hemodynamic stability and good urinary output. If there is quick vaginal delivery, there is prompt restoration of hemostatic mechanism. Clinically, evident coagulopathy resolves within 12 hours of delivery and order of normalization is first patient comes to normal then fibrinogen flowed by FDP and lastly platelets. One should also be vigilant for development of acute respiratory distress syndrome (ARDS).

PROGNOSIS

Most common complication of abruptio is prematurity. Other prognostic factors for fetal outcome are presence of fetal growth restriction. Prematurity and FGR cause raised perinatal mortality including fetal demise. Incidence of cesarean becomes more in fetal compromise. Fetal mortality varies from 20% to 40% and it comprises 10% of all stillbirths. Chance of recurrence in next pregnancy after one history of abruptio is 5-17% and after two incidence goes to 25%. It is also responsible for 6% of maternal deaths. Adverse perinatal outcome like periventricular leukomalacia, intraventricular hemorrhage, and cerebral palsy may also occur.[19] Sheehan's syndrome is also reported after abruptio of severe variety. A study was carried out to find out placental abruption as cause of fetal death in two different time periods by Cabar et al.[20] which shows since 1994-1997 incidence was 0.78% (n = 60) and in 2001-2005, it was 0.59% and there is no statistical significance. Incidence of concealed hemorrhage was 57.9 in dead fetus and 22% were live in 1994-97 whereas in 2001-5 tetany was higher in dead fetus 66.7% versus 29.3% in live fetus. Postpartum maternal complications were higher in fetal death in both groups.[20] In a cohort study, over 10 years 2003-2012[10] showed no maternal death. Amongst the feto maternal morbidities found in the study, maternal coagulation failure was found in 7.7%, 16.6% of mothers were given transfusion of blood and blood products, there was increased risk of fetal acidosis (OR 14.9; 95% CI 9.2-23.9) and neonatal resuscitation was higher (OR 4.6 95% CI 3.1-6.8). Perinatal mortality was 15.8% including 78% fetal deaths. Intrauterine fetal death (IUFD) and maternal shock have also shown to be significantly associated with coagulopathy in a recent African study.[21]

Abruptio placenta is an important cause of poor fetal and maternal outcome. Its incidence over the years is remaining the same. Till date, the cause is not fully understood although plenty of factors are thought to be responsible. Being a complex disease a lot of research is still needed to know the etiology of this dreaded disease of pregnancy.

KEY POINTS

- Cardiotocography is important in diagnosis of concealed abruptio—for 4 hours in minor motor vehicular accidents
- Continuous electronic fetal monitoring (EFM)—increased uterine activity, late deceleration, and sinusoidal pattern suggest abruptio
- Restoration of volume and early delivery prevent coagulopathy
- Changes of coagulation profile are often late
- Fetal death in abruptio leads to high maternal morbidity
- Treatment of atonic PPH in Couvelaire uterus is same as in others.

REFERENCES

1. Tikkanen M. Etiology, clinical manifestations and prediction of placental abruption. Acta Obstet Gynecol Scand. 2010;89:732-40
2. Bibi S, Ghaffar S, Pir MA, et al. Risk factors and clinical outcome of placental abruption: a retrospective analysis. J Pak Med Assoc. 2009; 59:672-4.
3. Ananth CV, oyelese Y, Yeo L, et al. Placental abruption in the United States 1979 through 2001: temporal trends and potential determinants. Am J Obstet Gynecol. 2005; 192:191-8.
4. Mukherjee S, Bawa AK, Sharma S, et al. Retrospective study of risk factors and maternal and fetal outcome in patients with abruptio placentae. J Nat Sci Bio Med. 2014;5(2):425-8.
5. Salafia CM, Lopez Zeno JA, Sherer DM, et al. Histologic evidence of old intrauterine bleeding is more frequent in prematurity. Am J Obstet Gynecol. 1995;173(4):1065-70.
6. Pariente G, Wiznitzer A. Sergienco R, et al. Placental abruption: Critical analysis of risk factors and perinatal outcomes. J Matern Fetal Neonatal Med. 2011;24:698-702.
7. Ananth CV, Savitz DA, Williams MA. Placental abruption and its association and prolonged rupture of membranes: A methodologic review and meta analysis. Obstet Gynecol. 1996;88:309-18.

8. Hung TH, Hsieh CC, Hsu JJ, et al. Risk factors for placental abruption in Asian population. Reprod Sci. 2007;14(1):59-65.
9. Sanchez SE, Pacora PN, Farfan JH, et al. Risk factors of abruptio placentae among Peruvian women. Am J Obstet Gynecol. 2006;194:225-30.
10. Boisrame T, Sananes N, Fritz G, et al. Placental abruption: Risk factors, management and fetal prognosis. Cohort study over 10 yrs. Eur J Obstet Gynecol Reprod Biol. 2014;179:100-4.
11. Jahronmi BN, Husseini Z. Pregnancy outcome at maternal age 40 and older. Taiwan J obstet Gynecol. 2008;47:318-21.
12. Rasmussen S, Irgens LM. Occurrence of placental abruption in relatives. BJOG 2009; 116(5):693-9.
13. Kaminski LM, Ananth CV, Prasad V, et al; New Jersy Placental abruption study investigators. The influence of maternal cigarette smoking on placental pathology in pregnancies complicated abruption. Am J Obstet Gynecol. 2007;197:275.el-5.
14. Dugoff L, Hobbins JC, Malone FD, et al. First trimester maternal serum PAPP-A and free beta subunits human chorionic gonadotropin concentration and nuchal translucency are associated with obstetric complication: a population based screening study (the FASTER trial). Am J Obstet Gynecol. 2004;191(4):1446-51.
15. Workalemahu T, Enquobahri DA, Williams M, et al. Placental telomere length and risk of placental abruption. J Matern Fetal Neonatal Med. 2016;29(17)2767-72.
16. Lindheheimer MD, Conrad KP, Karumanci SA. Renal physiology and disease in pregnancy. In: Alperin R (Ed). Seidin and Greisch's. The kidney. New York: Elsevier; 2007. pp. 2361.
17. Cali G, Minneci G. Placenta: From basic facts to highly sophisticated placenta accreta story. In: Kurjak A, Chervenak FA. Donald School Textbook of Ultrasound in Obstetrics & Gynaecology, 4th Edition. New Delhi: Jaypee Brothers Medical Publishers; 2017. pp. 435-53.
18. Matsuda Y, Kouno S, Hiroyama Y, et al. Intrauterine infection, magnesium sulphate exposure and cerebral palsy in infants born between 26-30 weeks of gestation. Eur J Obstet Gynecol. 2000;91(2):159-64.
19. Matsuda Y, Kouno S, Kouno S. Comparison of neonatal outcome including cerebral palsy between abruptio placentae and placenta praevia. Euro Jr Obstet Gynecol Reprod Biol. 2003;106(2):125-9.
20. Cabar FR, Nomura RM, Machado TR, et al. Feta death in abruption: comparison of two different time periods. Rev Assoc Med Bras. 2008;54(3):256-60.
21. Coleman J, Srofenyo EK, Ofori EK, et al. Maternal and fetal prognosis in abruptio placentae in Korle–Bu teaching hospital Ghana. Afr J Reprod Health. 2014;18(4):115-22.

Rupture Uterus: The Catastrophe Compendiously Summarized

Pratima Mittal, Sheeba Marwah

INTRODUCTION

Uterine rupture is a lethal surgical apocalypse complicating pregnancy, with grave fetomaternal outcomes. Maximum cases of uterine ruptures that have been narrated in literature, have occurred in resource poor settings like India, following trial of labor after cesarean delivery (TOLAC).[1]

DEFINITION

Uterine rupture is described as a defect in the uterine wall. Often the terms "rupture" and "dehiscence" are used interchangeably, though former denotes that all uterine muscle layers, including the serosa have given way, whereas latter implies clinically occult and incomplete disruption.

INCIDENCE

Uterine rupture in women with a previous cesarean is witnessed in 3/1,000 cases. It is more frequent in women undergoing a TOLAC, when juxtaposed with those undergoing planned repeat cesarean delivery (PRCD).[1,2] Rupture of the unscarred pregnant uterus is an infrequent event, occurring in 1/5,700-1/20,000 pregnancies.[2-5] Despite innovations and progresses in modern obstetric practice, the incidence of rupture in both scarred and unscarred uteri has amplified in recent decades,[6] especially in developing countries. This can be credited to a grander number of unbooked obstetric emergencies, often commencing from pastoral and country areas with poor or no antenatal care. In India, it still accounts for 5-10% of all maternal deaths.[2,6]

CLASSIFICATION

Rupture of uterus is typically classified as either:
- Complete uterine rupture—when all layers of the uterine wall are separated, with or without expulsion of the fetus (Fig. 1).
- Incomplete uterine rupture or dehiscence, when the uterine muscle gets separated but the visceral peritoneum is intact.

Uterine rupture is also categorized on the basis of previous uterine surgery resulting in a scar on the myometrium, into:
- Rupture of scarred uterus
- Rupture of unscarred uterus.

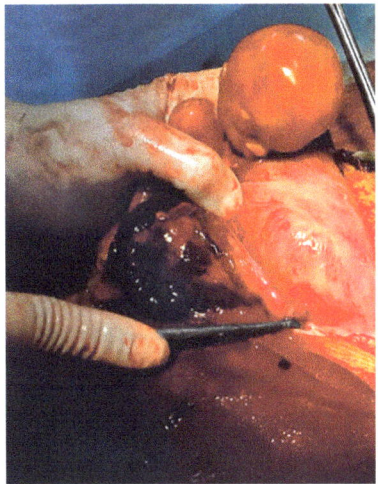

Fig. 1: Complete rupture of uterus with baby lying outside.

RISK FACTORS

Over the years, the world has turned the corner to this catastrophe—it has halted and begun to decrease the occurrence of rupture, which has gone from being a fatal intraoperative diagnosis, to a life threatening, but preventable clinical entity. This can largely be attributed to a better understanding of factors increasing the possibility of rupture. These include the following:

- *Previous lower segment cesarean section (LSCS):* Women with history of more than one prior cesarean may have a slightly higher rate of uterine rupture; the incidence being higher (1.9%) in parturient subjected to TOLAC.[2-9] However, noteworthy is the fact that history of previous vaginal delivery, any time before or following previous cesarean delivery has been found to considerably reduce the risk of uterine rupture in such women.[1-5]
- *Previous fundal or high vertical hysterotomy:* An elevated incidence of rupture is observed in women with a previous high vertical, especially fundal, hysterotomy (1–12%). This includes an inverted T, J incision, or an extended low transverse incision into the upper uterine segment. After a previous classical (fundal) cesarean hysterotomy, the reported risk of rupture varies to the tune of 1–12% in past literature reviews.[1-3]
- *Previous uterine rupture:* Rupture can recur in next pregnancy, so pregnancy after rupture in previous pregnancy should always keep an obstetrician at a very high alert.
- *Obstructed or unsupervised labor:* A poor cervical low Bishop scoring at time of admission to labor and delivery and dystocia, particularly at advanced dilation (>7 cm) might also amplify the possibility of rupture in parturient women.[5-7] Sluggish cervical dilation in the first stage of labor and a prolonged second stage are postulated to be other intrapartum risk factors.
- *Previous history of trauma to uterus/ perforation:* It might be caused by trauma or congenital (Ehlers-Danlos type IV) or acquired weakness of the myometrium.
- *Inadvertent use of oxytocin:* Myometrium gets weakened from long drawn-out labor in a woman or use of effective uterotonic drugs.[2-9]
- *Rupture of the unscarred uterus:* Risk factors associated with rupture of the unscarred uterus include high parity, exposure to uterotonic drugs, uterine anomalies, advancing maternal age, dystocia, macrosomia, multiple gestation, abnormal placentation (e.g. placenta accreta, increta, or percreta), or prior cerclage.[1,10-17]
- *Other probable risk factors* inconsistently bracketed with an increased risk of rupture include[9,10,18-20]—high maternal age, postdatism, macrosomia, and interdelivery interval <18–24 months.

Factors Decreasing the Risk of Rupture

A previous vaginal delivery, either before or after the prior cesarean delivery, has been significantly found to reduce the risk of uterine rupture.[1-5]

Prediction of Uterine Rupture

Unfortunately, once the clinical signs indicating rupture surface, major maternal and/or neonatal morbidity already may have already set in the patient. Numerous predictive paradigms for uterine rupture bringing into play an amalgamation of risk factors have been illustrated, but none has proven consistent or clinically reliable for the purpose.[4-9]

- *A History of* previous preterm LSCS, history of surgical site infection in last pregnancy, and short interpregnancy interval (below 18 months) following cesarean delivery seem to be associated with a greater probability of uterine rupture in women undergoing TOLAC.
- *On examination,* if previous scar has healed by secondary intention, one should suspect that the uterine scar may be weak.
- *Imaging for prediction of uterine rupture:*
  - *Antepartum imaging*—ultrasound (either transabdominal or vaginal) measurement of both the thickness of the residual myometrium in the lower uterine segment (LUS) and the dimensions of the hypoechoic uterine defect in place of the previous cesarean is the most scrutinized process to forecast the risk of rupture[12-16] and counsels women envisaging TOLAC.[12-16] LUS thickness on ultrasonography (USG) near term is contrariwise associated with the higher likelihood of uterine scar dehiscence or rupture at delivery. Notwithstanding its shortcomings, the greatest LUS thickness <2.0 mm (lowest value amongst minimum three measurements near term) has been found to be good predictor for rupture or dehiscence.[12-17]
  - *Interpregnancy imaging*—U or V wedge-shaped hypoechoic uterine defects (also called niches) in a region of the myometrial thinning[10-16] have been observed on imaging studies several months after delivery. Confirmation of the same on hysteroscopy is diagnostic.[10-16] Repair of such defects, including fibrotic tissue excision and closure of the anterior uterine wall vaginally or laparoscopically, is often advocated, followed by PRCD in next pregnancy.

CLINICAL PRESENTATION OF UTERINE RUPTURE

Given the potential grave fetomaternal upshots in the event of an intrapartum uterine rupture, each obstetrician must be acutely cognizant and well versed with the clinical signs related to uterine rupture.

- *Antepartum and intrapartum period:*
  - *Abnormal fetal heart rate (FHR)*: Sudden development of category II or III FHR patterns is consistently seen in patients with uterine rupture, though no FHR pattern is pathognomonic of rupture. The most frequent FHR abnormality is fetal bradycardia[13-16] that may be sudden or preceded by variable or prolonged decelerations.
  - *Abdominal pain:* Rupture may be associated with sudden onset of abdominal pain, but pain may be partially masked by neuraxial analgesia administered for management of labor pain, or epidural top ups in women undergoing TOLAC.
  - *Scar tenderness*: Dehiscence might manifest as pain in stitch line elicited as scar tenderness.
  - *Abnormal uterine contour:* Fundus may be hard and retracted, with fetal parts easily palpable.
  - *Vaginal bleeding:* Vaginal bleeding may befall, though it might be fairly small even with major intra-abdominal hemorrhage.
  - *Loss of station* of the presenting part of the fetus.
  - *Hematuria* in event of rupture extending into the bladder.

- *Hemodynamic instability:* It is often consequent to intra-abdominal hemorrhage.
- *Changes in contraction patterns*: Both increased uterine contractility and loss of uterine tone have been described.[13-16] Also, a plodding fall in the amplitude of consecutive contractions, the so-called "staircase sign" on external tocodynamometry[16] (Fig. 2).
- *Presentation in postpartum period*—in postpartum women, occult uterine rupture if would have occurred during delivery, presents as pain and/or unrelenting vaginal bleeding (regardless of use of uterotonics) and hematuria (following extension up to the bladder).
- *Presentation at laparotomy:* There may be complete or incomplete rupture. Incomplete rupture may show an intact thin layer of serosa or peritoneum with live or dead fetus in the uterine cavity. Complete rupture may show the fetus lying outside the uterine cavity partially or completely with intraperitoneal blood and liquor collection (Figs. 1 and 3).
- *Role of imaging for diagnosis of rupture uterus*: In hemodynamically stable women in labor with suspected rupture, focused assessment with sonography for obstetrics (FASO) imaging may be deployed for evidence of any hemoperitoneum.[11-14] Imaging studies in women not in labor might show disruption of the myometrium, a hematoma next to the hysterotomy scar, extrauterine fluid-distended fetal membranes, free peritoneal fluid, anhydramnios, an empty uterus, fetal parts outside the uterine cavity, and/or fetal demise.[2,5,11-14] Computed tomography or magnetic resonance imaging, if performed might detect peritoneal air, besides other pathology associated with rupture, like ileus or abscess.

DIFFERENTIAL DIAGNOSIS

The differential diagnosis of uterine rupture is centered around presenting signs and symptoms. Abruption manifesting as acute abdominal pain, bleeding, and category II or III FHR tracings is distinguished mostly during laparotomy.

Besides, one must differentiate hemodynamic instability owing to intra-abdominal bleeding from any source, including hepatic rupture following pre-eclampsia with severe features or HELLP syndrome (Hemolysis, Elevated Liver function tests, Low Platelets)

MANAGEMENT

- *Management of women with antepartum uterine rupture*: Hemodynamically unstable patients should be resuscitated

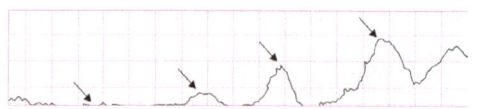

Fig. 2: CTG tracing showing staircase sign.

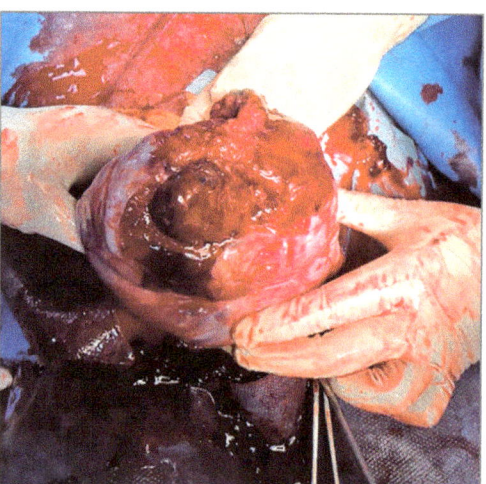

Fig. 3: Intraoperative findings of fundal rupture.

with pertinent fluids and blood transfusion, and prepared for cesarean delivery, mostly under general anesthesia. The choice of abdominal incision is guided by the clinical diagnosis, but as a rule, a midline incision is preferred as it provides wider exposure for an extensive abdominal exploration, involving the uterine fundus, and bowel, if need be.

- *Management of women with uterine rupture at laparotomy:*
  - *Delivery of fetus*: This is performed using conventional maneuvers, but delivery may be difficult if fetal parts have extruded through the site of rupture.[1-5,15-17,21,22] Providing adequate exposure and use of vacuum or other fetal extraction instruments may facilitate delivery.
  - *Repair versus hysterectomy*: Decision to save the uterus is taken keeping in mind parturient's obstetric history and future reproduction plans. Whichever closure technique is chosen during conservative repair, the key objectives targeted while undertaking conservative surgery are uterine defect reparation, curbing hemorrhage, recognizing damage to other organs (e.g. urinary tract), minimizing early postsurgical morbidity, and reducing the risk of complications in future pregnancies. If repair is contemplated, the uterine defect should be closed using a technique similar to that for traditional hysterotomy closure, with supplementary interventions (as required) to attain hemostasis (Fig. 4). Also, whenever repair is contemplated, tubal ligation advocates to prevent patient from further morbidity in next pregnancy. Hysterectomy most often might be a prompt, life-saving measure for her in critical condition, or when adequate closure and hemostasis is not achieved after attempted uterine repair. However, if an adequate closure and hemostasis does not seem feasible, hysterectomy should be performed.
  - *Management of coexistent complications*: Associated postpartum hemorrhage (PPH) arising due to uterine atony may result in persistent bleeding, which is coped following standard protocols.[22-25] If the uterine laceration extends to the bladder or a ureteral injury is suspected, an experienced urologist should be roped in and bladder repair done in two layers followed by urethral and/or suprapubic catheter placement for up to 14 days.[1-5,22-25] Injuries to blood vessels and other pelvic organs are repaired using standard techniques, involving a proficient pelvic/vascular or general surgeon.

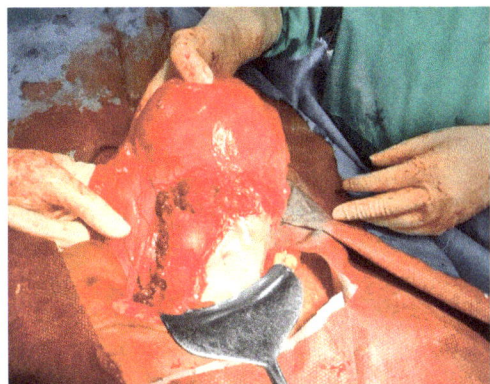

Fig. 4: Repair of previous uterine scar rupture with right lateral extension done on laparotomy.

OUTCOME

- *Maternal mortality and morbidity:* Up to one-third of women with a uterine rupture undergo hysterectomy; comorbidities of hysterectomy encompass operative

injuries such as urinary tract or bowel lacerations, blood transfusion, and postoperative infection.
- *Perinatal mortality and morbidity*: The perinatal death rate associated with uterine rupture is 5–26%,[2,11,16,17,21-25] mostly owing to neonatal hypoxic-ischemic encephalopathy following intrauterine hypoxia. The rate of occurrence of these outcomes is dependent on factors such as the size and location of the rupture (e.g. lateral is more morbid than anterior) and speed of intervention.

Recurrence Risk

Reports of the risk of recurrent rupture vary widely (range 0–100%),[22-25] the highest risk of recurrent rupture being when the previous rupture was in the fundus or longitudinal.

Management of Subsequent Pregnancies

In order to decrease the risk of recurrent rupture, most often a cesarean delivery is advocated for subsequent pregnancies, and the same is scheduled before the onset of labor.
- *Timing of delivery*: If the previous rupture occurred at term, during labor, and in the LUS, delivery is timed at 36+0 to 37+6 weeks of gestation considering the potential maternal and fetal consequences of recurrent rupture.[1-6,22-25] An earlier delivery, prior to 36+0 weeks gestation, is performed on a case-by-case basis, bearing in mind factors like preterm labor in the current pregnancy, or a history of preterm or antepartum rupture in a prior pregnancy.
- A course of *antenatal corticosteroids* 48 hours before planned preterm delivery is suggested for patients who have not received a previous course.
- In case, recurrent rupture is suspected, emergency cesarean delivery is indicated.

PREVENTION OF UTERINE RUPTURE

Good obstetrical practices like avoiding fundal pressure in the second stage of labor, gentle performance of procedures involving uterine manipulation, such as external cephalic version for malpresentation in a woman with a significant uterine anomaly, judicious utilization of uterotonic agents for induction and augmentation of labor, apposite and timely use of cesarean delivery for management of protraction, and besides exercising care in choosing candidates for TOLAC with meticulous intrapartum monitoring, go a long way in averting risk of rupture.

SHARING EXPERIENCE FROM OUR OWN HOSPITAL

Analyzing the last two year data (July 2016–June 2018) at Safdarjung Hospital, 61 cases of uterine rupture occurred, amongst 67,000 deliveries during this period, making it an incidence of 0.09%. Out of these 62.29% women were un-booked, with no antenatal supervision ever. Also, 56 cases occurred in previously scarred uterus; 2 cases followed vaginal delivery in postpartum period and in 2 cases rupture was in an unscarred uterus. While, only repair was done in 9.8% (6 cases) repair with ligation was performed in 63% (39 cases), 26% (16 cases) women had to undergo hysterectomy for the same, of which 8% (5 cases) had subtotal hysterectomy. Concomitant bladder repair was required in around 11.45% (7 cases). 94% women needed blood transfusion. It was associated with 85.24% stillbirths, whereas only 3 maternal deaths were noted as patients were referred in compromised state.

CONCLUSION

Uterine rupture is one of the most devastating complications of labor posing grave danger to life of both mother and fetus hence adding to the high maternal and perinatal mortality and morbidity. It can be either complete rupture or incomplete/dehiscence. Diagnosis of uterine rupture is based on clinical or radiologic findings. Laparotomy and urgent delivery are often indicated in patients because of nonreassuring FHR changes and/or hemodynamic instability. Definitive surgical management involves hysterectomy. Prompt clinical diagnosis and timely referral to tertiary center and facility level readiness to respond to obstetric and newborn emergencies are vital for the survival of women and their newborns, following rupture. Also optimum care around birth is quint essential in averting this catastrophe in high-risk women.

KEY POINTS

- Uterine rupture in pregnancy is a rare and often catastrophic complication with a high incidence of fetal and maternal morbidity and mortality.
- Uterine rupture is described as a defect in the uterine wall. Uterine rupture in women with a previous cesarean is witnessed in 3/1,000 cases. It is more frequent in women undergoing a TOLAC.
- Common risk factors identified for rupture uterus are—previous LSCS (most common), previous fundal or high vertical hysterotomy, previous uterine rupture, and obstructed or unsupervised labor. Previous history of trauma to uterus or perforation.
- Other risk factors are inadvertent use of oxytocin, high parity, exposure to uterotonic drugs, uterine anomalies, advancing maternal age, dystocia, macrosomia, multiple gestation, abnormal placentation (e.g. placenta accreta, increta, or percreta), or prior cerclage, birth weight >4,000 g, and interdelivery interval <18–24 months.
- History of previous preterm LSCS, surgical site infection in last pregnancy, interpregnancy interval less than 18 months following cesarean delivery, should be explored before deciding the mode of delivery.
- One should suspect rupture, if there are sudden developments of category II or III FHR patterns, abdominal pain, scar tenderness, abnormal uterine contour, vaginal bleeding, loss of station of the fetal presenting part, and changes in uterine contraction patterns. If patient has hematuria, bladder rupture is also suspected.
- Postpartum women with occult uterine rupture presents as pain and persistent vaginal bleeding (regardless of use of uterotonics) and hematuria (following extension up to the bladder).
- If rupture has occurred before delivery, hemodynamically unstable patients should be resuscitated and prepared for cesarean delivery, preferably under general anesthesia. Generally, a midline incision is preferred as it provides wider exposure.
- At laparotomy after delivery of fetus decision to save the uterus is taken on the basis of parturient's obstetric history, future reproduction plans, and feasibility of repair. Conservative surgery aims at repair of uterine defect, curbing hemorrhage, recognizing damage to other organs (e.g. urinary tract).
- Highest risk of recurrent rupture is observed when the previous rupture was at the fundus or the uterine scar was

longitudinal. In order to decrease the risk of recurrent rupture, a cesarean delivery is advocated for subsequent pregnancies and the same is scheduled before the onset of labor.

REFERENCES

1. Guise JM, Eden K, Emeis C, et al. Vaginal birth after cesarean: new insights. Evid Rep Technol Assess (Full Rep). 2010;(191):1-397.
2. Landon MB, Lynch CD. Optimal timing and mode of delivery after cesarean with previous classical incision or myomectomy: a review of the data. Semin Perinatol 2011;35:257-61.
3. Vachon-Marceau C, Demers S, Goyet M, et al. Labor dystocia and the risk of uterine rupture in women with prior cesarean. Am J Perinatol. 2016;33:577-83.
4. Harper LM, Cahill AG, Roehl KA, et al. The pattern of labor preceding uterine rupture. Am J Obstet Gynecol. 2012;207:210.e1-6.
5. Guise JM, Eden K, Emeis C, et al. Vaginal birth after cesarean: New insights. Evidence Report/Technology Assessment No.191. (Prepared by the Oregon Health & Science University Evidence-based Practice Center under Contract No. 290-2007-10057-I). AHRQ Publication No. 10-E003. Agency for Healthcare Research and Quality, Rockville, MD 2010. [online] Available from: http://www.ahrq.gov/sites/default/files/wysiwyg/research/findings/evidence-based-reports/vbacup-evidence-report.pdf. (Last accessed on July, 2019).
6. Landon MB. Predicting uterine rupture in women undergoing trial of labor after prior cesarean delivery. Semin Perinatol. 2010;34:267-71.
7. Roberge S, Chaillet N, Boutin A, et al. Single-versus double-layer closure of the hysterotomy incision during cesarean delivery and risk of uterine rupture. Int J Gynaecol Obstet 2011;115:5-10.
8. Tahseen S, Griffiths M. Vaginal birth after two caesarean sections (VBAC-2)-a systematic review with meta-analysis of success rate and adverse outcomes of VBAC-2 versus VBAC-1 and repeat (third) caesarean sections. BJOG. 2010;117:5-19.
9. Al-Zirqi I, Daltveit AK, Forsén L, et al. Risk factors for complete uterine rupture. Am J Obstet Gynecol. 2017;216:165.e1-165.
10. Jastrow N, Demers S, Chaillet N, et al. Lower uterine segment thickness to prevent uterine rupture and adverse perinatal outcomes: A multicenter prospective study. Am J Obstet Gynecol. 2016;215:604.e1-604.
11. Jastrow N, Vikhareva O, Gauthier RJ, et al. Can third-trimester assessment of uterine scar in women with prior Cesarean section predict uterine rupture? Ultrasound Obstet Gynecol. 2016;47:410-4.
12. Kok N, Wiersma IC, Opmeer BC, et al. Sonographic measurement of lower uterine segment thickness to predict uterine rupture during a trial of labor in women with previous Cesarean section: A meta-analysis. Ultrasound Obstet Gynecol. 2013;42:132-9.
13. Schepker N, Garcia-Rocha GJ, von Versen-Höynck F, et al. Clinical diagnosis and therapy of uterine scar defects after caesarean section in non-pregnant women. Arch Gynecol Obstet. 2015;291:1417-23.
14. Ridgeway JJ, Weyrich DL, Benedetti TJ. Fetal heart rate changes associated with uterine rupture. Obstet Gynecol. 2004;103:506-12.
15. Ayres AW, Johnson TR, Hayashi R. Characteristics of fetal heart rate tracings prior to uterine rupture. Int J Gynaecol Obstet. 2001;74:235-40.
16. Craver Pryor E, Mertz HL, Beaver BW, et al. Intrapartum predictors of uterine rupture. Am J Perinatol. 2007;24:317-21.
17. Matsuo K, Scanlon JT, Atlas RO, et al. Staircase sign: A newly described uterine contraction pattern seen in rupture of unscarred gravid uterus. J Obstet Gynaecol Res. 2008;34:100-4.
18. Roberge S, Demers S, Berghella V, et al. Impact of single-vs double-layer closure on adverse outcomes and uterine scar defect: A systematic review and meta-analysis. Am J Obstet Gynecol 2014;211:453-60.
19. Lannon SM, Guthrie KA, Vanderhoeven JP, et al. Uterine rupture risk after periviable cesarean delivery. Obstet Gynecol. 2015;125:1095-100.
20. Naji O, Abdallah Y, Bij De Vaate AJ, et al. Standardized approach for imaging and measuring Cesarean section scars using ultrasonography. Ultrasound Obstet Gynecol. 2012;39:252-9.

21. Fekih M, Memmi A, Nouri S, et al. Asymptomatic horn rudimentary pregnant uterine rupture with a viable fetus. Tunis Med. 2009;87:633-6.
22. Attarde VY, Patil P, Chaudhari R, et al. Sonographic findings of uterine rupture with expulsion of the fetus into broad ligament. J Clin Ultrasound. 2009;37:50-2.
23. Gerli S, Baiocchi G, Favilli A, et al. New treatment option for early spontaneous rupture of a postmyomectomy gravid uterus. Fertil Steril. 2011;96:e97-8.
24. Chibber R, El-Saleh E, Al Fadhli R, et al. Uterine rupture and subsequent pregnancy outcome--how safe is it? A 25-year study. J Matern Fetal Neonatal Med. 2010;23:421-4.
25. Fox NS, Gerber RS, Mourad M, et al. Pregnancy outcomes in patients with prior uterine rupture or dehiscence. Obstet Gynecol. 2014;123:785-9.

Chapter 11E

Expectant Management of Placenta Previa

Gomathy Narayanan, Narayanan R

■ INTRODUCTION

Way back in 1945, McAfee and Johnson postulated an expectant line of management of placenta previa with the aim to continue pregnancy for better fetal salvage, without compromising maternal health. It was an era when the facility of ultrasound imaging (USG) was not available. This line of management was recommended when patients arrived at the hospital before full term with a warning bout of painless vaginal bleeding.

In the present day clinical practice, where we perform first trimester nuchal translucency (NT) scan and an anomaly scan in the second trimester as a routine, reporting of placenta in the lower part of the uterine cavity as low lying or previa in asymptomatic women is not uncommon. This finding is more common in the first half of pregnancy. It is identified in 42% between 11 and 14 weeks, 3.9% in 20–24 weeks, and 1.9% at term. The shift or upward migration is due to the differential growth of lower segment. The average migration rate is said to be 1 mm per week. On an average, 10% of asymptomatic women who were diagnosed to have low lying of placenta or previa continue to progress to 38 weeks without vaginal bleeding. If there is overlap of more than 20 mm to the internal cervical os after 26 weeks, it is predictive of placenta previa. If the follow-up scan at 32 weeks still shows placenta previa, it remains so in 95% of cases till 38 weeks.

■ ASYMPTOMATIC PLACENTA PREVIA

Counseling is central to the management of all asymptomatic women with placenta previa. Factors such as age, parity index, previous history of cesarean section, associated conditions like pre-eclampsia, gestational diabetes mellitus (GDM), fetal growth restriction, multiple pregnancy, placenta accreta, abruption, preterm labor, and preterm premature rupture of membrane (PPROM) pose an absolute necessity for counseling and individualized obstetric care. These women must avoid all strenuous physical activity including lifting heavy weights (>5 kg), standing for more than 4 hours and long distance travel. They should refrain from any sexual activity and orgasm, which may precipitate vaginal bleeding and premature uterine contractions. Care must be taken to emphasize the importance of regular antenatal care, prevention, and correction of anemia and fetal surveillance. It is reported that the mean gestational age at the time of the first episode of vaginal bleeding is 29–32 week; one-third of cases bleed for the first time before 30 weeks, one-third from 32 to 36 weeks and the rest after 36 weeks. Therefore, in asymptomatic women, a follow-up scan at 32 weeks is indicated. If she remains asymptomatic, her subsequent scan can be delayed until 38 weeks. It is preferable that they reside within 5 kilometers of a tertiary center to seek emergency assistance.

With increased incidence of cesarean sections, there is increased risk of placenta previa. The number of cesarean sections a woman has undergone will increase the risk exponentially. With one cesarean it is 0.65% and with 4 previous cesareans, the risk mounts up to 10%. The recurrence rate of placenta previa is 12%.

Women with placenta previa are at increased risk (10%) of having a morbidly adherent placenta, especially if they have previously delivered by cesarean section and if placental implantation is on the anterior wall in the present pregnancy. 75% of adherent placentae are associated with placenta previa. A short interval between cesarean and conception further increases the risk and more so if the placental implantation is anterior. When there is suspicion in the abdominal ultrasound [transabdominal ultrasonography (TAS)] and Doppler examination, it must be confirmed with transvaginal sonography (TVS) or transperineal ultrasound. Transvaginal scan is reported as a safe procedure in several studies. If doubt persists, MRI will confirm the finding and also identify the extent of invasion.

Antenatal care in placenta accreta is similar to placenta previa, but during delivery, the problems may be manyfold in terms of hemorrhage. It is preferable to deliver these women by 37 weeks as an elective procedure. Preoperative consent for cesarean hysterectomy must be taken. If available, interventional radiology facility must be kept ready to arrest hemorrhage. Prolonged rest poses the risk of thromboembolism. Heparinization is contraindicated, but the use of antithrombotic stockings may be encouraged.

Prerequisites for expectant management:
- Gestational age <37 weeks
- Maternal vital signs stable
- Morphologically normal fetus without distress
- Managed in center with facility for cesarean section round the clock
- Blood for transfusion available

Asymptomatic placenta previa (diagnosed on USG):
- Avoid long distance travel/standing for >4 hours/lifting heavy weights (>5 kg)/sexual activity
- Maintain Hb% >10 g% and PCV >30
- Regular ANC
- Anomaly USG at 20 weeks
- Follow-up USG at 32 weeks
- Rule out placenta accreta
- USG at 38 weeks to decide on planned delivery

SYMPTOMATIC PLACENTA PREVIA

The first episode of painless vaginal bleeding usually occurs without any precipitating episode although strenuous physical activity, long travel or sexual intercourse may be the initiating factors. Complete placenta previa is more likely to present with vaginal bleeding earlier. The amount of bleeding in the first episode may be variable, although it is unlikely to be heavy enough to induce shock. A second episode is expected in 70% of cases and 10% may even have a third episode. The rest of the cases may have multiple episodes of bleeding. The amount of subsequent bleeding tends to be increasingly heavy as the cervix and lower segment change as pregnancy progresses and thinning of lower segment of uterus causes tears in the intervillous spaces of placenta.

Most of the patients stop bleeding with bed rest, particularly those in second trimester. Bleeding starts with bright red color and ends with brownish discharge. Once the bleeding stops, a per-speculum examination is necessary to rule out local lesions. Per-vaginal examination is contraindicated because it can result in massive hemorrhage.

Once the bleeding stops, the decision to retain her in the hospital until delivery will depend on individual factors such as extent of support at home, distance from the tertiary center, and her ability to reach the hospital within 20 minutes. She must be prepared to arrive at the hospital along with an attendant and all case records. While at home, she should be made aware of identifying fetal movements, uterine irritability, and vaginal bleeding.

When a patient reports with recurrent bouts of bleeding, she must be retained in the hospital even though there are a few recommendations to the contrary. The advantages of hospitalization are better monitoring and timely action, if bleeding occurs again.

Anti-D immunization must be given to all nonsensitized Rh negative women. With recurrent bout of vaginal bleeding, it should be repeated at 6 weekly intervals.

Warning bout of bleeding:
- Admit for rest
- Monitor mother and fetus
- Speculum examination after bleeding ceases to R/o local causes
- Steroid for lung maturity
- Anti-D if indicated
- Decide on hospital care or care at home

Prerequisites for home care:
- Easy accessibility to treatment center
- 24 hour care at home as in hospital
- Patient should be able to recognize fetal movements /uterine irritability/vaginal bleeding

PLACENTA PREVIA WITH MASSIVE HEMORRHAGE

When a patient arrives in a state of shock with massive bleeding, aggressive expectant management is required with prompt correction of shock, supportive treatment, and multiple blood transfusions. Such patients must be managed in a tertiary center. The blood loss is from the maternal compartment and hence the fetus is not in immediate jeopardy. The fetal heart rate (FHR) tracings may show signs of distress but it get corrected with maternal treatment. Expectant line of management may be continued if maternal stability is achieved and the fetal well-being is restored. A massive hemorrhage can initiate preterm uterine contractions and labor. The use of tocolytics as a preventive measure is not successful, but should be used when there is evidence of uterine irritability. Among the tocolytics, magnesium sulfate scores over the others because of less or no adverse effect on the mother and fetus. It has additional advantage of fetal neuroprotection. Beta-mimetics adversely affect the maternal cardiovascular system. Indomethacin inhibits platelet function and carries the risk of premature closure of fetal ductus arteriosus. There are very few studies confirming the advantage of cervical cerclage or vaginal pessaries to prevent preterm labor, when the cervix is short. Therefore, they are not advised.

Massive hemorrhage:
- Correction of shock
- Blood transfusion
- Fetal monitoring
- Hospital stay and rest till delivery
- Steroids as indicated
- Magnesium sulfate for tocolysis
- Antithrombotic stockings
- Anti-D if indicated
- Deliver by 36 weeks

Placenta previa is a potentially lethal complication of pregnancy. Its incidence is increasing significantly as a result of escalating incidence of cesarean sections. Imaging has revolutionized its management. If the principles of management are adhered to scrupulously, the expectant care enhances fetal salvage without compromising maternal health. If the prerequisites are met, some women with placenta previa can be managed at home successfully with its inherent advantages of cost effectiveness and comfort. Aggressive expectant management of placenta previa associated with profuse hemorrhage is a novel concept, which yields encouraging outcome.

SUGGESTED READING

1. Drostes K. Expectant line of management: Hospitalization or outpatient bed rest. Am J Obstet Gynecol. 1994;170(5P61):1254-7.
2. D'antonio F, Timor-Tritsch IE, Palacios-Jaraquemada J, et al. First trimester detection of abnormally invasive placenta in high risk women: Systematic review and meta analysis. Ultrasound Obstet Gynecol. 2018;51:176-83.
3. Familiari A, Liberati M, Lirn P, et al. Diagnostic accuracy of magnetic resonance imaging in detecting severity of abnormal invasive placenta: Systematic review and meta-analysis. Acta Obstet Gynecol Scand. 2018;97(5):507-520.
4. Gowri G, Snigdha P, Divya S. Antepartum Haemorrhage. Clinical Obstetrics Case Based Approach 2018. New Delhi: Jaypee Brothers Medical Publisher Pvt. Ltd.; 2018.
5. Johnson HW. The conservative management of some varieties of placenta praevia. Am J Obstet Gynecol. 1945;50:398.
6. Kay HH. Placenta praevia and abruption. In: Ronald S. Gibbs RS (Ed). Danforth's Obstetrics and Gynecology, 10th edition. Philadelphia: Lippincott Williams & Wilkins; 2010. pp. 385-99.
7. Moveir JR. Conservative management: inpatient vs outpatient. Am J Obstet Gynecol.1994;170 (6):1683-5.
8. Oppenheimer I, Homes P, Samson N, et al. Diagnosis of low lying placenta can migrate in third trimester. Ultrasound Obstet Gynecol. 2001;18:100-2.
9. Oppenheimer I. Diagnosis and management of placenta praevia. Obstet Gynecol Can. 2007;29(3):261-6.
10. RCOG Green-top Guidelines No. 22. Anti- D immunization should be given to all non sensitized Rh-negative women with APH in spite of routine prophylactic anti-D; 2011.
11. RCOG Green-top Guidelines No. 27. Cervical cerclage or prophylactic tocolysis to prevent bleeding and preterm labour in women with placenta praevia has no role; 2011.
12. RCOG Green-top Guidelines No.63. With increased number of prior caesarean sections there is increased risk of placenta praevia; 2011.
13. RCOG Green-top Guidelines No.7. Corticosteroids should be given to women between 24 to 34 weeks gestation; 2011.
14. Shaaban OM, Ahmed HA, Ali MK, et al. Evolution of second trimester low implanted placenta to praevia at term: A prospective cohort study. Int J Reprod Contracept Obstet Gynecol. 2018;7 (11):4330-5.
15. Silver R, Depp R, Sabbagha RE, et al. Placenta praevia: Aggressive expectant management. Am J Obstet Gynecol. 1984;150(1):15-22.
16. Warshak CR, Eskandu R, Hull AD, et al. Accuracy of ultrasonography and magnetic resonance imaging in diagnosis of placenta praevia accreta. Obstet Gynecol. 2006;108: 573-81.
17. Wing DA, Paul RH, Miller LK. Outpatient management of symptomatic placenta praevia appears to be an acceptable alternative to traditional conservative expectant inpatient management. AmJ Obstet Gynecol. 1996;175(4p1-1):806-11.
18. Yang Q, We S, Oppenheimer I, et al. Association of caesarean delivery for first birth with placenta praevia. BJOG. 2007;114(5):609-13.

Chapter 11F

Morbidly Adherent Placenta (Placenta Accreta Spectrum): Prearm and Perform

VP Paily

INTRODUCTION

Morbidly adherent placenta has gained much importance in recent times as it is emerging as a major cause of maternal mortality and morbidity. The incidence of placenta accreta spectrum (PAS) is rapidly increasing because of the rising cesarean section rate across the globe, especially the developing countries. Pregnancies following cesarean section have higher chance of implanting over the scar. As pregnancy advances, it presents as morbidly adherent placenta with its serious consequences.

NOMENCLATURE

There are different names to describe the condition, morbidly adherent placenta being only one of them. Earlier we used to differentiate morbidly adherent placenta depending on the depth of invasion—accreta when the invasion was into the basalis layer of decidua, increta when it involves the myometrium and percreta when it has reached the serosa and beyond. The grouping under these categories becomes meaningless as the depth of invasion can vary in different areas of the placenta in the same woman. It would be more logical to designate it depending on the deepest level of invasion in an individual.

The FIGO (International Federation of Obstetrics and Gynaecology) has recently recommended the name PAS, which reflects the fact that a range of invasion is possible in a given situation. However, it has the drawback that it clubs together all different depths of invasion and does not stress the importance of the percreta variety, which is the most dangerous. Comparing outcomes of management in different centers becomes less reliable unless the percentage of percreta placenta is mentioned.

PATHOGENESIS

Why in some women the placenta invades deeper than the stratum spongiosum, is not clearly understood. Behavior of the trophoblast is governed by various factors. Usually, the invasion stops at the stratum spongiosum of the deciduas as it provides a network of blood vessels, which can be invaded by the trophoblast to create the sinuses of maternal blood from which the fetus draws oxygen and nutrients. If there is deficiency of decidua as happens over the scar tissue, the trophoblast invades deeper leading to abnormal implantation. The more the number of previous cesareans, the more the chance of abnormally invading placenta (AIP). In the current pregnancy, if the placenta is previa, the incidence of AIP will be 3.3% with one previous cesarean section, 11% with two, 40% with three 61% with four, and 67% with five previous cesarean sections.

If the abnormal invasion is in the lower segment, a percreta placenta will invade the bladder wall. But even if it is not percreta, the blood supply to the lower segment increases. There will be new blood vessels from the bladder and vagina reaching the lower segment, making any attempt to separate the bladder from the placenta very bloody. Here in lies the danger in tackling placenta previa accreta. The bleeding can be so torrential that the tissues will be submerged in the pool of blood. Further dissection in this field with compromised visibility leads to injury to the bladder and ureter. The rapid loss of blood volume will lead to circulatory collapse and shock and even cardiac arrest.

The logical approach to tackle this problem is to prevent this exsanguination in the first place and be armed to replenish circulatory blood volume as and when the bleeding occurs. The strategies we have developed are based on these principles. We cut off blood supply to the pelvis with special clamps (see below) and make sure that adequate wide bore intravenous lines are inserted before starting the procedure. In addition, if one has the facilities for cell salvage that will be an added advantage.

DIAGNOSIS

Because of the association of AIP to previous trauma to the uterus, in every woman with a history of previous surgery on the uterus, AIP should be suspected and looked for. In clinical practice, the most common settings to consider are pregnancies in women with history of previous cesarean section or myomectomy. Adenomyosis, endometriosis, hysteroscopic surgery for uterine septa, and genital tuberculosis are some of the other conditions that can predispose to AIP.

Ordinary 2D gray scale ultrasound scan is the most commonly employed tool to diagnose. It helps to diagnose the site of implantation and depth of invasion. Color Doppler if available will help to assess the degree and extend of vascularity.

The diagnostic points to look for are:
- Is the sonolucent layer between the placenta and uterine wall maintained?
- Are there lacunae (lakes) inside the placental substance with turbulent flow?
- Are there blood vessels bridging between uterus/placenta and the bladder?
- Is the retroplacental myometrium thinned out (less than one millimeter)?
- Is there bulge of placenta into bladder cavity?

These findings may start to appear in the second trimester itself.

Picking up AIP early is critical in planning the management. The Kerala Federation of Obstetrics and Gynaecology (KFOG) recommends that every pregnant woman with a previous cesarean delivery should have a scan done at 32 weeks of pregnancy specially aimed at finding the location of placenta and whether it is accreta. The recommendation is that if the placenta is overlying the uterine scar, such cases should be treated only in a center with facilities to tackle placenta accreta. This is because all cases of accreta need not be picked up by the ultrasound scan or even by magnetic resonance imaging (MRI). We take MRI as complementary to ultrasound scan in the diagnosis of placenta accreta. This is especially valuable, if the placenta is situated on the posterior wall of the uterus. The features to look for are similar to the ultrasound findings mentioned above.

HOW DOES PLACENTA ACCRETA PRESENT?

A woman with placenta accreta can remain asymptomatic throughout pregnancy. However, it is a wrong notion that placenta accreta cases do not bleed during pregnancy. In fact, those cases of placenta accreta that present with antepartum hemorrhage have more predilection for bleeding during surgery as the lower segment may be more congested due to the possible bacterial invasion.

COUNSELING THE WOMAN AND FAMILY

It is important to forewarn the woman and family about the potential serious problems that can occur during cesarean delivery.

Excess bleeding which can progress to torrential unmanageable bleeding is the main threat. The second problem to be discussed is the possibility of injury to viscera like bladder and ureter. A sketch showing the uterus with the adjacent bladder and the placenta in the area of the scar will help the woman and family understand the problem. One has to be factual in explaining the anticipated problems without frightening the woman and family. The need for massive transfusions, stay in the intensive care unit and urinary catheter insertion for a few days should be explained in advance.

The preoperative assessment form should, in addition to the above points, mention the need for hysterectomy.

PREPARATION FOR DELIVERY

It is always desirable to have a planned cesarean section in these women. As the chance of spontaneous onset of labor and presenting as an emergency is higher as expected date of delivery approaches, a policy of elective cesarean section at 34–37 weeks is recommended. With a view to avoid neonatal intensive care unit (ICU) care for the baby, we prefer a policy of electively delivering between 36 and 37 weeks. These women would have received antenatal corticosteroid for fetal lung maturity at 28-32 weeks. An additional single shot of 12 mg IM is recommended preoperatively.

Adequate amount of cross-matched blood and components should be reserved. We usually keep four units of cross-matched packed red blood cells (RBCs) and four units of plasma.

If the hemoglobin level is low (e.g. below 11 g) antenatally, we build up the hemoglobin with parenteral iron if necessary.

TEAM BUILDING

The team to deal with the problem should be identified beforehand. In the West, the practice is to direct all cases of placenta previa accreta to designated referral centers in the antenatal period itself. This is not an established practice in our country even though it is highly desirable.

The team to carry out the surgery should include an experienced obstetrician and anesthesiologist. We usually have a urologist informed and on standby for help if urinary tract injury is not manageable by us.

In the West, other specialists are involved in the management. They include usually oncosurgeon, vascular surgeon, interventional radiologist, blood transfusion specialist, and their support staff. If cell salvage machine is to be operated, staff required for it also has to be available in the theater. Adequate number of experienced nurses and the neonatology team are the other additional manpower required.

ON THE DAY OF SURGERY

The woman is prepared as for any other surgery. In cases known to have percreta placenta or lateral extension of placenta to broad ligament, we prefer to put ureteric catheters before start of surgery. This helps to identify the ureters during surgery so that inadvertent injury to the ureter can be prevented. A Foley catheter also is introduced. It is fixed in such a way that the inflated bulb is free to be moved around inside the bladder. This helps to identify the upper border of the bladder, before separating it from the surface of the bladder or uterus as the case may be.

We insert the ureteric catheter under epidural, and leave the distal end of the catheter outside the urethra to be pulled out at the end of surgery. The Foley catheter is left in situ for postoperative urinary drainage.

Intravenous lines have to be inserted first, we usually put two 14 or 16 G intravenous lines and a central line plus arterial catheter.

STEPS TO REDUCE INTRAOPERATIVE BLEEDING

There are different techniques employed to reduce the blood flow to the placental site. In the West insertion of balloon in common iliac arteries or the aorta is the prevalent method. The balloon is inserted preoperatively and inflated after the fetus is out, before attempting placental separation. Ideally, it needs a hybrid theater with facilities for interventional radiology. In a developing country setting this is not an easy option.

In many of the resource-constrained settings, people rely on ligation of internal iliac arteries after the fetus is delivered. This is technically challenging and may not give the desired effect as the blood supply to the placental site might have developed extensive collaterals with vessels from anterior and posterior abdominal walls, bladder, and the bowels. We tried initially bilateral internal iliac artery ligation but found it inadequate to control the bleeding. Hence, we developed temporary clamps to occlude the common iliac arteries (Fig. 1). It was later found that occlusion of the lower end of aorta is easier and better than occluding the common iliac arteries. This has the advantage of cutting off the blood flow through the middle sacral artery, which may develop collaterals with uterine arteries through the uterosacral ligaments and posterior vaginal walls.

The clamp is specially designed to be used without dissecting the peritoneum and isolating the aorta. It has smooth surface on the inside of the blades and a guard at the tip to prevent the vessel from slipping out of the clamp.

The procedure is simple. After the fetus is delivered, the uterus is kept exteriorized and the bowels are packed upward, exposing the lower end of aorta. Its position is confirmed by palpating both common iliac arteries. A Babcock forceps is used to pull up the lower end of aorta. The aorta clamp is then inserted to get the aorta fully within the blades and is clamped. Even on maximum tightening of the ratchet, the blades will not crush the walls of the aorta because there is a built in gap between the blades (Fig. 1).

ANESTHESIA

Our preferred anesthesia is epidural with general or epidural with spinal anesthesia.

SURGICAL PROCEDURE

The abdomen is prepared just as for any other laparotomy. We prefer the supine position with left lateral tilt. The preferred incision is vertical midline, which may have to extend 4-5 cm above the umbilicus. As almost always there may be a previous scar on the anterior abdominal wall, one has to keep in mind the possibility of adhesions, especially for the bladder to be at a higher level.

Prior knowledge of the location of the placenta will help to avoid putting incision on

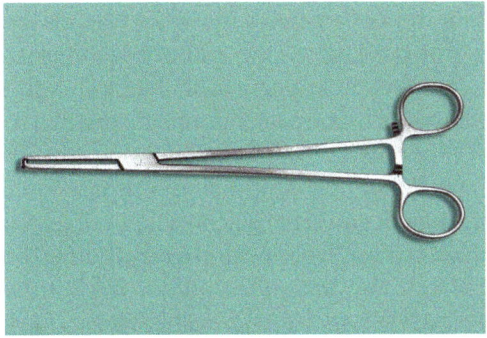

Fig. 1: Aorta clamp.

the placental site. One should strive to keep away from the placental site as otherwise it can lead to profuse bleeding even before the fetus is delivered. Some even recommend the use of intraoperative ultrasound examination.

The incision on the uterus can be vertical or transverse. It can even be over the fundus, if the patient is for hysterectomy.

Once the uterus is incised and fetus handed over for resuscitation, one has to take a decision regarding further steps. The choices are:
- Hysterectomy with placenta in situ.
- Removal of placenta, excising any localized deeply invading area with the uterine wall and reconstructing the uterus.
- To tie and cut the cord short and leave the placenta in situ for autolysis. Close the uterus as after any cesarean section.
- If the morbid adhesion to uterine wall is localized and is not going through the muscle of the uterine wall, the placenta can be removed from that area by sharp dissection. Bleeding from that area can be stopped by tying off the feeder vessels to that area.

The choice should depend on the woman's wishes, need for further children, type of placental implantation, etc. By and large we prefer hysterectomy unless the patient desires further pregnancies. It may be inevitable, if the placental extrusion is over a large area and removal of placenta with intact uterine wall is not possible. Some authors recommend excision of the segment of bladder wall, which is invaded by the placenta and reconstruct the bladder. We are not in favor of this step. We have found that almost always separation of the bladder from the placenta is possible even though it may leave behind a very thinned out bladder wall that needs reinforcing sutures. Postoperatively catheter will have to be kept for a long period (e.g. 10–14 days).

Steps of Hysterectomy

Having got the fetus delivered, the cord is clamped and cut. The edges of uterine wound may bleed briskly. Green Armytage clamps can be applied to the uterine edges to temporarily arrest the bleeding. The volume of fluid in suction bottle is noted at this point so that subsequent addition can be considered as the amount of blood loss. In addition, a sterile double-sided absorbent mat with central hole is kept on the abdomen to soak up any spilled blood from the operative field.

The uterus is exteriorized and the bowels packed off to apply the clamp to the lower end of aorta as described above. One should palpate and confirm that the common iliac artery pulsation on both sides has disappeared. Once the aorta clamp is applied, the time is announced loud and a person is entrusted to announce the elapsed time every 5 minutes. The surgeon has to be conscious of the time the clamp is in situ and try to proceed as fast as possible but should not compromise safety in an attempt to complete the surgery fast.

Clamps are then applied to both cornual pedicles so that the blood supply from upper aorta through ovarian arteries is also occluded. By sequential clamping one can take care of the upper pedicles up to the uterine arteries. At this point, the Foley bulb is moved inside the bladder to outline the upper borders of the bladder. The uterovesical fold of peritoneum extending from the bladder to uterus is then picked up with Allis forceps and separated from the underlying tissue. If the placenta is percreta, there will be a thin layer of coagulum on the surface of the placenta giving it the look of the fetal surface of the placenta. One has to take care not to break this coagulum as otherwise it will start bleeding. If there are vessels seen crossing from bladder surface to placenta/uterus, they can be coagulated or tied.

Once the bladder has been separated below the level of the uterine arteries, the clamps can be applied on the side of the uterus. If ureteric catheters had been passed at the beginning, palpation of that catheter will reassure and help the surgeon to remain at a safe distance from the ureter.

Unlike in the usual hysterectomies, taking care of the uterine arteries does not guarantee cessation of bleeding. One has to patiently separate the bladder below the level of the extruded placenta. Once that has been achieved clamps can be put on both sides of the isthmus of the uterus and across the cervix, to remove the uterus with the placenta in situ. Palpating the lower part of the uterus from front to back will help one to find out whether the dissection has reached below the level of the placenta. We strongly recommend that the dissection should not be carried below that level to reach the vagina so as to do a total hysterectomy as it will lead to excessive bleeding from the bladder base and vagina. The cervical stump is closed with full thickness mattress stitches. The upper pedicles on the side of uterus are doubly secured.

Once the uterus is removed, the bladder base and surface of the vagina are searched for any bleeding vessels and taken care of.

The aorta clamp is then unclamped but left in position so that it can be reclamped if there is profuse bleeding from the bladder base. The total duration of application of the clamp occluding the aorta is noted down. The anesthesiologist is informed when clamp is released so that he can monitor for any change due to influx of metabolites from the lower part of the body when circulation is reestablished.

Once satisfactory hemostasis is achieved, a wide-bore drain is kept at the bladder base and brought out through the anterior abdominal wall lateral to the inferior epigastric artery.

The total blood loss is noted by adding the collected amount in the suction bottles and the increase in the weight of the mops and the estimated blood loss seen on the floor. The increase in weight of the absorbent mat kept n the abdomen after the fetus is removed is also added to calculate the total blood loss.

Postoperatively we give low molecular heparin as prophylaxis till the woman is ambulant. Antibiotics are given for 48 hours. Continuous bladder drainage is kept for 48 hours and longer, if the bladder wall was thinned out or torn.

The second option is to resect the part of the uterine wall with the adherent placenta and reconstruct the uterus. This should be possible when there is only focal accreta.

The third option is to leave the placenta in situ for autolysis. In this case, one should not disturb the placenta at all. The cord is cut short and uterus is closed in layers. Subsequently, there is risk of secondary postpartum hemorrhage, infection and need for relaparotomy. About 25% of women who had such a conservative approach had to have relaparotomy.

The fourth option of removing segmental accreta placenta and leaving the uterus intact should be considered only if there is need for future child bearing and the placental invasion is not deep into the uterine wall. Removal of the placental cotyledons will leave a raw area on the uterine wall. Brisk bleeding can occur. Stitches can be put around the area to control the bleeding. In these cases, we usually do prophylactic ligation of the uterine arteries on both sides.

CONCLUSION

Morbidly adherent placenta (PAS) is emerging as a major threat to maternal safety in current obstetric practice. However, with suitable instruments and techniques it is possible to address the issue and reduce maternal mortality and morbidity.

Section 4: Postpartum Hemorrhage

- **Golden Hour Concept and First Response**
  Sheela V Mane, Garima Kachhawa, Asmita Kaundal
- **Atonic Postpartum Hemorrhage**
  Srinivas Krishna Jois
- **Traumatic Postpartum Hemorrhage**
  Padmalatha Venkataram, Srimathy Raman
- **Secondary Postpartum Hemorrhage**
  Jyothika A Desai, Ashakiran T Rathod
- **Vascular Interventions in Postpartum Hemorrhage**
  Indusekhara S, Vidya Bhargavi
- **Newer Approaches in Management of Postpartum Hemorrhage**
  Savvas Argyridis, Sabaratnam Arulkumaran

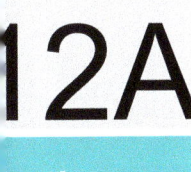

Golden Hour Concept and First Response

Sheela V Mane, Garima Kachhawa, Asmita Kaundal

INTRODUCTION

"Golden hour—the first 60 minutes from the time of recognition of postpartum hemorrhage (PPH). This is the most crucial time. To achieve the maximum survival, resuscitation must start now."

Postpartum hemorrhage is one of the leading causes of maternal death worldwide.[1] In India, hemorrhage alone accounts for 27% of the maternal deaths.[2] Most of the deaths occur within first 24 hours of delivery and are avoidable, if the healthcare team is vigilant. Some are at increased risk of having PPH so a detailed history, examination, and review of the antenatal records is helpful in categorizing who are at risk.[3] Said so, it is important to remember that anyone can have PPH so it is important to be prepared all the time.

At term, the blood flow to the uterus is 10–12 fold (700–800 mL/min) increased to that of the nonpregnant uterus which means, the uterus can bleed to death in a very short time hence need for quick action at the very first sign of it—Golden hour starts now.

BEING PREPARED

Management of the PPH starts from the very first time woman meets her healthcare provider. This preparedness is the key to the success of the management during golden hour.

Identify Who are at Risk

Patient should be thoroughly evaluated and categorized as "at risk" of having PPH at the very first visit and reevaluation should be done at all further visits. The antenatal card of such patients should have Red flag, which makes it easier for the clinician to recognize, follow-up and plan for the management of the woman. Patient who is screened at primary health center should be referred at this stage only for their booking in higher centers for delivery.

As soon as such patient enters the labor ward for delivery, all her previous records should be reviewed. A thorough general physical and systemic examination along with obstetric examination should be done and all the team should be altered. Hemoglobin should be checked again and blood should be arranged. Patient needs meticulous monitoring throughout the labor and postpartum period. Table 1 shows list of risk factors associated with PPH.

Iron and Folic Acid Supplementation

Nonanemic pregnant women should receive 60 mg of elemental iron with 400 μg of folic acid daily to prevent anemia in pregnancy along with the diet rich in iron.[4,5] Alternately World Health Organization (WHO) also recommends 120 mg of elemental iron plus 2,800 μg of folic acid weekly to pregnant women who are not anemic.[5]

Treat Anemia

Anemic woman tolerates even a little blood loss poorly and can collapse even when the blood loss is well within the normal limit than those for PPH. Moreover, these patients are

TABLE 1: Risk factors for PPH.			
Tone	*Trauma*	*Tissue*	*Thrombin (Coagulopathy)*
• Previous PPH	• Episiotomy	• Retained placenta	• Pre-eclampsia
• Multiple pregnancy	• Perineal lacerations	• Placenta accreta	• HELLP
• Grand multiparity	• Operative delivery		• Bleeding disorder
• Fetal macrosomia			• Sepsis
• Polyhydramnios			• Drugs (aspirin and heparin)
• Failure to progress in second stage			
• Prolonged third stage of labor			
• Fibroid uterus			
• Intrauterine in section			
• General anesthesia			

(HELLP: hemolysis, elevated liver enzyme levels, and low platelet level; PPH: postpartum hemorrhage)

at risk for having PPH. So, patients should be screened for and treated for anemia during the antenatal period so that they have adequate stores to tolerate the losses at the time of delivery. Those who are diagnosed to have anemia during the early pregnancy should be given 200 mg of elemental iron until her hemoglobin rises to 11 g% and subsequently she can continue the standard maintenance dose, i.e. 60 mg of elemental iron to prevent the recurrence.[5]

Trained Staff

Clinician as well as the staff at the labor ward should be adequately trained. So that they are able to identify the "at risk" patient and are able to manage and help in management of PPH, if the need arises. It is advisable to have frequent small PPH workshops and PPH drills at these centers to keep the healthcare providers updated so that the first-line management can be provided to the patients whenever needed before they are transferred to higher centers for further management.

Active Management of the Third Stage of Labor[6-8]

Active management of third stage of labor (AMTSL) is an essential step in the prevention of PPH. If the care provider and the woman regard a small reduction in blood loss and duration of third stage of labor as important—AMTSL is an answer. FOGSI (Federation of Obstetric and Gynaecological Societies of India) recommends AMTSL should be offered to all the women during childbirth since it reduces the incidence of PPH due to uterine atony.

Components of AMTSL

- Oxytocin 10 U (IM/IV) is the recommended uterotonic drug for the prevention of PPH (FOGSI even recommends use of 600 µg of misoprostol if oxytocin is not available).
- In the settings where the skilled birth attendants are available, controlled cord traction (CCT) is recommended. If the birth attendant is not skilled, CCT should not be practiced.

- Sustained uterine massage is no longer recommended as a routine intervention to prevent PPH in woman who has received oxytocin; postpartum abdominal assessment of uterus tone for early recognition of uterine atony is recommended.

Labor Ward Preparedness

- Labor ward should be clean, well-lighted space, having oxygen supply, and with easy accessibility to the blood bank, operation theater, and intensive care unit.
- Adequate staff should be appointed in the labor room ward.
- Essential drugs and instruments should be made available and they should be regularly checked and replaced immediately if used.
- An emergency obstetric tray containing intravenous (IV) cannula no. 14/16 gauge, blood sample bottles, syringes, cotton swabs, spirit, plaster to fix the 3 way cannula, sterile gloves, blood set, infusion set, IV fluid (Ringer lactate), Foley catheter no. 16, uro bag, oxygen mask, and airway should be ready.
- Postpartum hemorrhage tray containing two Sims speculum, anterior wall retractor, sponge holder at least 4 in number, 4 ribbon gauze for packing, allies clamp, needed holder, and suture should be made available. PPH tray should also contain bakri balloon or condom with Foley's catheter for balloon tamponade.

Referral to Higher Center

All those women who are categorized as "at risk" should be refereed to higher center with adequate facility for the management of PPH, operation theaters, intensive care unit, blood bank, well within time to avoid last moment panic, and rush. Also there should be provision for the transfer of the woman to higher center in emergency in case required. All these arrangements should be done before hand.

MANAGEMENT OF POSTPARTUM HEMORRHAGE

Postpartum hemorrhage is defined as blood loss of more than 500 mL in vaginal and more than 1,000 mL in case of cesarean section. As soon as there is suspicion of PPH raise an alarm to call for help. Start resuscitation measure immediately. More the time between the point of incident to start of resuscitation the survival rate decreases significantly. Quickly assess the blood loss, check vitals of the patients, start oxygen @ 6-8 L/minutes, ask the assistant to put two large IV lines 14/16 Gauge and take blood for cross matching, complete blood count, coagulation profile, insert Foley catheter to empty the bladder, and maintain the input and output record. Start IV fluids, initially 2 liters of prewarmed crystalloids to be given fast. Give uterotonics— injection oxytocin 10 units intramuscular (IM) or 5 units IV bolus, if not given previously else start 20 units in 1,000 mL RL @ 40-60 drops per minutes. Arrange at least 4 units of blood and if required transfuse. Start bimanual massage. Look for the cause of bleeding. All this should be done simultaneously. Communicate with the patient and her relatives about what is happening and the proposed management.

Stepwise Management of PPH (Flowchart 1)

- *Shout for help:* This is the first and most important step in the management of any emergency. Always have adequate hands to help you manage an emergency. While you are assessing the patient an assistant

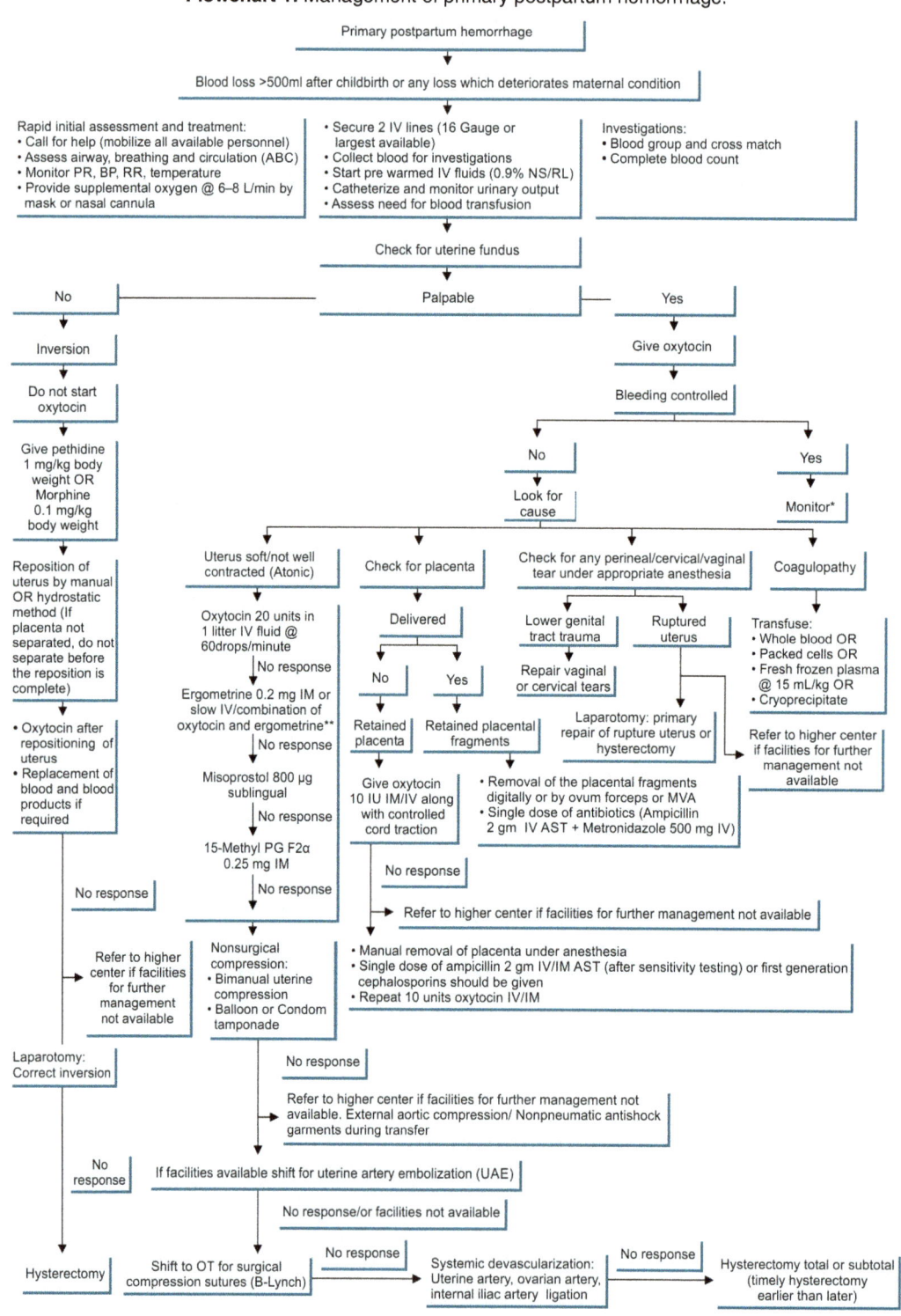

Flowchart 1: Management of primary postpartum hemorrhage.

Contd...

Contd...

Monitoring after postpartum hemorrhage:
- Check vitals and bleeding per vaginam every 15 minutes for first one hour followed by every 1 hour for next 4 hours and then every 6 hourly for next 24 hours
- Monitor urine output until the women is stable (≥30 mL/hr)

Follow up:
- Check for anemia after the bleeding is stopped for 24 hrs.
- Arrange for blood transfusion if required
- Supplement with oral ferrous sulfate or fumarate plus folic acid

**Ergometrine—Contraindications:
- Heart disease
- Hypertension

can put IV lines and draw sample. Other assistant can monitor the vitals, someone can arrange for blood and another, one can help in documentation of the events and communicate to the relative of the patient. Raise alarm and intimidate senior obstetrician, anesthetist, operation theater staff, blood blank, and intensive care unit.

- *Record vitals—Pulse rate (PR), blood pressure (BP), respiration rate (RR) and temperature.* It is recommended to have continuous vital monitoring in case of major hemorrhage. In case, the facility is not available, vitals should be monitored every 15 minutes.
- *Keep the woman warm:* Remove all the wet drapes and put the dry sheets. Put extra blanket, if needed. Use electric blanket, if available.
- *Start oxygen* by mask @ 6-8 L/min.
- *Assess blood loss:* Visual inspection does not give an accurate estimation of the blood loss still it is the first thing to be done. So the care provider needs to be experienced. Visual inspection should be correlated with the clinical signs to have a fairly good idea of the blood loss (Table 2).
- Send blood sample for blood group and cross match, complete blood count, and coagulation profile including fibrinogen levels.
- *Start IV fluids:* Crystalloid infusion to replace the blood loss till the time blood is being arranged. Up to 3.5 liters of prewarmed fluid can be given. Give 2 liters of isotonic crystalloids and further resuscitation can continue with either crystalloid or colloid.
- Empty bladder and leave the catheter in situ for output monitoring.
- Transfuse blood and blood products if required.
- Administer 10 units of oxytocin, if not given previously.
- *Look for the cause:* Cause for PPH can be divided into four categories and can be easily remembered as 4Ts:
  1. *Tone:* Uterine atony.
  2. *Tissue:* Retained placenta or placental tissue.
  3. *Trauma:* Episiotomy, vaginal or cervical lacerations or tears, and rupture uterus.
  4. *Thrombin:* Coagulation disorders.

Atonic PPH

Most common cause of PPH is atonic PPH.[9] Although with the increasing practice of AMTSL, the incidence of atonic PPH is decreasing worldwide still it remains the most common cause of hemorrhage. So the first step in the management of PPH is to palpate the fundus of the uterus to see whether it is contracted or not.
- Palpate for the fundus of the uterus. If the uterus feels soft the bleeding is because of atonic uterus.

TABLE 2: Assessment of blood loss.

	Class I—compensated	Class II—mild	Class III—moderate	Class IV—severe
% Blood loss	15% (500–1,000 mL)	20–25% (1,000–1,500 mL)	30–35% (1,500–2,000 mL)	40% (>2,000 mL)
Pulse	Normal	100 bpm	120 bpm	140 bpm
Systolic blood pressure	Normal	Normal	70–80 mm Hg	60 mm Hg
Mean arterial pressure	80–90 mm Hg	80–90 mm Hg	50–70 mm Hg	50 mm Hg
Tissue perfusion	Postural hypotension	Peripheral vasoconstriction	Pallor, restlessness, and oliguria	Collapse, anuria, and air hunger

- Rub the uterus to stimulate contraction.
- Empty the bladder.
- Give oxytocin 10 unit intramuscular, if not given previously (during active management of third stage of labor), else start oxytocin infusion 20 units in 1,000 mL of isotonic crystalloid @ 125 mL/hour unless fluid is restricted. Continue uterine massage.
- Give ergometrine 0.5 mg intramuscular or slow intravenous, if the patient is still bleeding.
- If bleeding is still not controlled give carboprost 0.25 mg intramuscular repeated every 15 minutes, if required maximum 8 doses.
- Give 800 μg misoprostol sublingually if still bleeding. Continue uterine massage.
- If still bleeding give injection tranexamic acid 1 g IV @ 1 mL/min over 10 minutes. Second dose of 1 g tranexamic acid can be given in case bleeding continues even after 30 minutes or stops but restarts after 24 hours.[9,10] Continue uterine massage. Table 3 enlists the drugs used for the management of PPH.
- If bleeding stops at any point during the medical management patient should be either shifted to intensive care unit or high dependency unit in the delivery room for continuous monitoring.
- In case medical management fails, clinician should proceed with the surgical method. Balloon tamponade is the first-line surgical intervention. Specialized balloons or condom catheter is inserted in the uterus and the balloon is inflated using 300-500 mL of normal saline. Position of the balloon is checked. And it is left in situ (several hours to 2 days). Continue oxytocin 20 units in 500 mL of normal saline. Balloon tamponade helps in controlling the bleeding by providing mechanical pressure to the walls of uterus raising the intrauterine pressure to more than the systemic arterial pressure. Balloon tamponade is successful in arresting 80-90% of PPH cases. Failing this, woman should be shifted to the operation theater for second-line methods.
- Aortic compression is temporary but effective method to stop bleeding and buy some time for the shifting of the patient to operation theater or arranging blood and blood products for transfusion. Aortic compression is applied just above the umbilicus and slightly toward the left side by the fist of the care provider where the thumb is kept outside the fist. Aortic pulsation can be easily felt through the anterior abdominal wall in the immediate postpartum period. Pressure is applied directly over these pulsations. With the other hand, palpate the femoral pulse with four fingers parallel to and just below

TABLE 3: Pharmacological management of PPH.

Drug	Oxytocin	Ergometrine	15-Methyl-prostaglandin F2α	Misoprostol	Tranexamic acid
Dose and route	Infuse 20 units in 1,000 mL of isotonic crystalloid @ 60 drops per minute	IM or IV slow 0.2 mg	IM 0.25 mg	Sublingual 800 µg	1 g @ 1 mL/min over 10 minutes
Maintenance dose	Infuse 20 units in 1,000 mL of isotonic crystalloid @ 40 drops per minute	• Repeat 0.2 mg after 15 minutes • If need 0.2 mg can be repeated 4 hourly	0.25 mg every 15 minutes		1 g if bleeding continues even after 30 minutes or stops but restarts after 24 hours
Maximum dose	Not more than 3 L of oxytocin containing IV fluid	5 doses (maximum 1 g)	8 doses (maximum 2 g)		
Precautions and contraindications	Do not give IV bolus	Pre-eclampsia, hypertension, and heart disease	Asthma	Asthma	

the inguinal ligament to check for the adequacy of compression. If the femoral pulsation is not obliterated that means the pressure exerted is not adequate.

- *Nonpneumatic antishock garment (NASG):* This is a life-saving garment, which can be used in case of uncontrolled hemorrhage. It stops bleeding, reverses shock, and stabilizes the patient's condition so that patient can be transferred to the higher center safely. NSAG is effective in reducing blood loss by 50–78%.
- *Apply hemostatic compression sutures:* These hemostatic sutures provide compression to the uterine vascular system hence help in controlling the bleeding.
- If bleeding is still uncontrolled, systemic devascularization of uterine artery, ovarian arteries, internal iliac arteries should be done.
- Decision for hysterectomy should be taken, if the woman is still bleeding. A second experienced clinician should be involved in if decision for hysterectomy is taken. Decision for hysterectomy should be taken earlier than late.

Inversion of Uterus

If the fundus of the uterus is not palpable or a cupping is felt at fundus then it is suggestive of inversion of uterus. Do not start oxytocin or stop infusion if already started. If placenta is still not separated do not separate at this point. Replace the fundus of the uterus manually, if fails do it by hydrostatic method. Once the uterus is replaced, start oxytocin 40 units in 500 mL of isotonic crystalloid. Continue bimanual uterine massage. Once, the uterus is contracted then the continue oxytocin drip. In case the inversion is not corrected manually or by hydrostatics method, laparotomy followed by surgical management is needed.

Retained Placenta or Placental Tissue

Third common cause of PPH is retained placenta or placental tissue. Check for the placenta whether delivered or not. If delivered check for its completeness. In case the placenta is not delivered, start oxytocin infusion 40 units in 500 mL of isotonic crystalloids and deliver the placenta by CCT. If still not delivered, one can try injecting 10 units of oxytocin in the umbilical cord and then removing the placenta. If the placenta is still undelivered, patient should be shifted to operation theater and manual removal of placenta under general anesthesia should be attempted. A single shot of ampicillin or third generation cephalosporins should be given, if manual removal of placenta is attempted. Care should be taken in case the patient has previous cesarean or history of surgical abortion as it can be placenta accreta/percreta.

In case the placenta is delivered but a piece of it is missing, the same can be removed digitally or using sponge holder.

Trauma to the Genital Tract

If episiotomy was given, look for the site if it is repaired properly or not. Look for vaginal or cervical lacerations or tears and repair as required. Labor wards should have good lights for this purpose. In case patient is not able to cooperate for examination or the tear is deep to be seen in labor ward, the bleeding site should be packed and woman should be shifted to the operation theater for visualization of the tear and repair under anesthesia.

Coagulopathy

If all the other causes are ruled out or the coagulation profile is deranged that means the bleeding is due to coagulation failure. Woman should receive adequate blood products for correction.

■ MAIN THERAPEUTIC GOALS OF MANAGEMENT OF MASSIVE HEMORRHAGE[11]

- Hemoglobin (Hb) > 8 g/dL
- Platelet count > 50,000/L
- Prothrombin time (PT) less than 1.5 times normal
- Activated partial thromboplastin time (APTT) less than 1.5 times normal
- Fibrinogen > 2 g/L.

TABLE 4: Fluid and blood component therapy.[3]

Nature of fluid	
Crystalloid	Up to 2 liters of prewarmed isotonic crystalloid
Colloid	Up to 1.5 liters of colloid until blood is available
Blood	Group specific red cells as soon as possible in case of immediate transfusion group O, RhD –ve, and K –ve red cell units
Fresh frozen plasma	If prothrombin time (PT) or activated prothrombin time (APTT) is prolonged and hemorrhage is ongoing, administer 12–15 mL/kg of FFPs If hemorrhage continues after 4 units of red blood cell transfusion administer 4 units of FFPs even if hemostats tests are not available (1:1 protocol)
Platelets	if platelet count is less than 75 × 10^9/L Or if hemorrhage is ongoing give one pool platelets
Cryoprecipitates	Administer 2 pools of if hemorrhage is still ongoing and fibrinogen is < 2 g/L

CHAPTER 12A: Golden Hour Concept and First Response

Box 1: Measures to be taken during minor PPH (blood loss 500–1000 mL) without clinical shock.

- Intravenous access (one IV cannula 14 gauge)
- Blood sample at least 20 mL for blood group, complete blood count, and coagulation profile
- Vital charting (PR, BP, RR, and temperature) charting every 15 minutes
- Start crystalloid infusion

(BP: blood pressure; PPH: postpartum hemorrhage; PR: pulse rate; RR: respiratory rate)

Box 2: Measures to be taken during major PPH (blood loss greater than 1,000 mL) and continuing to bleed or clinical shock.

- Assess airway, breathing, and circulation
- Position the woman flat
- Keep the woman warm
- Continuous vital monitoring (PR, BP, and RR) and checking for temperature every 15 minutes
- Oxygen by mask (high concentration 10–15 L/min)
- Secure IV lines (2 large bore cannula 14/16 gauge), once appropriately trained staff is available, consider arterial line for monitoring
- Take 20 mL of blood sample for blood group and cross matching (at least 4 units of blood), complete blood count, coagulation profile, renal, and liver function test)
- Catheterize to empty the bladder and to monitor the output
- Transfuse blood and blood products as soon as possible
- While waiting for blood start IV fluids, infuse up to 3.5 liters of warmed clear fluids (initially 2 liters of warmed isotonic crystalloids, further resuscitation can continue with additional isotonic crystalloids or colloids)
- Once the bleeding is controlled, consider transfer to intensive care unit or high dependency unit in delivery suit for monitoring
- Proper documentation of fluid balance, blood, blood products, and procedures

(BP: blood pressure; PPH: postpartum hemorrhage; PR: pulse rate; RR: respiratory rate)

Box 3: Key points to remember.

- PPH is most common but avoidable cause of maternal deaths worldwide
- Every woman is at risk of PPH though some are at greater risk
- Active management of third stage should be universally practiced to avoid PPH
- Too little and too late is the cause of mortality. Too little uterotonics, blood, and fluid replacement. Too late diagnosis of PPH, call to the senior clinician and decision for surgical management to arrest bleeding
- One should not wait for laboratory results to start blood, it should be based upon clinical assessment
- Decision for hysterectomy should be taken in time and a second experienced surgeon should be involved in decision making
- Sooner the resuscitation starts more are the chances of survival

Fluid replacement is the most crucial component of the PPH management. Around 3.5 liters of fluid should be infused while awaiting for the blood. Initial 2.5 liters should be prewarmed isotonic crystalloids which should be infused as fast as it can be followed by up to 1.5 liters of colloids while waiting for the blood (Table 4).

Blood transfusion is guided by the clinical assessment and the laboratory parameters. But one should not wait for the laboratory results to start blood. Blood should be transfused as early as possible (Table 4 and Boxes 1 to 3).

If the bleeding is still continuing and the laboratory results are not available then after 4 units of blood FFPs should be transfused @ 12–15 mL/kg until the laboratory results are not available. Early transfusion of FFPs should be considered in case of suspected coagulopathy like in cases of abruption, amniotic fluid embolism, or where the diagnosis of PPH was delayed. In case the PT/APTT is more than 1.5 times, the normal FFPs should be transfused more vigorously @ 15 mL/kg.

Platelet transfusion should be considered when the platelet count is less than 75×10^9/L.

Cryoprecipitates should be transfused to maintain the fibrinogen level above 2 g/L.

CONCLUSION

Though certain women are at increased risk of PPH it can happen to any women so the health care provider need to be vigilant all the time. Early detection, prior preparedness and timely management is the key to the success.

REFERENCES

1. Say L, Chou D, Gemmill A, et al. Global causes of maternal death: A WHO systematic analysis. Lancet Glob Health. 2014;2:e323-33.
2. Montgomery AL, Ram U, Kumar R, et al.; For the Million Death Study Collaborators. Maternal Mortality in India: Cause and healthcare service use based on national reprsentative survey. PLoS ONE. 2014;9(1): e83331.
3. RCOG. (2016). Prevention and management of postpartum haemorrhage, green top guidelines No.52, December 2016. [online] Available from: https://obgyn.onlinelibrary.wiley.com/doi/epdf/10.1111/1471-0528.14178 [Last accessed July, 2019].
4. WHO. (2016). Recommendations on antenatal care a positive pregnancy experience. [online] Available from: https://www.who.int/reproductivehealth/publications/maternal_perinatal_health/anc-positive-pregnancy-experience/en/ [Last accessed July, 2019].
5. WHO. (2016). Intermittent iron and folic acid supplementation in non anaemic pregnant women 2016. [online] Available from: https://www.who.int/elena/titles/intermittent_iron_pregnancy_malaria/en/ [Last accessed July, 2019].
6. WHO. (2012). Active management of third stage of labour 2012. [online] Available from: https://apps.who.int/iris/bitstream/handle/10665/119831/WHO_RHR_14.18_eng.pdf?sequence=1 [Last accessed July, 2019].
7. Gulmezoglu AM, Lumbiganon P, Landoulsi S, et al. Active management of third stage of labour with or without controlled cord traction: A randomised, controlled, non infertility trial. Lancet. 2012;379(9827):1721-7.
8. WHO. (2018). Recommendation on Intrapartum care for a positivee pregnancy experience, 2018. [online] Available from: https://www.who.int/reproductivehealth/publications/intrapartum-care-guidelines/en/ [Last accessed July, 2019].
9. WHO. (2012). Recommendation for the prevention and treatment of postpartum haemorrhage. Geneva: WHO. [online] Available from: https://www.who.int/reproductivehealth/publications/maternal_perinatal_health/9789241548502/en/ [Last accessed July, 2019].
10. WOMAN trial collaborates. Effect of early tranexamic acid administration on mortality, morbidity, hystrectomy, and other morbidities in women with postpartum haemorrhage (WOMAN): An international, randomised, double-blind, placebo-controlled trial. Lancet. 2017;389:2105-16.
11. Hunt BJ, Allard S, Keeling D, et al.; British Committee for Standards in Haematology. A practical guideline for the management of major haemorrhage. Br J Haematol. 2015;170: 788-803.

12B Atonic Postpartum Hemorrhage

Srinivas Krishna Jois

INTRODUCTION

Across the globe, preventable causes kill around 830 women per day during pregnancy and childbirth of which 99% happen in developing countries.[1] There is almost a 20 times difference in maternal mortality ratio between developing and developed countries (12/1L versus 239/1L).

The major causes for about 75% of these maternal deaths are:[2]
- Hemorrhage [mostly postpartum hemorrhage (PPH)] around 40%
- Sepsis—10%
- Hypertensive disorders of pregnancy—5%
- Intrapartum complications—5%
- Complications of unsafe abortions—8%
- Others—32%.

Some of the facts about PPH are:
- Unpredictable in 60% cases (no identifiable risk factors)
- Occurs in 2–11% (may be up to 20%) of deliveries
- Of the 14 million per annum case fatality is 1%
- Most common cause is atony and severe PPH occurs in 1/1,000 deliveries.

DEFINITION

- Loss of more than 500 mL of blood from the genital tract after vaginal delivery or 1,000 mL of blood following cesarean section is defined as PPH (after 20 weeks of gestation and 24 hours of delivery)
- Any hemorrhage that warrants transfusion
- Hemorrhage resulting in a 10% drop in hemoglobin (Hb)
- Any amount of blood loss after delivery, which alters the vital parameters [pulse, blood pressure (BP), and respiration]—this could be a practical definition.

Classification of the PPH as given by Royal College of Obstetricians and Gynaecologists (RCOG) is:
- Minor—500–1,000 mL loss
- Moderate—1–2 L
- Major (> 1 L)
- Severe—>2 L.

Another clinically applicable classification has been shown in the following Table 1, which has been proposed by Benedetti.[3] The classification also highlights the management option for them.

ETIOLOGY

The famous 4 'T's for the etiology of PPH[4] are tone (70%), tissue (10%), trauma (20%), and thrombin (1%).

An analysis of various risk factors for PPH shows that many of the antenatal factors (Table 2) and some of the intranatal factors (Table 3) can be considered as predictors of PPH, though PPH is not predictable in 60% of cases.

The strongest predictors are previous PPH, emergency cesarean delivery, oxytocin augmentation, general anesthesia, mediolateral episiotomy, macrosomia (when baby >4.5 kg), and prolonged 3rd stage.

TABLE 1: Proposed classification.

Hemorrhage class	Estimated blood loss (mL)	Blood volume loss (%)	Clinical signs and symptoms
0 (normal loss)	<500	<10	None
		ALERT LINE	
1	500–1000	15	Minimal
		CTTONLINE	
2	1200–1500	20–25	↓ urine output ↑ pulse rate ↑ respiratory rate Postural hypontension Narrow pulse pressure
3	1800–2100	30–35	Hypotension Tachycardia Cold clammy Tachypnea
4	> 2400	>40	Profound shock

Need observation ± replacement therapy
Replacement therapy and oxytocics
Urgent active management
Critical active management (50% mortality if not managed actively)

Source: Benedetti

TABLE 2: Antenatal risk factors for PPH.

Antenatal risk factors	odd's ratio
Age >35 years[5]	1.5 (95% CI; 1.2–1.9) for vaginal delivery 1.8 (95% CI; 1.2–2.7) for cesarean delivery
Asian ethnicity[6]	1.8 (95% CI; 1.4–2.2)
BMI > 30[7]	1.5 (95% CI; 1.2–1.8)
Grand multiparity[8]	No association
Primiparity[5]	1.6 (95% CI; 1.4–1.9)
Prolonged pregnancy[7]	1.37 (95% CI; 1.28–1.46)
Macrosomia[9] Baby weight: • 4,000–4,499 g • 4,501–4,999 g • 5,000 g and more	 1.69 (95% CI; 1.58–1.82) 2.15 (95% CI; 1.86–2.48) 2.03 (95% CI; 1.33–3.09)
Multiple pregnancy[10]	RR 1.88 (95% CI; 1.81–1.95)
Leiomyoma[11]	1.9 (95% CI; 1.2–3.1)
APH[6]	1.8 (95% CI; 1.3–2.3)
Past PPH[6]	2.2 (95% CI; 1.7–2.9)
Previous cesarean delivery[5]	3.1 (95% CI; 2.1–4.4)
Multiple pregnancy[12]	3.30 (1.00–10.60)

(APH: antepartum hemorrhage; BMI: body mass index; PPH: postpartum hemorrhage)

TABLE 3: Intrapartum risk factors for postpartum hemorrhage.

Factors	Odd's ratio
Induced labor[5]	1.5 (95% CI; 1.2–1.7)
Prolonged labor[5]	1.6 (95% CI; 1 to 1.6)
Prolonged 2nd stage[5]	1.6 (95% CI; 1.1–2.1)
3rd stage:[13]	
• 10 min	2.1 (95% CI; 1.6–2.6)
• 20 min	4.3 (95% CI; 3.3–5.5)
• 30 min	6.2 (95% CI; 4.6–8.2)
Epidural analgesia[5]	1.3; but the 95% CI extended from 1 to 1.63
Operative vaginal delivery[12]	1.66 (95% CI; 1.06–2.60)
Sequential instrument usage[5]	1.9 (95% CI; 1.1–3.2)
Elective versus emergency CS	No significant difference
Mediolateral episiotomy[12]	4.67 (95% CI; 2.59–8.43)
Chorioamnionitis[14]	1.3 (95% CI; 1.1–1.7) at vaginal birth to 2.69 (95% CI; 1.44–5.03) at cesarean section
Oxytocin augmentation[15]	3.32 (95% CI; 2.05–5.93)
Emergency CS[15]	4.75 (95% CI; 1.32–12.96)
General anesthesia[14]	2.90 (1.90–4.50)

(CS: cesarean section)

PREVENTION

It is always very ideal to prevent PPH from occurring. The strategy could be:
- Look at the predictors, assess the risk and if modifiable or treatable like anemia correct them
- Keep the general condition of the woman and hemoglobin at an optimal level
- Plan the delivery in an comprehensive emergency obstetric care (CEmOC) facility, if probability of PPH is high
- Judicious use of induction and augmentation
- Avoid bladder distention
- Beware of uterine relaxants used concurrently, e.g. magnesium sulfate and nifedipine in pre-eclampsia
- Use of instrumental delivery by experts
- Restricted episiotomy
- Active management of 3rd stage of labor—10 U oxytocin intramuscular/intravenous (IM/IV) within 1 minute of delivery of the baby [World Health Organization (WHO)]. Controlled cord traction is used when delivery is conducted by skilled birth attendant
- If oxytocin not available other agents may be used for prophylaxis, e.g. 600 µg misoprostol orally (WHO)
- Carbetocin is licensed for the prevention of PPH during cesarean section
- Uterine massaging is not recommended for prophylaxis of PPH (WHO and RCOG)
- Consider the use of IV tranexamic acid (0.5–1.0 g), in addition to oxytocin, during cesarean section to reduce blood loss in women at increased risk of PPH[16]
- Cord traction is recommended during cesarean for prevention of PPH (WHO).

PREPARATION

In spite of all prediction and preventive measures being followed, the inevitable is always hanging like a sword on the obstetrician. So preparedness is very important for an individual, team, and the institution.
- Periodic drills, daily scrutiny of the drugs, equipment, their availability, and operational details are very important.
- Updating staff about the emergency care for a bleeding woman has to be done often in the form of skill drills, at least once in 6–12 months (RCOG).
- High dependency unit (HDU) and intensive care unit (ICU) availability too is very crucial.
- Availability of blood and blood products and daily updates provided by the blood bank officer to the obstetricians regarding the availability of blood of different groups are desirable.
- An uninterrupted supply of group O, Rh negative blood can be really life saving.
- Also an emergency bell in the labor room, which alerts the team for an effective and energetic management assures a timely care and averts deaths.
- An early involvement of senior doctor can make a difference in the outcome most of the times.
- Multidisciplinary team approach is a key to success.
- Clinical estimation of the blood loss is sufficient and other methods for quantitative assessment of blood loss need not be resorted to.

So, the preparedness of the team helps in saving mothers from this catastrophe.

PROCEED WITH THE TREATMENT

The intention of any of the interventions for PPH aims at achieving hemostasis—arrest of bleeding. Thus, the pneumonic hemostasis has evolved to streamline the management of PPH.

Further discussion here is mainly on the management of atonic PPH.

The options for the obstetrician while dealing with a case of PPH differ in a setting where postvaginal delivery PPH has been encountered and in cases of PPH following a cesarean delivery.

Postvaginal Delivery PPH

- The following facts need to be considered when a case of PPH is encountered following vaginal delivery.
- An important dictum in the management of PPH does not underestimate the blood loss.
- It has been seen that a person who conducts delivery always is reluctant to accept that there is PPH, so always go for a 2nd opinion in doubtful cases.
- Blood loss estimation is not always accurate and no one method can be recommended as the best.
- There could be a component of traumatic PPH too hence a routine examination of the genital tract is mandatory.
- With continued blood loss coagulation disorder can slowly creep in making the situation more complex.
- Early replacement of lost blood and arrest of continuing loss are the most important aspects of treatment.

The management may be discussed under:
- General management:
  - *Call for help*: People to help for interventions of every kind, so need to call senior obstetricians, junior doctors, staff nurses, group D workers, messengers to blood bank, etc.
  - Catheterize the bladder, secure 2 IV lines with No 14 (orange) or 16

(gray) gauge IV cannula, oxygen administration at a rate of 5-10 L/min, start on IV fluids (warmed crystalloids), if using colloids avoid hydroxyethyl starch,[16] send the blood for CBC, coagulation screen, renal function tests, grouping and cross matching, initiate the massive transfusion protocol (MTP) if the bleeding is heavy and continuing [inform the blood bank officer regarding the need for MTP and the blood bank will arrange for 4 units each of packed cells, FFP (fresh frozen plasma), and platelets].
- If prothrombin time (PT) and activated partial thromboplastin time (APTT) are prolonged by more than 1.5 times then FFP is required in excess of 12-15 mL/kg body weight.[16]
- Intensive care unit care if required.
- Target Hb% is 8 g%, platelets—50,000/mL and PT and APTT should be <1.5, and fibrinogen >2 g/L.[16]
- Monitoring the vitals frequently or continuously
- *Assessment of patient*: Patient has to be assessed for the amount of blood loss, general condition which may be done in the following ways (Table 4).
- *Evaluation:* Evaluate for the cause of bleeding. Of the four 'T's, find out the cause.
- *Ecbolics:* Oxytocin, misoprostol, methylergometrine, syntometrine, and Prostaglandin F2 alpha (PGF2α). The details of the dosage and frequency of administration are shown in Table 5. The recommendations for the use of uterotonics have been shown in Table 6.

TABLE 4: Methods of assessment.

Method	Parameters to be assessed
Vital parameters	Pulse, blood pressure (BP), respiratory rate—a systolic BP below 80 mm Hg, associated with worsening tachycardia, tachypnea and altered mental state, usually indicates a PPH in excess of 1500 mL[17]
Rule of 30	If there is a fall of *systolic BP* by 30 mm of Hg, if the *pulse* rate raises by 30 beats/min, if the *urine output* is <30 mL/hour, if the *respiratory rate* is >30/min, if the *hematocrit* is <30%, the amount of blood loss is >30% of the whole blood volume
Shock index	Pulse rate/systolic BP, if >1, it indicates that the patient is in shock

TABLE 5: Administration of uterotonic or hemostat drugs, dose, and frequency.

Drug	Dose	Frequency	Maximum
Oxytocin	5-10 U IM/IV stat and infusion	125 mL/hr of 20-40 U in 500 mL saline	About 100 U
Methylergometrine	0.2 mg IV if no contraindications	1st dose repeated after 15 minutes rest 2-4 hourly	5 doses
PGF2 Alpha	250 µg IM or intramyometrial	15 minutes once	8 doses
Misoprostol	600-1000 µg oral/sublingual/rectal	One time	-
Tranexamic acid	1 g slow IV	1 g for 8 hours	-

TABLE 6: Recommendations for the management of PPH.

	IV oxytocin	Methylergometrine	Carboprost	Misoprostol
WHO[18]	Strongly recommended	Can be used	Can be used	2nd choice if others not available
RCOG[19]	1st line—5 U IV, may be repeated. 40 U in 500 mL saline infusion at 125 mL/hr	1st line—ergometrine 0.5 mg IV after ruling out contraindications	250 µg, IM or intramyometrial	800 µg sublingual
ACOG[20]	10 U IM, 10–40 U as infusion in 500–1,000 mL	0.2 mg IM	250 µg IM/ intramyometrial	600–1,000 µg

(ACOG: American College of Obstetrics and Gynecology; PPH: postpartum hemorrhage; RCOG: Royal College of Obstetricians and Gynaecologists; WHO: World Health Organization)

- *Massaging* the uterus—not found to be useful for prevention but for management of atonic PPH, this is recommended as the first line.
- *Operation theater (OT) shifting/continuing oxytocin:* When the general and medical measures fail to control PPH, decision needs to be taken by a senior obstetrician regarding further course of action. If controlled, continue oxytocics for about 8 hours and assess the need for blood and blood product transfusion. When bleeding continues, the mechanical methods—tamponade to be considered.
- *Tamponade:* Many a times by this time the parturient is exhausted and repeated instrumentation of vagina, uterine explorations and other interventions may be very uncomfortable to the patient and also an anesthetist may be of immense help in stabilizing the hemodynamic state of the woman. Hence, it may be ideal to carry further interventions in the OT. Bimanual compression could be a good method though uncomfortable both for the patient and the obstetrician.
- *The physiological basis of all the tamponade methods, devascularization or compression sutures is that, they slow down the circulation, decrease the pressure in uterines and thus encourage clotting.* It may be the observations of many of us that often an atonic uterus is encountered during cesarean with no bleeding which suggests that clots have already formed in the vessels arresting the bleeding. But an essential prerequisite for all these is adequacy of platelets and fibrinogen levels. In disseminated intravascular coagulation (DIC) thus no method helps to control bleeding.
- Tamponade could be with Bakri balloon (Fig. 1) ideally, or other methods like using condoms, Sengstaken Blackmurray tube, double balloon catheter, and multiple Foley's catheters may be used. American College of Obstetrics and Gynecology (ACOG) also recommends using uterine packing.
- When the patient stops to bleed with tamponade, continue the same for 12-24 hours with continuation of oxytocics also.
- During an episode of PPH after a vaginal delivery, when these conservative measures fail, there is a need for surgical interventions, which requires laparotomy (Table 7).

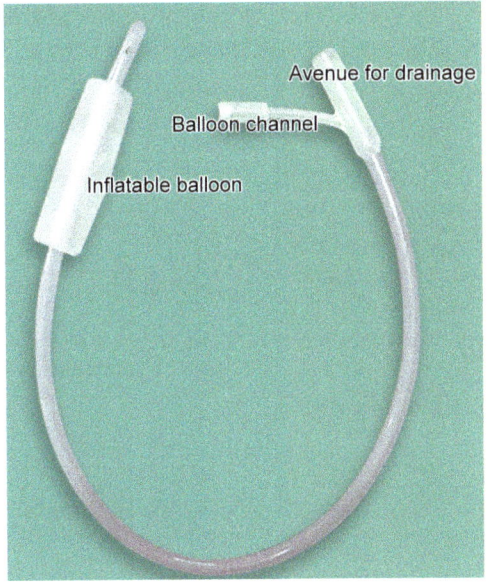

Fig. 1: Bakri balloon.

- But if there is availability of interventional radiology services, it may be prudent to consider *uterine artery embolization* at this point.
- But while managing a case of PPH, the *mode of treatment is not dictated by the protocol but the severity of the clinical situation.* Hence, it may be necessary to do a quick hysterectomy in a woman who is deteriorating fast and in whom conservative measures would take her to DIC quickly and the situation may go out of hand.
- Surgical measures are discussed under management of PPH during cesarean section.

PPH DURING CESAREAN DELIVERY

This situation clearly provides a better scenario for an obstetrician for the following reasons:

- Patient is anesthetized so exploration and interventions are easier
- Help of the anesthetist, staff nurses and monitoring are available
- Administration of uterotonics much easier, including intramyometrial carboprost option
- Intravenous line, and many a times in cases with predictors, blood also may be available
- Early surgical interventions can conserve the uterus and the life of the mother
- An assistant is available and prioritizing the options could be more rationally done (as the stress of PPH management sometimes may reduce the mental capacity of the surgeon).

General Measures

- These are usually in place like IV fluids, bladder drainage, monitoring vitals, etc.
- Others are the same as it is during a vaginal delivery
- Uterotonics and bimanual compression of the uterus are tried
- Assessment for the cause of bleeding is done.

Others

- Tamponade can be done through the uterine incision and the other end of the tamponade gadget is passed out through the cervix. One caution to be taken is to inflate the bulb of the gadget after closing the uterine incision so that the inflated balloon is not damaged during suturing.
- When the manual compression of the uterus successfully stops the bleeding that is an indication that this hemorrhage will respond to tamponade or compression sutures.
  - *Compression sutures*—varieties of compression sutures all attempting to compress the anterior uterine wall to the posterior wall are in practice.

TABLE 7: Recommendations on conservative interventions.

	WHO[18]	RCOG[19]	ACOG[20]
Massaging	Recommended	First method	First method
Colloids		May be used after initial resuscitation up to 1.5 L till blood is available, do not use hydroxyethyl starch	
Crystalloids	During initial resuscitation	Initial resuscitation with 2 L of warmed isotonic crystalloid—continue	
Balloon tamponade	PPH is refractory or when uterotonics not available	First-line mechanical method	Foley or Bakri balloon when compression fails
Aortic compression	As a temporary measure	Temporary but effective	
Bimanual compression	As a temporary measure		First method with massaging
Uterine packing	Not recommended		4 inch gauze soaked in 5,000 U of thrombin in 5 mL saline used
UAE	If persistent bleeding and resources available	If available	When tamponade fails and facilities available
NASG	As a temporary measure		
Surgical interventions	Persistent bleeding with failure of conservative measures	After 3rd dose of carboprost, depending on clinical situation	Decided based on clinical situation

Blank areas indicate no mention of the intervention in the guidelines as recommendations

(ACOG: American College of Obstetrics and Gynecology; NASG: nonpneumatic antishock garment; UAE: uterine artery embolization; PPH: postpartum hemorrhage; RCOG: Royal College of Obstetricians and Gynaecologists; WHO: World Health Organization)

- One of the most popular compression sutures, which is very comfortable to place during a cesarean section is B-Lynch compression sutures (Figs. 2A and B).[21]
- Most of the professional organizations recommend this during a cesarean section PPH, as this requires an opening in the uterus. If this needs to be applied following a vaginal delivery PPH, uterus needs to be opened with an incision similar to Kerr's incision.
- A delayed absorbable suture like Vicryl No 1 may be used for this purpose.
- A modification of this called Hayman's stitch (Figs. 3A and B) is an alternative which does not require opening of the uterus.[22] So postvaginal delivery PPH and postcesarean PPH in which it is found that uterus is atonic after closure of the uterine incision, Hayman's suture may be ideal.
- Occasionally, when a small segment of the uterus is noncontractile especially at the site of the placental bed, square stitches (Cho's) may be useful (Figs. 4A and B).[23] Multiple square stitches also may be used in atonic uterus.

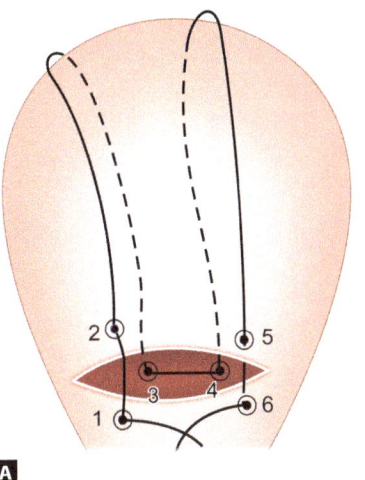
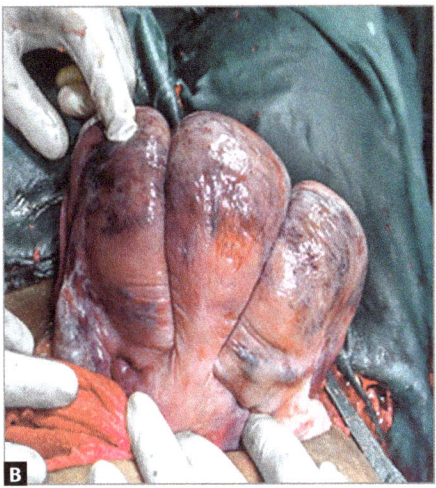

Point 1—3 cm below the incision on right side and 4 cm medial to the lateral border of uterus (on the left point 6). Point 2—3 cm above the incision on right side and 4 cm medial to the lateral border of uterus (on the left point 5). Point 3 and 4—on the posterior wall of the uterus at the isthmus.

Go through the anterior wall at 1, exit out through 2, brace the right side, and go posteriorly enter the cavity through point 3, exit through point 4 posterior to anterior brace the uterus, enter the cavity through 5 on left side, and exit out at 6. The cut ends at 1 and 6 are tied over lower segment with an assistant compressing the uterus cephalocaudally.

Figs. 2A and B: B-Lynch sutures—diagrammatic representation and picture.

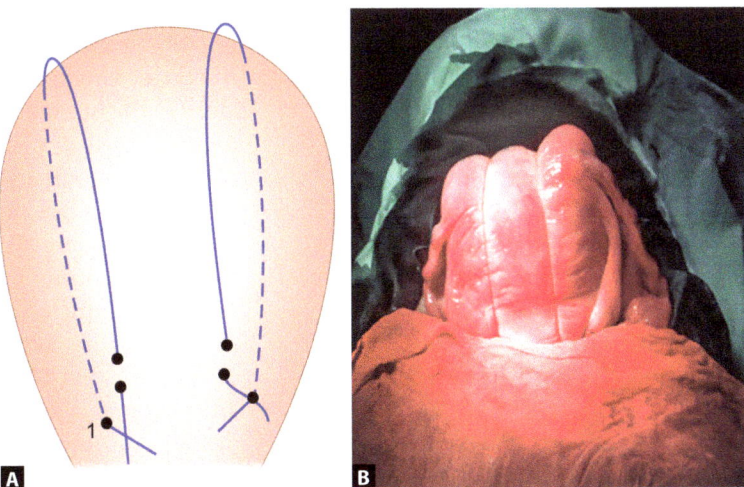

Go through point 1 about 2–3 cm from the lateral wall of the uterus in the lower segment, exit through the posterior wall. Take the suture material on to the fundus like a brace and bring it to the point 1. Same stitch is repeated on the left side too. Cut ends of the first stitch and later the second one are tied after the assistant holds the uterus compressing the uterus in a cephalocaudal direction.

Figs. 3A and B: Hayman's sutures—diagrammatic representation and picture.

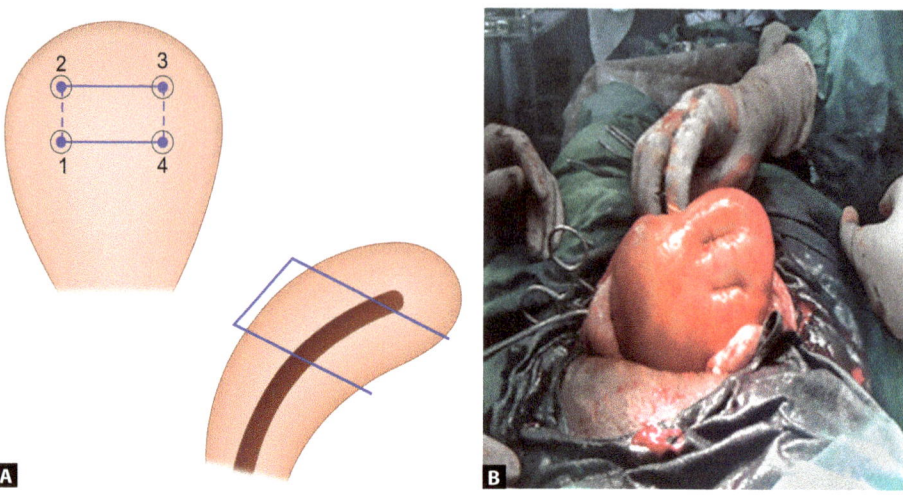

Cho's square stitch:
At point 1 pierce through both anterior and posterior walls and at point 2 come from posterior to anterior wall. Go through both the walls at point 3 and come out anteriorly through point 4. Tie the free ends.

Figs. 4A and B: Cho's square sutures—diagrammatic representation and picture.

- For lower segment bleeding specially in placenta previa, a cervicoisthmic apposition stitches[21] have been tried successfully (Figs. 5A to C).[24]
- A comparison of various suturing methods has shown success to the tune of 95–100% in various studies.[22] So to decide about the type of compression suture,[25] it is at the discretion of the surgeon depending on the experience, exposure, and expertise.
- *Stepwise devascularization*: This is another option for controlling PPH either during a cesarean section or during a vaginal delivery, especially when the conservation of the uterus is very important.
    - Its principle is that, when the principle arterial supply to the uterus is cut off, the whole system behaves like venous system with a slow and low pressure circulation which substantially reduces bleeding and also encourages formation of capillary clots.
    - Initially, uterine artery ligation at a site on the lateral wall of the uterus close to the incision site including a small portion of myometrium can be done initially on one side, later on both sides. Lower segment bleeding may benefit from ligation of the descending branch also. It does not require dissecting the uterine artery as shown in the photograph (Fig. 6).
    - The next step is to ligate the utero-ovarian anastomosis at the corneal region in the broad ligament. Again both sides one after the other if required (Fig. 7).
    - Internal iliac artery (anterior division) ligation is the last resort amongst devascularization

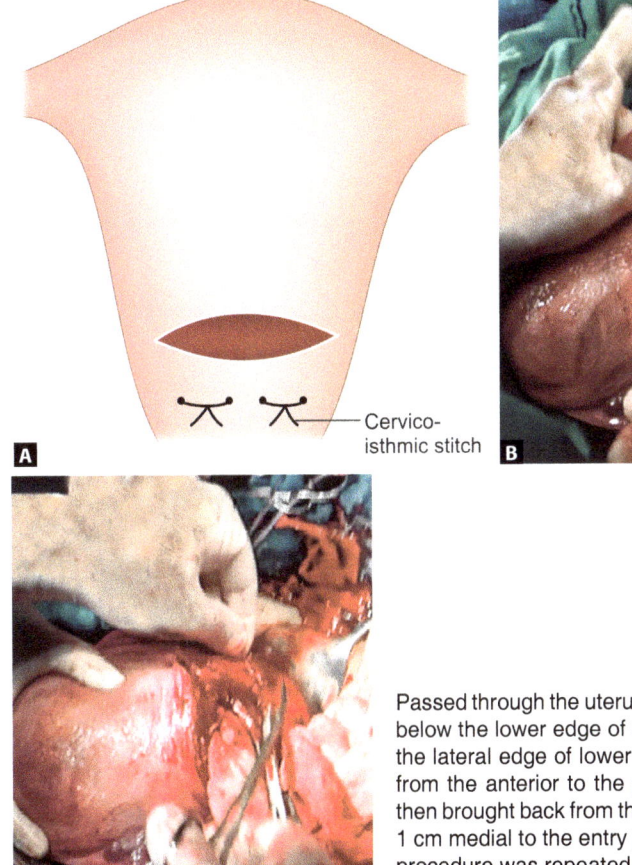

Cervico-isthmic stitch

Passed through the uterus above the bladder reflection, 3 cm below the lower edge of uterine incision and 2 cm medial to the lateral edge of lower segment. The needle was passed from the anterior to the posterior aspect of the uterus and then brought back from the posterior through the anterior wall 1 cm medial to the entry point and tied anteriorly. The same procedure was repeated on the other side.

Figs. 5A to C: Cervicoisthmic apposition sutures—diagrammatic representation and picture.

techniques and requires expertise. Proper identification of the artery is very important (Figs. 8A to C).

Both compression sutures and devascularization measures have been shown not to compromise the future fertility of the woman by various studies.

HYSTERECTOMY

Hysterectomy though should be the last resort in atonic PPH, it should never be delayed if it could be life saving. The decision needs to be taken as early as required dictated by the condition of the patient, availability of resources for conservative management, expertise of the surgeon, and not as per the stepwise approach in the management of atonic PPH.

The golden hour concept is most important in these patients and hysterectomy could become the first option in many patients.

Whenever resorted to, it should preferably be a sub-total hysterectomy unless the bleeding is from the lower segment. This may be facilitated by the approach of "clamp-cut,

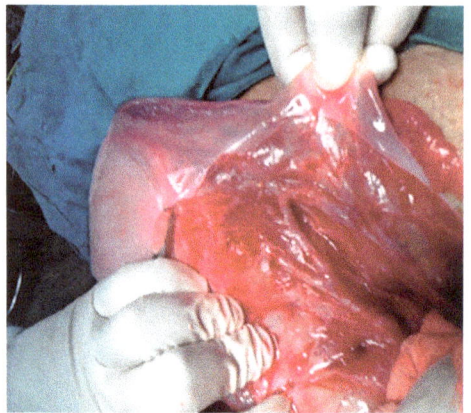

Fig. 6: Uterine artery dissected in a case of supralevator hematoma due to bleeding from descending branch.

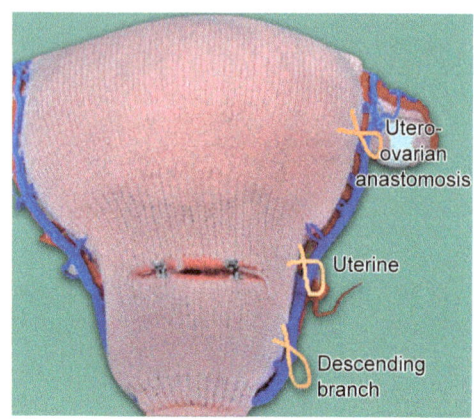

Fig. 7: Sites of devascularization.

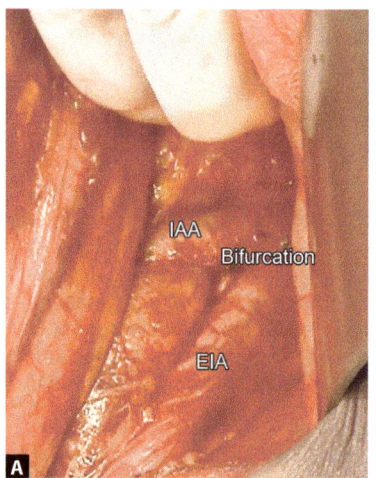

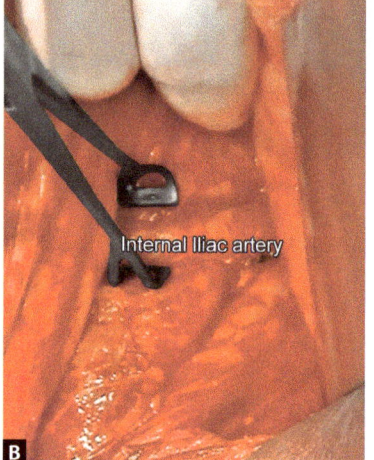

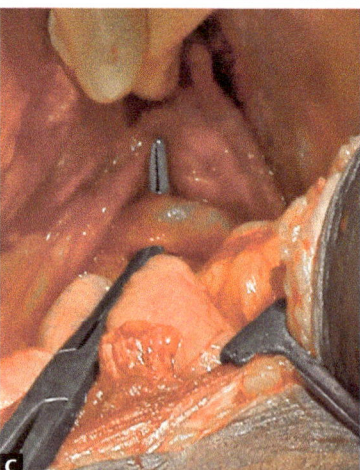

Figs. 8A to C: Internal iliac artery dissected and identified the bifurcation of common iliac artery (IAA—internal artery-anterior branch and EIA—external iliac artery), held with Babcock's, and ready for ligation.

clamp-cut and after uterines are clamped and cut, ligate the stumps" rather than the policy of "clamp-cut-ligate".

When resorted to, hysterectomy needs opinions from two qualified gynecologists, documentation of this is very important.

Total hysterectomy, if becomes necessary; identification of vagina and limit of dissection are difficult and a senior person has to be involved for this.

USE OF BLOOD AND BLOOD PRODUCTS[19]

In cases of PPH, a very important aspect of management is replacement of blood and clotting factors:

- Though the initial resuscitation involved rapid infusion of 2 L of isotonic crystalloids (normal saline), followed by colloids up to 1.5 L if blood is not available.
- Replacement of blood is the most appropriate therapy in this situation.
- There are no defined criteria to define the level at which transfusion is to be initiated. But if Hb is <6 g% transfusion is necessary and if >10 g most often not necessary.
- For dire emergency, group O, Rh negative, and if feasible K negative blood should be used.
- Cross-matched blood should be arranged as soon as possible.
- Continued bleeding with the coagulation results awaited, consider transfusion of FFP (12–15 mL/kg body weight) after transfusing 4 units of packed cells.
- If PT and APTT are prolonged for more than 1.5 times higher doses of FFP are required. Coagulation tests may have to be repeated once in half an hour, if bleeding is continuing.
- Consider early use of FFP in cases of PPH associated with abruption placenta, intrauterine fetal demise (IUFD), and amniotic fluid embolism.
- Cryoprecipitate is the best when fibrinogen levels are very low.
- If even with 8 units of packed cells, bleeding continues and the coagulation results are yet to arrive, cryoprecipitate has to be used along with 1 pool of platelets.
- Platelets are transfused with a level of 75,000/cu mm during PPH.
- The target levels are Hb—8 g; platelets—50,000/cu mm; and PT and APTT—<1.5.

SPECIAL CONSIDERATIONS

Recombinant Factor VIIa

- Recombinant factor VIIa has been used successfully in many cases and some studies have reported good results. The prerequisites for the action of this is normal pH, normal level of platelets, and fibrinogen; and hypothermia reduces its efficacy.
- The limiting factor is its cost.
- It is not recommended for routine use.

Cell Salvage[19]

In this process, the blood during any bleeding episode is collected, filtered and washed, and used for the same patient.

If equipment and facilities are available, this should be considered especially during cesarean section and also during vaginal delivery. It is very useful in women refusing transfusion (Jehova's witness).

Massive Transfusion Protocols[19]

In massive hemorrhage, initiate MTP, which involves packed cells, FFP, and platelets given in the ratio of 1:1:1.

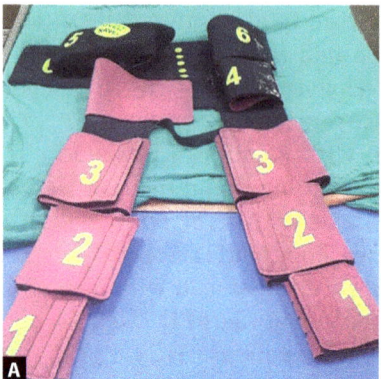 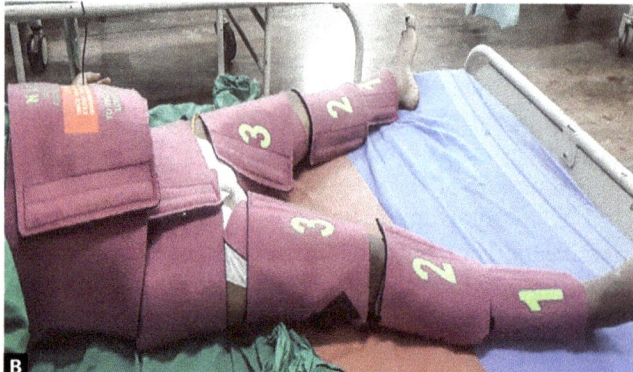

Figs. 9A and B: (A) Nonpneumatic antishock garment (NASG); (B) NASG applied to a patient with PPH.

One should be cautious about transfusion-associated circulatory overload (TACO) and transfusion-associated lung injury (TRALI) when MTP is initiated early in PPH.

Pulmonary edema could be a problem.

Nonpneumatic Antishock Garment

Nonpneumatic antishock garment is a temporary wrap for the lower half of the body which helps to decrease the blood supply to the lower half of the body and maintains perfusion to the vital organs (Figs. 9A and B).

It provides some time, especially while transferring a patient from the labor room to the OT, from one center to the other.

CONCLUSION AND KEY POINTS

- Postpartum hemorrhage is a nightmare for an obstetrician.
- Should be managed energetically at the earliest opportunity—"golden hour".
- Management is not dictated by any hierarchy in the management protocol.
- Involvement of a senior obstetrician makes a difference in the outcome.
- Drills should happen so that the team is in an alert state always, as the catastrophe most often in unpredictable.
- Blood and blood products should be judiciously used.
- Death of a woman due to PPH is one of the preventable deaths and all efforts should be made by every individual and institutions to avert this tragedy.
- Hysterectomy to be resorted to with a second opinion.
- Blood transfusion protocols should be adhered to.
- Onsite blood availability makes a great difference.
- Multidisciplinary team approach in cases of severe acute maternal morbidity resulting from PPH can save lives.
- Active management of third stage of labor can prevent about 60% of PPH.
- Every obstetrician should be individualizing the tamponade method, compression sutures, and devascularization methods as per his ability, exposure, competence, and availability of resources.
- Do not waste precious time for total hysterectomy, resort to subtotal hysterectomy except in cases with lower segment bleeding.

REFERENCES

1. WHO. (2018). factsheet on Maternal mortality 16th Feb 2018. [online] Available from: https://

1. www.who.int/news-room/fact-sheets/detail/maternal-mortality [Last accessed July, 2019].
2. Say L, Chou D, Gemmill A, Tunçalp Ö, et al. Global causes of maternal death: A WHO systematic analysis. Lancet Glob Health. 2014;2(6):e323-33.
3. Benedetti T. Obstetric haemorrhage. In: Gabbe SG, Niebyl JR, Simpson JL (Eds). A Pocket Companion to Obstetrics, 4th edition. New York: Churchill Livingstone; 2002.
4. Anderson J, Etches D, Smith D. Postpartum haemorrhage. In: Damos JR, Eisinger SH, (Eds). Advanced Life Support in Obstetrics (ALSO) Provider Course Manual. Kansas: American Academy of Family Physicians; 2000. pp. 1-15.
5. Ohkuchi A, Onagawa T, Usui R, et al. Effect of maternal age on blood loss during parturition: a retrospective multivariate analysis of 10,053 cases. J Perinat Med. 2003;31:209-15.
6. Magann EF, Evans S, Hutchinson M, et al. Postpartum hemorrhage after vaginal birth: an analysis of risk factors. S Med J. 2005;98:419-22.
7. Usha KT, Hemmadi S, Bethel J, et al. Outcome of pregnancy in a woman with an increased body mass index. Br J Obstet Gynaecol. 2005;112:768-72.
8. Humphrey MD. Is grand multiparity an independent predictor of pregnancy risk? A retrospective observational study. Med J Aust. 2003;179:294-6.
9. Stotland NE, Caughey AB, Breed EM, et al. Risk factors and obstetric complications associated with macrosomia. Int J Gynaecol Obstet. 2004;87:220-6.
10. Walker MC, Murphy KE, Pan S, et al. Adverse maternal outcomes in multifetal pregnancies. Br J Obstet Gynaecol. 2004;111:1294-6.
11. Akrivis C, Varras M, Bellou A, et al. Primary postpartum haemorrhage due to a large submucosal nonpedunculated uterine leiomyoma: a case report and review of the literature. Clin Exp Obstet Gynecol. 2003;30:156-8.
12. Combs CA, Murphy EL, Laros RK Jr. Factors associated with postpartum hemorrhage with vaginal birth. Obstet Gynecol. 1991;77:69-76.
13. Magann EF, Evans S, Chauhan SP, et al. The length of the third stage of labor and the risk of postpartum hemorrhage. Obstet Gynecol 2005;105:290-3.
14. Combs CA, Murphy EL, Laros RK Jr. Factors associated with hemorrhage in cesarean deliveries. Obstet Gynecol. 1991;77:77-82.
15. Ekin A, Gezer C, Solmaz U, et al. Predictors of severity in primary postpartum hemorrhage. Arch Gynecol Obstet. 2015;292(6):1247-54.
16. Mavrides E, Allard S, Chandraharan E, et al.; on behalf of the Royal College of Obstetricians and Gynaecologists. Prevention and management of postpartum haemorrhage. BJOG. 2016;124: e106-49.
17. Allgöwer M, Burri C. Shock index. Dtsch Med Wochenschr. 1967;92:1947-50.
18. WHO. (2012). WHO recommendations for the prevention and treatment of postpartum haemorrhage. [online] Available from: https://apps.who.int/iris/bitstream/handle/10665/75411/9789241548502_eng.pdf?sequence=1 [Last accessed July, 2019].
19. RCOG. (2016).Prevention and management of post partum haemorrhage—Green top guidelines No 52, Dec 2016. [online] Available from: https://obgyn.onlinelibrary.wiley.com/doi/full/10.1111/1471-0528.14178 [Last accessed July, 2019].
20. Committee on Practice Bulletins-Obstetrics. ACOG practice bulletin No 183: Postpartum hemorrhage. Obstet Gynecol. 2017;130(4): e168-86.
21. B-Lynch C, Coker A, Lawal AH, et al. The B-Lynch surgical technique for the control of massive postpartum haemorrhage: an alternative to hysterectomy? Five cases reported. Br J Obstetrical Gynaecol. 1997;104:372-5.
22. Ghezzi F, Cromi A, Uccella S, et al. The Hayman technique: a simple method to treat postpartum haemorrhage. BJOG. 2007;114:362-5.
23. Cho JH, Jun HS, Lee CN. Hemostatic suturing technique for uterine bleeding during cesarean delivery. Obstet Gynecol. 2000;96:129-31.
24. Das C, Mukherjee P, Choudhury N, et al. Isthmic-cervical apposition suture—an effective method to control postpartum hemorrhage during cesarean section for placenta previa. J Obstet Gynecol India. 2005;55(4)322-4.
25. Matsubara S, Yano H, Ohkuchi A, et al. Uterine compression sutures for postpartum hemorrhage: an overview. Acta Obstet Gynecol Scand. 2013;92:378-85.

Chapter 12C

Traumatic Postpartum Hemorrhage

Padmalatha Venkataram, Srimathy Raman

■ MAGNITUDE OF THE PROBLEM

Postpartum hemorrhage (PPH) is an important contributor to adverse maternal outcomes.[1] Prompt recognition and appropriate management in a timely manner by trained personnel are important to ensure good outcomes.[2] Although atonic PPH is the most common, 10-20% of PPH can be due to lower genital tract bleeding.[3,4] Maternal deaths due to PPH occurring because of lower genital tract bleeding are rare in the developed world. It is very difficult to get accurate figures but they can play a significant role especially if there is a poorly resourced maternity infrastructure.[5] The pneumonic PPH stands good even for traumatic PPH—prediction, prevention, and management of hemorrhage.

■ IDENTIFICATION OF POSTPARTUM HEMORRHAGE

Traumatic causes should be suspected and looked for when there is PPH and the uterus is found to be well-contracted.[2] Also if patients present with symptoms and signs of hypovolemic shock not correlating with the degree of external bleeding, it is important to exclude hematomas. Combination of atonic and traumatic PPH is not uncommon and can occur especially in women who have had prolonged labor followed by instrumental delivery. Careful and well-documented observations after delivery, i.e. 4th stage of labor are important as in patients with continued oozing blood loss estimation can be inaccurate and underestimated. This can happen in atonic PPH as well as in traumatic causes.

■ CAUSES OF TRAUMATIC POSTPARTUM HEMORRHAGE

This discussion excludes uterine rupture and inversion of the uterus since they are covered elsewhere. The various causes of lower genital tract bleeding include episiotomies and perineal tears, periurethral and periclitoral tears, vaginal lacerations, and cervical tears which can also present with hematomas. Increased vascularity which occurs in pregnancy increases the risk of developing tears and hematomas due to the stress of labor.[6] Tears and hematomas can happen both spontaneously or due to the interventions in labor.[5] Hematomas may also occur due to incomplete suturing of vaginal lacerations or episiotomy wherein the bleeding vessel or the apex has not been identified. They can also present with no obvious trauma after a normal delivery with intact vaginal epithelium.[7]

Pelvic hematomas may be divided into four types—vaginal, vulvar, vulvovaginal, broad ligament and retroperitoneal.[7] Generally, they can be classified into supra- and infralevator hematomas. Infralevator hematomas occur below the levator ani muscle while supralevator (broad ligament, retroperitoneal) occurs above the levator ani. Recognition of supralevator hematomas is difficult as they may not be obvious on genital tract examination. They may present with massive bleeding in the retroperitoneal space and they are also difficult to manage and so they are more worrisome.

RISK FACTORS

Assisted delivery (forceps or vacuum extraction), prolonged labor or precipitate labor, maternal obesity, large baby, and episiotomy are important risk factors for lower genital tract hemorrhage.[6-8] Rotational forceps increases the risk of occurrence of spiral vaginal tears.

Malpresentation, twins, shoulder dystocia, and presence of vulval varicosities all increase the risks of lower genital trauma. Coagulation disorders also predispose to increased occurrence of bleeding and hematoma.

PREVENTION OF POSTPARTUM HEMORRHAGE

A proactive approach is needed as with all obstetric complications. This includes correction of antenatal comorbidities such as anemia[1] as well as careful management of the different stages of labor. Labor management techniques such as use of partogram, identification, and correction of slow progress with adequate attention to hydration, pain relief, and support are important to prevent labor complications including PPH. It is important that adequate time is given in second stage. Also ensuring that cervix is fully dilated and provision of adequate perineal support with appropriate use of optimal episiotomy helps in decreasing the chances of traumatic PPH.[5]

Adequate postpartum care with modified early obstetric warning system (MEOWS) and when excessive blood loss is suspected or identified, immediate resuscitation steps should be commenced. Adequate and appropriate fluid replacement along with steps to tackle the bleeding by identifying the cause of bleeding is important.

Generally, the need for operative delivery/episiotomy increases the risk of PPH. It is important that adequate support and care are provided to reduce the need for these procedures so that the chance of bleeding is decreased. Availability of skilled and trained personnel especially in difficult deliveries is important both to prevent and manage complications appropriately. Coagulation defects should be suspected and identified and appropriate measures to correct them should be undertaken early.

DIAGNOSIS

Close monitoring in the 4th stage of labor—MEOWS chart is mandatory to identify problems early. Tachycardia and hypotension should be promptly identified and acted upon. Prompt general and abdominal examination should be performed. Distension of the abdomen and excessive tenderness might indicate intraperitoneal/broad ligament bleed especially with rupture uterus or forniceal tears. Height of the uterus should be noted and marked if vaginal hematomas are suspected. The uterus might be shifted to a side in case of broad ligament hematoma. Also many a time, there can be a combination of atonic and traumatic PPH as was mentioned earlier.

Bleeding which happens with the uterus well-contracted and especially following a difficult or instrumental vaginal delivery is an indication for a thorough and systematic examination of the upper genital tract. The characteristic feature of this trauma is steady fresh blood loss.

Systematic examination in the lithotomy position and if needed in theater is important. It is essential to have good relaxation and adequate lighting. Proper assistance and use of long, flat-bladed vaginal retractors are required in these patients to exclude upper vaginal and cervical tears. The entire vagina from perineum to cervix including the fornices should be examined for lacerations.[5,7]

If the source of bleeding is not identified and addressed promptly and adequately, there is always a risk of patient developing coagulation failure and its resultant comorbidities.

It is also important to do a complete examination especially after a rotational forceps delivery, as this is known to be associated with upper vaginal and cervical tears.

The examination involves placing one ring forceps to the anterior lip and grasping the cervix at the 2-o'clock position with a second ring forceps, and then progressively leap-frogging to ensure that the full circumference has been inspected.[5,7]

MANAGEMENT OF TRAUMATIC POSTPARTUM HEMORRHAGE

General Principles

Once the extent of the tear is identified, immediate steps to control the bleeding are important. Availability of senior personnel along with blood and blood products is important as with management of atonic PPH. Hospital protocols for management of PPH are needed and they need to be followed when extensive bleeding is identified. Also using an obstetric emergency box and a PPH kit can save time and lives. Staff training and skills drills help in effective team work in all obstetric emergency situations. External aortic compression[1] and use of Nonpneumatic antishock garment (NASG)[9] are other techniques to consider helping in stabilizing the patient while attempts to tackle bleeding are being done.

The initial steps in the management as in all emergencies include—call for help, assess airway, breathing, and circulation; commencing oxygen; and lying the patient flat, ensuring intravenous (IV) access with bloods drawn for investigations and commencing fluids and blood replacement as needed.[1] Early administration of tranexamic acid[10] and simultaneous measures to manage coexisting problems like atony is important. If unstable or source of bleeding difficult to identify, tight vaginal packing with 4 inch ribbon gauze before transferring to theater may help in decreasing the blood loss. Topical hemostatic agents (absorbable gelatin matrix and fibrin sealants) have a limited role in controlling traumatic PPH.[5] Continued bleeding despite all hemostatic measures may be a pointer to coagulopathy and it is important that the obstetrician triggers a massive blood transfusion protocol early.

Adequate anesthesia with regional techniques or general anesthesia in theater is needed to repair tears which have extended higher into the vagina or cervix.[2] Here we will only concentrate on the management of traumatic PPH.

Also after treatment, these women need to be closely monitored in a high dependency unit (HDU) setting with MEOWS chart. Due consideration to thromboembolism prophylaxis as well as being aware of complications of massive bleeding and transfusion including development of multiorgan failure is paramount. Multidisciplinary involvement with senior anesthetists and intensivist with support from hematologist is crucial especially in an unstable patient.[1]

Management of Tears

Perineal Tear Repair

The principles of repair are that the suturing of the tear/episiotomy is commenced proximal to the apex. It is important to use a continuous technique and the preferred suture material is polyglactin/polyglycolic acid. Also all dead spaces need to be obliterated and if unable to do so, a vaginal pack may be needed. Any identified third or fourth degree tears should be repaired as per the Royal College of Obstetricians and Gynaecologists (RCOG) guidelines.[11]

Episiotomy

Episiotomy increases the risk of PPH by four to five times and they can bleed heavily.[5] Hence, it is important to practice restrictive and selective use of episiotomy. Application of hemostat to the active bleeders to promote hemostasis should be a routine. Applying pressure with gauze on the area of bleeding till the sutures are taken can significantly reduce the bleeding.

Periurethral and Periclitoral Lacerations

Small periurethral and periclitoral lacerations can happen commonly especially in nulliparous woman when episiotomy is not performed because of the pressure to the anterior part by the presenting part. These may be managed with pressure for a couple of minutes and left unsutured if not bleeding. However, if there is significant bleeding they need to be repaired with a fine continuous suture after inserting a urethral catheter in order to avoid placement of sutures inadvertently in the urethra.[7]

Vaginal Tear Repair

There can be various different patterns of tears. There may be one or two tears of the vagina which are amenable to simple corrective suturing. Or there may be multiple tears which may make individual suturing difficult. Alternatively, the sutures may pull through the edematous tissue thereby causing more bleeding. The other possibility is that there is a deep vaginal tear extending into the abdominal cavity causing a retroperitoneal hematoma.

Superficial vaginal tears are repaired in a similar technique to perineal repair. An absorbable, suture material reaching the full depth of the tear ensures that there is no subsequent hematomas.[5,7]

It is also important to identify and ligate any bleeding vessels especially for deeper tears. Taking the suture as high as feasible on the vaginal wall, applying gentle traction and working cranially suturing the vaginal walls till the apex is reached is another useful method for repairing deep vaginal lacerations/extensions of the episiotomy. Vaginal packing may be needed in friable vaginal walls where suturing may be hard and also with unobliterable dead spaces as discussed earlier.[5,7] Repair of deep and extensive lacerations needs to be performed with adequate anesthesia and preferably in theater.

Lacerations which are higher and involve the vaginal vault or cervix may also be associated with tears in the uterus or result in broad ligament or retroperitoneal hematomas. The anatomical relation of the ureters and the bladder base to the lateral and anterior vaginal fornices and the rectum in posterior tears must be borne in mind when these tears are repaired. In such patients where a high extension is noted, a laparotomy may be needed and simultaneous abdominal and vaginal approach will facilitate repair while avoiding damage to these structures as these can lead to genitourinary fistulas. It is important to place an indwelling Foley and rectal examination is needed to prevent any suture placement in the rectum.

Vaginal packing with 4 inch ribbon gauze may be needed for 24–36 h to achieve vaginal tamponade. The technique is similar to uterine packing ensuring that the entire vaginal wall is packed (application on sides, front, back, top, and bottom). Thrombin-soaked or povidone iodine-soaked vaginal packs are an alternative which can be used. Sterile plastic drapes can be used to cover the pack and this aids easy removal and prevents bleeding from raw surfaces when the pack is removed. Insertion of a urinary Foley catheter and administration of broad-spectrum antibiotics are essential when pack is in situ.[5,7] Rüsch or Bakri balloon catheters and Blakemore-Sengstaken tubes also help in provision of tamponade.

Ventouse-related lacerations often are circular in nature and occur due to inadvertent incorporation of vaginal tissue into the ventouse when it slips or if not applied correctly. These are not linear but present as an area of missing vaginal tissue which has been denuded. As the tissues are friable, vaginal packing is generally advocated. Rectal and bladder injuries are rare but may occur with instrumental vaginal deliveries and identification is important as nonrecognition of a bladder or rectal laceration will result in fistula formation.

Cervical Tear

Minor cervical tears are common and may not even be detected. If the cervical lacerations are small and if not bleeding, they can be left alone. However, if they are bleeding or if they are longer than 2 cm, they need to be sutured. An absorbable suture is to be used and with a tapered needle. Suturing can be done either as an interrupted or with a figure-of-eight stitch after grasping the caudal edges of the laceration with a ring forceps (sponge holder). The suture can be held and used for retraction and further stitches taken cranially till the apex. It is important to ensure hemostasis has been achieved and if needed the ring forceps can be applied for some time to control oozing.[5,7]

Annular detachment of the cervix is extremely rare and occurs usually with a rigid or scarred cervix.[7] It is rare but small "bucket-handle" tears and small areas of detachment may be encountered in situations where delivery happens with a cervical stitch in situ or prolonged labor and unless bleeding, these tears may be left alone.

Selective arterial embolization can be tried if the bleeding from cervical and vaginal vault lacerations is not controlled by suturing. Hematomas also may need to be controlled by this technique. Laparotomy may be necessary, if the tear in the cervix is high, i.e. going beyond the internal os.

MANAGEMENT OF HEMATOMAS

Minor self-limiting infralevator/vulva hematomas happen commonly. Fortunately, massive hematomas are rare but when they happen, can be serious. They are classified, as we discussed earlier based on their location with reference to levator ani.

Infralevator Hematomas

They are usually due to injury to branches of the pudendal artery. They present with development of a tense mass covered by skin. They can also present with rectal pressure.

Initial management consists of resuscitation measures as discussed earlier. Small nonexpanding hematomas, which are less than 5 cm, can be managed conservatively with observation, treatment with icepacks, and adequate analgesia. It is; however; helpful to map the extent of the hematoma so that it can be used to check if there is increase in size.

In unstable patients or if the hematoma is expanding or is bigger than 5 cm, surgical exploration is necessary. It is always a good practice to make the incision in the vagina as this helps in decreasing any scarring.[5-7]

It is important to identify the bleeding points and once identified, figure-of-eight stitches are taken to achieve hemostasis. As discussed earlier, consideration for a vaginal pack and possibly a drain should be done, if there is any bleeding or cavity. These should be left for 24 hours along with a Foley catheter.

Supralevator Hematomas

This bleeding mainly comes from the descending branch of the uterine artery and the vaginal artery.[5,6]

These may present either immediately after delivery (around 50%) or can have a delayed presentation in the rest half of the cases. The presentation is varied and can range from lower abdominal pain to even shock in severe cases. Expectant management is appropriate for these broad ligament and retroperitoneal hematomas in stable patients with nonexpanding hematomas. Diagnostic techniques like ultrasound, CT, or MRI may be necessary to delineate the size and position of these hematomas.

Expectant management with careful monitoring of vitals can be considered. However, adequate resuscitation with IV fluids, blood, and blood products is needed along with administration of antibiotics. Packing of the vagina or balloon tamponade also can be attempted. However, if the patient becomes unstable, active intervention is indicated.[5-7]

The options include surgical exploration-laparotomy and proceed or radiological intervention in the form of selective arterial embolization.

- *Surgical management-Laparotomy and proceed:* This is indicated when there is a suspicion of an extension of cervical tear to the uterus or a uterine rupture as the cause of supralevator/broad ligament hematomas. Consideration can be given to internal iliac artery ligation and if unable to perform so or continued bleeding, hysterectomy may have to be considered to gain access to the vault and lateral pelvic walls.[7] Despite hysterectomy, persistent bleeding, and oozing may need tamponade with pelvic gauze packing or balloon tamponade which can be lifesaving.[6] To avoid a repeat laparotomy and to facilitate easy removal of pack through the vault, the distal end can be brought out through the vault.
- *Interventional radiology-Selective arterial embolization:* When the supralevator hematoma, which has no cervical or uterine extension is continuing to expand, these techniques can be used. This avoids the need for laparotomy with its attendant risks especially on an already unstable patient. The technique of selective arterial embolization may be employed but there are risks associated with the radiological procedure as well and the limited availability of expertise limits its widespread usage.

SUMMARY

Lower genital tract trauma as a cause of PPH should be suspected and looked for if there is ongoing bleeding with the uterus well contracted. Traumatic PPH is easy to tackle, if identified and controlled especially in lower genital bleeding. Volume replacement and correction of anemia, acidosis, and prevention of hypothermia are also paramount along with steps to control bleeding.

Early recognition by regular assessments preferably with MEOWS chart in the 4th stage of labor, early intervention, a proactive approach, protocol-based management, and clear documentation are vital to obtain a good outcome.

REFERENCES

1. Mavrides E, Allard S, Chandraharan E, et al. The Royal College of Obstetricians and Gynaecologists. Prevention and management of postpartum haemorrhage. BJOG. 2016;124: e106-49.
2. Chestnut D, Wong C, Tsen L, et al. Chestnut's obstetric anaesthesia: Principles and Practice, 5th edition. Philadelphia: Saunders; 2014.
3. Bhau U, Kaul I. Recent Advances in management of PPH. JK Science. 2008;10(4).
4. Hiralal Konar. DC Dutta, 6th edition: 2004 27-411,412
5. Arulkumaran S, Karoshi M, Keith LG, et al. A comprehensive Textbook of Postpartum Haemorrhage, 2nd edition. England: Sapiens Publishing; 2012.
6. Alturki F, Ponette V, Boucher LM. Spontaneous Retroperitoneal Hematomas Following Uncomplicated Vaginal Deliveries: A Case Report and Literature Review. J Obstet Gynaecol Can. 2018;40(6):712-5.
7. Arulkumaran S, Baskett T, Calder A. Munro Kerr's operative obstetrics, 12th edition. Philadelphia: Saunders Ltd; 2014.
8. NICE. (2017). Intrapartum care for healthy women and babies. NICE Clinical Guideline CG 190. Feb 2017. [online] Available from: https://www.nice.org.uk/guidance/cg190 [Last Accessed July, 2019].
9. Miller S, Martin HB, Morris JL. Anti-shock garment in postpartum haemorrhage. Safe motherhood programs. Best Prac Res Clin Obstet Gynaecol. 2008;22(6):1057-74.
10. WOMAN trial collaborators. Effect of early tranexamic acid administration on mortality, hysterectomy, and other morbidities in women with post-partum haemorrhage (WOMAN): an international, randomised, double-blind, placebo-controlled trial. Lancet. 2017;389: 2105-16.
11. RCOG. (2015). The Management of Third- and Fourth-Degree Perineal Tears. RCOG Greentop Guideline No. 29. June 2015. [online] Available from: https://www.rcog.org.uk/en/guidelines-research-services/guidelines/gtg29/ [Last accessed July, 2019].

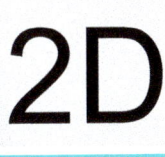

Secondary Postpartum Hemorrhage

Jyothika A Desai, Ashakiran T Rathod

INTRODUCTION

Secondary postpartum hemorrhage (PPH) is any abnormal or excessive bleeding from the birth canal occurring after 24 hours and before 12 weeks after birth.[1] The above definition does not include the amount of blood loss which may range from mild to massive hemorrhage. Hence, it is a subjective diagnosis. If the woman perceives the bleeding to be more than normal, then she will present herself to the obstetrician. Since how much is abnormal is not defined, all such cases are considered as secondary PPH. Sometimes, it leads to unnecessary evaluation. Since the mortality associated with secondary PPH is not as high as in primary PPH, not many randomized control studies are available. The pathogenesis is thought to be subinvolution at the placental site. The two common causes of subinvolution are retained placental tissue and uterine infection.

INCIDENCE

In developed countries, it is 1–2%. No data is available from developing countries.[1]

ETIOLOGY

- Retained placental tissue
- Uterine infection
- Uterine pathology
- Bleeding disorders
- Choriocarcinoma.

Retained Placental Tissue

This occurs if there is:
- Incomplete expulsion of placenta or membranes after vaginal delivery
- Retained succenturiate lobe
- Adherent placenta, where the placenta is left behind for resorption. This may happen naturally with time or with additional treatment of injectable methotrexate
- Placental polyp.

Retained products can cause hemorrhage by preventing the uterus from involuting and by secondary infection leading to endometritis or endomyometritis.

Uterine Infection

It can occur with or without retained products. The infected cesarean section scar can slough and bleed into the uterine cavity, cervicovaginal lacerations, and episiotomy wound can get infected and bleed or bleeding can be from the granulation tissue of these wounds.

Uterine Pathology

- Cervical lesions like polyp and carcinoma can bleed in the puerperium.
- Uterine lesions like fibroids can cause subinvolution and hemorrhage; infection and necrosis in a submucous fibroid can cause bleeding.
- Puerperal inversion of the uterus.

- Uterine arteriovenous malformations (AVMs) and uterine artery aneurysm are rare conditions but can cause catastrophic hemorrhage and should be considered in differential diagnosis. These conditions should be suspected, if bleeding occurs after cesarean section. Uterine AVMs are multiple communications between myometrial arteries and veins. They can be congenital or acquired. Acquired AVMs occur more commonly following uterine curettage, uterine surgery (cesarean section), or trauma to the uterus. A pseudoaneurysm is due to a defect in the arterial wall through which blood collects extraluminally and is connected to the artery through the defect. It does not contain all the three layers of the arterial wall unlike a true aneurysm. The formation of such arterial pseudoaneurysms are rare and can occur as a complication secondary to pelvic surgery, vascular trauma during C-section, or after uterine curettage.
- In vaginal birth after cesarean, scar dehiscence/rupture can present with delayed PPH.

Choriocarcinoma

Usually manifests more than 4 weeks after delivery.

Bleeding Disorders

Postpartum hemorrhage can occur in women with von Willebrand's disease, hemophilia A or B carriers, and in factor XI deficiency. In undetected cases, PPH might be the first symptom. They are more prone for secondary PPH because in primary PPH the main contributory factor is uterine atony. The arrest of bleeding after delivery is mainly by contraction of the uterine muscles. Another reason is that the hypercoagulable state of pregnancy starts to normalize 1 week after delivery. Patients on anticoagulants also can present with both primary and secondary PPH.

Secondary PPH to some extent can be predicted. Table 1 shows the risk factors.

■ CLINICAL FEATURES

Majority (41%) of the patients present between 8 and 14 days after delivery, followed by 23% of cases presenting between 15 and 21 days.[2] Bleeding per vagina can be mild not requiring admission to massive hemorrhage with the patient presenting in shock.

Pain abdomen can be present either due to infection or retained products. Fever and offensive vaginal bleeding indicate uterine infection. History of bleeding disorders should be taken.

TABLE 1: Risk factors for secondary PPH.[1]

Prepregnancy risk factors	Antenatal complications	Labor complications	Postpartum complications
Maternal smoking	Prelabor rupture of membranes	Delivery by cesarean section	Primary postpartum hemorrhage
Previous history of secondary PPH	Threatened miscarriage	Precipitate labor of less than 2 hours	Not breastfeeding
Multiparous women	Multiple pregnancy	Prolonged third stage	Postnatal sepsis
	Antepartum hemorrhage	Incomplete placenta or membranes	
	Hospital admission during the third trimester		

ASSESSMENT

General condition should be assessed. Look for uterine size and tenderness. Inspection of cesarean and episiotomy wound should be done along with a speculum examination to rule out local lesions in the cervix.

INVESTIGATIONS

Depending on history and examination:
1. Hemoglobin, erythrocyte sedimentation rate (ESR), total and differential count.
2. C-reactive protein if infection is suspected.
3. Blood culture in suspected sepsis.
4. High and low vaginal swabs for culture.
5. Swabs for culture/sensitivity should be sent from the infected wound.
6. *Ultrasound examination for retained placental tissue*: Neill et al. studied 53 women undergoing ultrasound with secondary PPH. The diagnosis was confirmed by histopathological examination of the products of conception and also by assuming absence of retained tissue, if vaginal bleeding decreased within 1 week in women managed conservatively. They concluded that the positive predictive value of ultrasound in diagnosing retained products is 46%, the negative predictive value being 96%, with a sensitivity of 93% and specificity of 62%.[3] They also proposed a standardized system for reporting postpartum ultrasound scan (Box 1). Ultrasound is an important tool in the evaluation of secondary PPH because it has a good negative predictive value but at the same time over diagnosis may lead to unnecessary surgical intervention.
7. Color Doppler is to be considered to diagnose uterine AVM and uterine artery aneurysms and pseudoaneurysm. It also helps to distinguish between clots and retained placental tissue, the placental tissue usually retains the blood supply unlike clots. In color flow Doppler, to-and-fro sign is seen in the neck and yin-yang sign in the body of the pseudoaneurysm. AVMs show marked aliasing on color flow Doppler and spectral Doppler shows arterialized venous flow.[4]
8. Serum β-human chorionic gonadotropin (hCG), if choriocarcinoma is suspected. Additionally chest X-ray and computed tomography (CT) scan may be required to rule out metastasis.
9. Coagulation profile, if bleeding disorders are suspected.
10. Magnetic resonance imaging (MRI) in suspected cases of placenta accreta/percreta/increta.
11. Pelvic angiography may help if bleeding site is unknown.

Box 1: A proposed standardized system for reporting postpartum.
- Normal endometrial cavity
- Endometrial cavity containing fluid only
- Endometrial cavity enlarged [anteroposterior (AP) depth >1 cm]. Maximum AP dimensions noted
- Endometrial cavity containing echogenic foci. Dimensions of largest foci noted. Doppler evaluation of blood flow in foci

Source: Ultrasound scan Adapted from Neill et al. 2002.

TREATMENT

There are no randomized controlled trials for management of secondary PPH. The goals of treatment are to improve the general condition, control hemorrhage, and treat the cause.

Resuscitation (Volume Replacement/Inotropic Drugs, etc.)

Massive hemorrhage is seen in approximately 10% of cases and requires quick action.[3] Two large bore intravenous (IV) lines should be started. Fluid, blood, and blood products are given as required. The evaluation of case and formulating the plan of management is done along with the senior obstetrician. Some patients may require inotropic and ventilator support.

Antibiotics

The two major causes of secondary PPH are retained placenta and endometritis. Retained placenta invariably has some degree of infection. So a majority of women are given antibiotics even though the infection may not be confirmed in all cases. The organisms identified include group B Streptococcus, *Bacteroides* species, *E. coli, Clostridium perfringens,* and group D Streptococcus. Recommended antibiotics are amoxicillin and clavulanic acid[5] and a combination of amoxicillin, metronidazole, and gentamicin.[6]

Uterotonics

Oxytocin, prostaglandin F2 alpha (PGf2α), methylergometrine, and misoprostol are used as in primary PPH. One study shows that uterotonics given when the clot or debris in the uterine cavity is more than 2 cm reduced the rate of surgical intervention.

Uterine Evacuation

This procedure is done if retained products are suspected either clinically or on ultrasound. IV antibiotics should be given at least 1 hour before the procedure. 24 hours antibiotic cover prior to the procedure would be better. During evacuation oxytocin may be used. Histological evidence is seen in only 36% of cases.[5] No specific method has been found to be superior and safe for evacuation. There is a risk of uterine perforation in the postpartum period. In some cases, flare up of preexisting sepsis is seen to occur. The risk of Asherman's is increased. The products should be sent for histopathological examination.

Uterine Tamponade

Intrauterine balloon tamponade can be used as in primary PPH.

Surgical procedures like uterine compression sutures and internal iliac artery ligation have been described in many cases of secondary PPH.

Selective Pelvic Artery Embolization

Ongoing hemorrhage can be diagnosed by pelvic angiography and the specific bleeding vessel embolized. Bilateral uterine artery embolization helps in almost all cases. In adherent placenta when conservative management is done and the placenta left behind, uterine artery embolization is effective in the prevention as well as in the treatment of secondary PPH. In Arteriovenous malformations and false aneurysms of uterine artery, uterine artery embolization is very effective to control hemorrhage.

Hysterectomy

It is usually done as a last resort, but early decision should be taken to prevent mortality and morbidity. If patient is already in disseminated intravascular coagulation (DIC) because of massive hemorrhage, doing hysterectomy may not help.

Role of Tranexamic Acid[7]

Tranexamic acid reduces blood loss in both primary and secondary PPH.

Role of Recombinant Factor VIIa[8]

Its use has been reported for primary PPH and may help in secondary PPH too.

Local Vasopressin[9]

The use of intrauterine vasopressin to control hemorrhage in secondary PPH has been reported in coagulopathies.

In known coagulation disorders, prophylactic desdeamino vasopressin and clotting factor concentrates should be given, if clotting factors are less than 50IU/dL.[10] The use of tranexamic acid[11] and oral contraceptive pills[10] are also reported in such conditions. In women on anticoagulants, vitamin K and fresh frozen plasma are given if patient is on warfarin and protamine sulfate in patients on heparin.

■ REFERENCES

1. Alexander J, Thomas PW, Sanghera J. Treatments for secondary postpartum haemorrhage (Review). Cochrane Database Syst Rev. 2002;(1):CD002867.
2. Hoveyda F, MacKenzie IZ. Secondary postpartum haemorrhage: incidence, morbidity, and current management. BJOG. 2001;108:927-30.
3. Neill AC, Nixon RM, Thornton S. A comparison of clinical assessment with ultrasound in the management of secondary postpartum haemorrhage. Eur J Obstet Gynecol Reprod Biol. 2002;104:113-5.
4. Nanjundan P, Rohilla M, Raveendran A, et al. Pseudoaneurysm of uterine artery: a rare cause of secondary postpartum hemorrhage, managed with uterine artery embolisation. J Clin Imaging Sci. 2011;1:14.
5. King PA, Duthie SJ, Dong ZG, et al. Secondary postpartum haemorrhage. Aust N Z J Obstet Gynaecol. 1989;29:394-8.
6. Ledee N, Ville Y, Musset D, et al. Management in intractable obstetric haemorrhage: an audit study on 61 cases. Eur J Obstet Gynecol Reprod Biol. 2001;94:189-96.
7. Alok K, Hagen P, Webb JB. Tranexamic acid in the management of postpartum haemorrhage. BJOG. 1996;103:1250-1.
8. Boehlen F, Morales MA, Fontana P, et al. Prolonged treatment of massive postpartum haemorrhage with recombinant factor VIIa: case report and review of the literature. BJOG. 2004;111:284-7.
9. Lurie S, Appleman Z, Katz Z. Subendometrial vasopressin to control intractable placental bleeding. Lancet. 1997;349:698.
10. Economides DL, Kadir RA, Lee CA. Inherited bleeding disorders in obstetrics and gynaecology. Br J Obstet Gynaecol. 1999;106:5-13.
11. Bonnar J, Guillebaud J, Kasonde JM, et al. Clinical applications of fibrinolytic inhibition in gynaecology. J Clin Pathol Suppl (R Coll Pathol). 1980;14:55-9.

12E Chapter

Vascular Interventions in Postpartum Hemorrhage

Indusekhara S, Vidya Bhargavi

INTRODUCTION

Being the most life-threatening obstetric emergency, postpartum hemorrhages (PPH) require prompt response. PPH is responsible for approximately 25% of global maternal mortality and is a predominant cause of maternal morbidity. With prompt recognition and timely intervention, PPH remains as a preventable cause of maternal mortality. Most cases of PPH are minor, requiring conservative management with minimal morbidity; however, if unnoticed can lead to major morbidity and serious catastrophic events. Refractory PPH requires multidisciplinary approach. Interventional radiology (IR) techniques for management of PPH consist of uterine arterial embolization (UAE) and arterial balloon occlusion. IR has a potential role in PPH because of its accuracy in localization of bleeding site, high technical success with prompt hemostasis, minimally invasive nature, low complication rates, and the possibility of maintaining fertility.

DEFINITION

Postpartum hemorrhage is traditionally defined as blood loss of more than 500 mL with vaginal birth and 1,000 mL with cesarean section.[1]

Accurate PPH diagnosis is subjective due to inaccurate estimates of blood loss and physiological plasma volume increases during pregnancy obscuring the symptoms of hemorrhage. Any amount of bleeding that threatens the hemodynamic stability of the woman [heart rate >110, blood pressure (BP) < 85/45, O_2 sat <95% or suspicion of disseminated intravascular coagulation (DIC)] should be considered as PPH.

CLASSIFICATION

- Primary—within 24 hours of birth
- Secondary—between 24 hours of birth and 12 weeks postpartum.

ETIOLOGY

4Ts—Tone, Trauma, Tissue and Thrombin (Table 1).

ENDOVASCULAR MANAGEMENT OF POSTPARTUM HEMORRHAGES

Interventional radiology is a therapeutic and diagnostic specialty that performs minimally invasive procedures under image guidance [digital subtraction angiography (DSA), ultrasound, computed tomography (CT) or magnetic resonance imaging (MRI)] to allow precise diagnosis and treatment of diseases. IR techniques for management of PPH primarily include UAE and temporary arterial occlusion of internal iliac artery.

Initially in 1960s, transarterial angiography was used as a diagnostic tool to establish the sites of hemorrhage after an attempt of failed surgical exploration. UAE to control PPH was first reported by Brown and Heaston et al. in 1979,[2] in a patient with

TABLE 1: Postpartum hemorrhage etiology.	
Uterine Atony (Tone)	• Prolonged labor, especially prolonged 2nd stage of labor • Increasing parity • Oxytocin withdrawal: – Uterine overdistension Multiple pregnancy, polyhydramnios, and macrosomia • Instrumental birth
Trauma	• Uterine rupture, cervical tear, vaginal tear, and perineal tear
Tissue related factors	• Retained products of conception • Invasive placenta (accreta, percreta, and increta) • Uterine inversion
Thrombosis	• Thrombocytopenia • Coagulation disorders • Disseminated intravascular coagulation—severe preeclampsia, placental abruption, sepsis, and amniotic fluid embolism • Hereditary bleeding disorders • Dengue hemorrhagic fever

postbilateral internal iliac arterial ligation and posthysterectomy status. Since then numerous cases of transcatheter arterial embolization for postpartum bleeding have been reported with excellent technical and clinical outcomes.

Uterine arterial embolization is a procedure to control bleeding by administering embolic agent into the bleeding arterial branches through the catheter. Arterial balloon occlusion involves temporary inflation of balloon in the bleeding arteries through transarterial introduction of balloon catheter to achieve immediate hemostasis.

INDICATIONS FOR ENDOVASCULAR MANAGEMENT[3]

- Uterine atony subsequent to normal/prolonged labor, with or without cesarean section
- Surgical trauma or uterine tears during cesarean section
- Bleeding subsequent to normal vaginal delivery or a cesarean section
- Bleeding subsequent to hysterectomy
- Prophylactically in a known or suspected case of invasive placenta or previous cesarean section scar
- Hemorrhage from ectopic pregnancy either prophylactically or after surgical removal of the ectopic fetus
- Secondary PPH due to uterine arteriovenous malformations.

The severity or the type of PPH does not preclude the use of UAE. UAE has high success rates for atonic bleeding. IR is the management option of choice for atonic bleeding. In case of massive bleeding from the invasive placenta or trauma, timely temporary balloon occlusion of the internal iliac artery can restore and maintain the hemodynamic status during surgery or UAE.

CONTRAINDICATIONS

There are no absolute contraindications in life-threatening hemorrhage. Relative contraindications include allergy or reactions to contrast media, renal insufficiency, severe hypertension, uncorrectable bleeding disorders or coagulation parameters, acute/chronic pelvic infection, and use of vasoconstrictors causing spasm of arteries.

VASCULAR ANATOMY RELEVANT TO POSTPARTUM HEMORRHAGE

Precise understanding of angiographic images, technical success, and safe embolization requires detailed anatomical knowledge.[4] The common iliac arteries arise from the aorta at L4 vertebral level, course anterior to the common iliac veins, and inferior vena cava; divide into the external (EIA) and internal iliac (IIA) arteries. The IIA divides into anterior and posterior branches. The posterior division branches are the iliolumbar, the lateral sacral, and the superior gluteal arteries. The anterior division branches are variable and include the uterine artery (UA), the middle and inferior hemorrhoidal arteries, the vesicular, the internal pudendal, the obturator, and the inferior gluteal arteries.

The UA branch is most pertinent to transcatheter embolization in PPH. The UA is a proximal branch of IIA and can be the first branch, or trifurcate with the superior and inferior gluteal arteries, or arise from the inferior gluteal artery. In minority, the anatomy of the UA is variable, and can originate from the ovarian artery. The UA typically has a hairpin curve as it passes through the cardinal ligament and proceeds cephalad along the body of the uterine body at the level of the cervix. The cervicovaginal artery originates from the proximal UA. Anastomoses between the ovarian artery and UA and between the right and left uterine arteries are present in majority of the women.

Collateral branches to the uterus can be a source of bleeding and usually arise from the ovarian, inferior mesenteric, round ligament, and internal pudendal arteries.[5] The ovarian arteries originate from the anterolateral aspect of the aorta, below the renal arteries. In minority, the ovarian arteries can arise from the renal arteries. Ovarian arteries have a corkscrew appearance as they run along the psoas muscle toward the suspensory ligament of the ovary. From the ligament, the ovarian artery penetrates the broad ligament and mesovarium to reach the ovary. The artery to the round ligament of the uterus originates either from the inferior epigastric artery or directly from the external iliac artery.

The vaginal artery originates from the anterior division of the IIA just below the origin of the UA or from the UA and supplies anterior and lateral surface of the vagina. Branches from the inferior vesical, the internal pudendal, and the middle rectal arteries supply the vagina. Therefore, these branches can be a source of bleeding in vaginal laceration.

A persistent sciatic artery is a rare vascular anomaly with a high potential risk to cause irreversible ischemic damage of the lower limb during UAE for PPH.[6] The persistent sciatic artery begins at the IIA and travels through the greater sciatic foramen, from where its course becomes closer to the sciatic nerve. Reflux of embolic material can lead to ischemic damage of lower limb.

■ PREPROCEDURAL REQUISITES

Prior to IR procedure, it is crucial to assess vital signs, understand the cause and amount of bleeding, previous treatment (e.g. ligation, hysterectomy, and intrauterine balloon tamponade), and amount of blood transfusions. Informed consent to be taken after discussing in detail about the possible risks and benefits with the patient and family. Initial assessment of the peripheral vascular system and recent imaging and laboratory studies should be done. Coagulation parameters and serum creatinine levels should be reviewed.[7]

Appropriate decisions have to be made on selection of introducer sheath size, approach, and management option. Volume restoration with crystalloid and colloids to be initiated prior to angiography and blood products arranged. Adequate replacement of coagulation factors is essential whenever there is a significant alteration of coagulation parameters. Prophylactic intravenous antibiotics can be administered prior to the procedure.

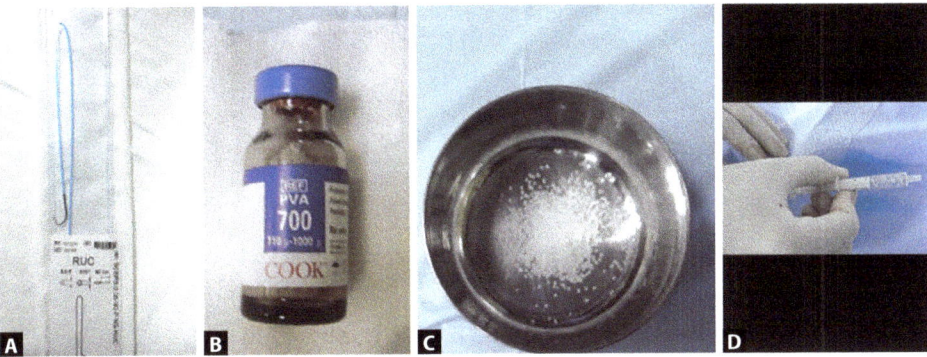

Figs. 1A to D: RUC catheter and PVA particles.

TECHNIQUE OF UTERINE ARTERIAL EMBOLIZATION

Initial angiography of the pelvic and uterine arteries is obtained with a 5F introducer sheath through arterial access from right or left femoral artery. A 4F sidewinder, renal curve, or Robertson uterine artery (RUC) catheter is introduced into the iliac arteries crossing over aortic bifurcation through the vascular sheath. The RUC catheter is preferred by the author as it allows catheterization of bilateral uterine arteries easily. An initial digital angiography is obtained with the catheter in common iliac artery to study the anatomy of pelvic vessels, further the catheter is directed into UA slowly. Selective angiography is then obtained to identify the uterine arterial branches and any leaking areas. Embolization of the abnormal vessel is performed either with polyvinyl alcohol (PVA) particles or gel foam scrapings and pledgets (Figs. 1 A to D).

Embolization is performed by injecting PVA particles in small quantities suspended in dilute contrast till the flow into the capillary bed of uterine wall is stopped and there is reduction of flow in the main UA. This ensures adequate vascular supply to the uterine musculature and prevents necrosis of uterine wall. Any evidence of contrast leak from a UA

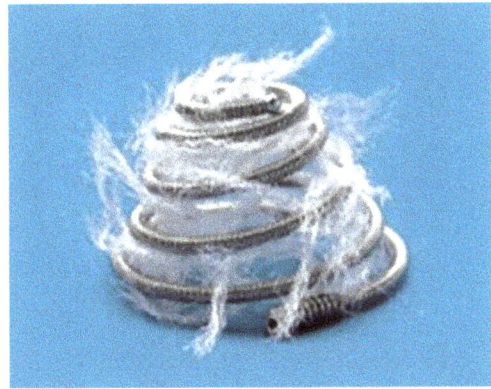

Fig. 2: Embolization coil.

branch requires super selective catheterization of the branch (with a coaxial microcatheter) and deployment of embolization coils to completely arrest bleeding (Fig. 2).

SPECIAL CLINICAL SETTINGS

1. *Uterine atony:* UAE should be the treatment of choice in atonic uterine bleeding.[8] Angiography generally reveals dilated and tortuous bilateral uterine and arcuate arteries with hypervascularity. Embolization with PVA particles and Gelfoam pledgets would control the bleeding sufficiently (Figs. 3A to D).
2. *Trauma to the genital tract*: Though surgical repair is the definitive treatment

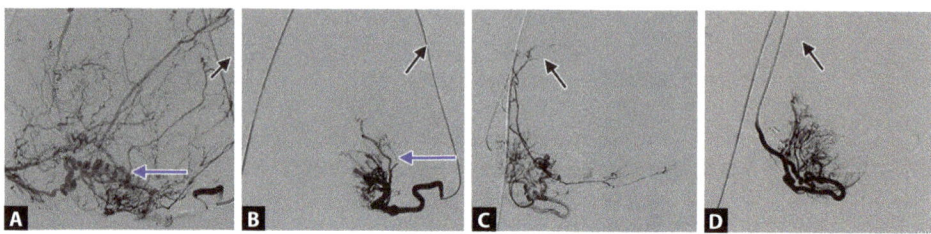

Figs. 3A to D: (A) Left uterine artery angiography of a case with atonic PPH prior to embolization. (B) Postembolization picture (C and D) same patient right uterine artery angiogram pre- and postembolization. Patient had complete recovery with no further bleeding P/V.
Note: Small arrows—catheter, long arrows—vascular network in the uterine wall.

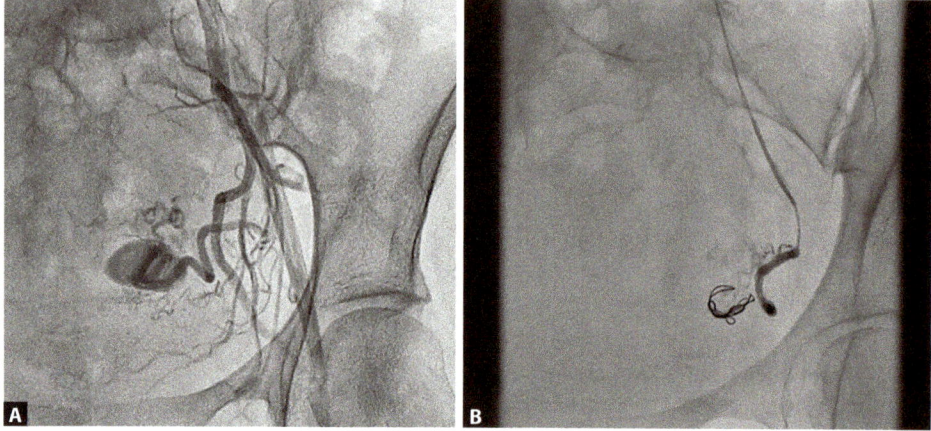

Figs. 4A and B: (A) PPH due to leaking uterine artery branch; (B) embolization with Nestor embolization coil, pre-, and postembolization pictures.

for hemostasis in trauma of the genital tract, UAE as a first-line treatment provides a clear visual field for the repairing the trauma by reducing the bleeding.[9] Angiography of the uterine vessels and pelvic floor vasculature can quickly assess vascular injury. The arteries most frequently injured are the uterine, internal pudendal, and vaginal arteries, which manifest as a pseudoaneurysm and/or contrast extravasation. Preferable embolic agents are coils and liquid embolic agents like n-butyl 2-cyanoacrylate glue (Figs. 4A and B).

3. *Placental abnormality*: Prophylactic occlusion of the iliac artery with balloon catheter can maintain the hemodynamic stability during hysterectomy. UAE immediately or on-demand after delivery effectively controls the bleeding and accentuates the degree of uterine preservation. Angiography shows dilated vascular channels scattered throughout the remaining placenta, thus suggesting trophoblastic vascularization primarily from the UA.[10] Collateral blood supply other than that of the UA, such as that of the ovarian artery, internal pudendal, or vesical artery, can contribute blood supply to the placenta. Particulate embolic agents like PVA and Gelatin sponge particles are preferred (Figs. 5A to D).

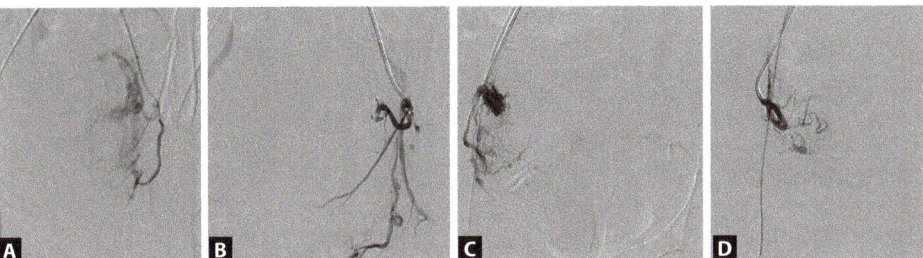

Figs. 5A to D: This patient had obstetric hysterectomy for placenta increta. 7th postoperative day developed bleeding P/V and intraperitoneal bleeding with drop in hemoglobin. Emergency embolization was done for remaining branches of uterine artery with PVA particles. (A and B) left uterine artery before and after embolization; (C and D) right uterine artery.

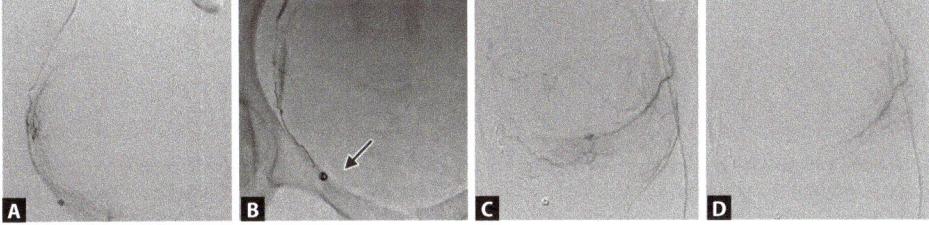

Figs. 6A to D: Young primi diagnosed with dengue hemorrhagic fever and liver failure, developed severe vaginal bleeding 24 hours postdelivery and was on ventilator. Initially managed conservatively with transfusion and blood products, progressed to acute renal failure requiring dialysis. Continued to bleed hence considered for UAE with coils (arrow) and PVA particles. (A and B) Right uterine artery before and after embolization; (C and D) left uterine artery before and after embolization.

4. *Factors related to coagulopathy*: UAE helps to achieve immediate hemostasis and reduces the excessive blood loss and need of blood transfusions (Figs. 6A to D).
5. *Secondary PPH from uterine arteriovenous malformation*: UAE is the first line of management. Preprocedural imaging is helpful for evaluating possible extrauterine feeders.[11] Angiography shows hypertrophied, dilated, and tortuous uterine arteries entangled into a mass and early drainage from the arteriovenous malformation to pelvic veins. Particulate and liquid embolic agents like n-butyl 2-cyanoacrylate glue are preferred (Figs. 7A to F).

ARTERIAL BALLOON OCCLUSION

Antepartum arterial balloon occlusion is another interventional technique which is occasionally used in cases of high-risk pregnancy with placenta accreta or increta. For this close coordination of obstetrician, interventional radiologist and anesthesiologist are necessary.

Prior to C-section, the patient undergoes positioning of compliant balloons in both internal iliac arteries under fluoroscopic imaging either in the catheterization lab or in the OT with C-arm machine. The bilateral femoral arteries are accessed with two vascular sheaths. After this, guidewire and catheter combination used to cross over the aortic bifurcation to enter contralateral iliac arteries. Over the guidewire, suitable compliant balloons are threaded and positioned in internal iliac arteries on both sides. The shafts of both balloons are secured and connected to saline infusions to prevent thrombosis.

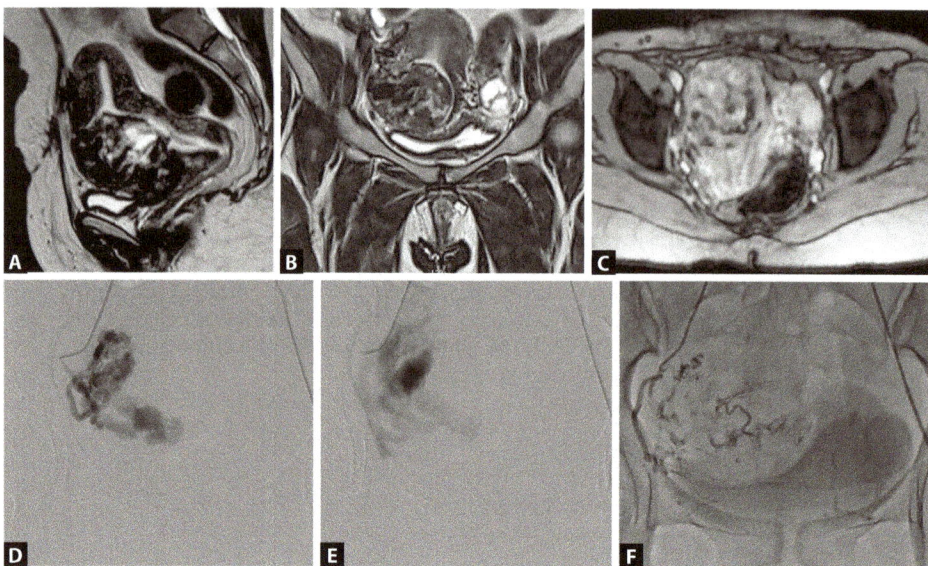

Figs. 7A to F: Secondary postpartum hemorrhage due to acquired AV fistula. (A) T2 weighted sagittal (B) and coronal (C) images demonstrating heterogeneous signal intensity mass with flow voids in the anteroinferior wall of uterus causing distortion of endometrial cavity with multiple foci of blooming on axial T2* images. (D) Right uterine artery with high flow and early filling of veins; (E) venous phase of same angiogram; (F) Postembolization image with cast of cyanoacrylate glue and lipiodol mixture.

After the delivery of the baby, before removal of placenta the balloons are inflated to arrest the circulation temporarily. Once the placenta separates, after ensuring stoppage of bleeding into the uterus, the balloons are deflated and a recheck is done. If there is no further bleeding, the closure is done and following this the balloons and sheaths are removed. It is preferable to avoid anticoagulation during the procedure hence the introducer sheaths are perfused with saline continuously.

COMPLICATIONS

Major complications are rare, overall complication rate being less than 7%.[12] Most of the complications are related to the hemorrhage itself or to subsequent surgical intervention. Complications related to PPH embolization occur either secondary to angiographic procedure (vessel dissection, hematoma at the puncture site and contrast associated allergy, or nephrotoxicity) or secondary to embolization. The most common complication is self-limiting postembolization syndrome identified by pain, fever, nausea, and leukocytosis.

Ischemic complications include necrosis of uterus and bladder and ovarian dysfunction due to nontarget embolization through utero-ovarian anastomoses.[13]

Neurologic complications are rare due to arterial communications between IIA branches and the arterial branches of spinal cord, sciatic nerve, and femoral nerve.

Complications related to balloon catheters include maternal thromboembolic events leading to acute lower limb ischemia, necessitating surgical or radiologic interventions, and other complications like arterial pseudoaneurysms, dissection, and arterial rupture[14] are also reported.

OUTCOMES

Clinical success rate ranges from 86.5% to 95.0%. Factors resulting in unsuccessful embolization include DIC, hemodynamic instability, hemoglobin level below 8 g/dL, and extravasation detected on angiography.[15]

Prophylactic placement of balloon catheters decreases the overall surgical morbidity, as measured by decreased mean estimated blood loss (EBL), less cases with EBL above 2,500 mL and lesser blood transfusions.[16]

FERTILITY AFTER UTERINE ARTERIAL EMBOLIZATION

Uterine arterial embolization is a uterus sparing procedure and it preserves the childbearing potential of the women.[17,18] Menstruation and fertility following UAE are retained in 97.3% women among most studies. Full-term pregnancies have been reported in patients with previous UAE. Some studies report premature labor as a complication among women with previous UAE, which may be related to pre-existent conditions associated with PPH. However, UAE can result in ovarian dysfunction, though rare and affect the menstruation and fertility.

RADIATION EXPOSURE

The dose of radiation to the ovaries is large as the radiation beam has a directly impact on the ovaries and it cannot be guarded through the entire procedure. The estimated mean absorbed radiation dose for an ovary in transcatheter arterial embolization (TAE) of up to 58.6 cGy (range: 20–73 cGy) has been reported. However, there are no events of UAE induced skin reactions, or consecutive babies being born with anomalies. To lower the radiation dose, multiple DSA, the field of view, magnification fluoroscopy, fluoroscopy time, pulse rate frequency, and the distance between the patient and image intensifier should all be reduced.[19,20]

ADVANTAGES OF INTERVENTIONAL RADIOLOGY

Interventional radiology techniques are minimally invasive, safe, with high success, and low complication rates. Usually done under local anesthesia and with very minimal pain. Immediate prompt hemostasis can be achieved with possibility of repeat procedure if required. Morbidity following IR techniques is also minimal with reduced need for blood transfusions and hospital stay. Preservation of fertility is a greatest benefit of IR in PPH.

CONCLUSION

Interventional radiology and UAE should be considered early in the multidisciplinary algorithms of PPH management. IR achieves prompt hemostasis, thus significantly reducing maternal mortality and morbidity rates with additional benefit of preserving women's fertility.

KEY POINTS

- Uterine arterial embolization is the management of choice for atonic bleeding.
- In case of massive bleeding from the invasive placenta or trauma, timely temporary balloon occlusion of the IIA can restore and maintain the hemodynamic status during surgery or UAE.
- Precise understanding of angiographic images, technical success, and safe embolization requires detailed anatomical knowledge.
- Factors resulting in unsuccessful embolization include DIC, hemodynamic instability, hemoglobin level below 8 g/dL, and extravasation detected on angiography.

- Uterine arterial embolization can result in ovarian dysfunction, though rare and affect the menstruation and fertility.
- To lower the radiation dose, multiple DSA, the field of view, magnification fluoroscopy, fluoroscopy time, pulse rate frequency, and the distance between the patient and image intensifier should all be reduced.

REFERENCES

1. Rath WH. Postpartum hemorrhage—update on problems of definitions and diagnosis. Acta Obstet Gynecol Scand. 2011;90:421-8.
2. Heaston DK, Mineau DE, Brown BJ, et al. Transcatheter arterial embolization for control of persistent massive puerperal hemorrhage after bilateral surgical hypogastric artery ligation. AJR Am J Roentgenol. 1979;133:152-4.
3. RCOG. (2007). The role of emergency and elective interventional radiology in postpartum haemorrhage; (Good Practice no 6). [online] Available from: https://www.rcog.org.uk/globalassets/documents/guidelines/goodpractice6roleemergency2007.pdf [Last accessed July, 2019].
4. Chen C, Lee SM, Kim JW, et al. Recent update of embolization of postpartum hemorrhage. Korean J Radiol. 2018;19(4):586-96.
5. Soyer P, Dohan A, Dautry R, et al. Transcatheter arterial embolization for postpartum hemorrhage: indications, technique, results, and complications. Cardiovasc Intervent Radiol. 2015;38:1068-81.
6. Soyer P, Boudiaf M, Jacob D, et al. Bilateral persistent sciatic artery: a potential risk in pelvic arterial embolization for primary postpartum hemorrhage. Acta Obstet Gynecol Scand. 2005;84:604-5.
7. Salazar GM, Petrozza JC, Walker TG. Transcatheter endovascular techniques for management of obstetrical and gynecologic emergencies. Tech Vasc Interv Radiol. 2009;12(2):139-47.
8. Salomon LJ, deTayrac R, Castaigne-Meary V, et al. Fertility and pregnancy outcome following pelvic arterial embolization for severe postpartum haemorrhage. A cohort study. Hum Reprod. 2003;18:849-52.
9. Fargeaudou Y, Soyer P, Morel O, et al. Severe primary postpartum hemorrhage due to genital tract laceration after operative vaginal delivery: successful treatment with transcatheter arterial embolization. Eur Radiol. 2009;19:2197-203.
10. Soyer P, Morel O, Fargeaudou Y, et al. Value of pelvic embolization in the management of severe postpartum hemorrhage due to placenta accreta, increta or percreta. Eur J Radiol. 2011;80:729-35.
11. Kim T, Shin JH, Kim J, et al. Management of bleeding uterine arteriovenous malformation with bilateral uterine artery embolization. Yonsei Med J. 2014;55:367-73.
12. Kachura JR. The role of interventional radiology in obstetrics. Fetal Matern Med Rev. 2004;15:145-80.
13. Courbiere B, Jauffret C, Provansal M, et al. Failure of conservative management in postpartum haemorrhage: uterine necrosis and hysterectomy after angiographic selective embolization with Gelfoam. Eur J Obstet Gynecol Reprod Biol. 2008;140:291-3.
14. Dilauro MD, Dason S, Athreya S. Prophylactic balloon occlusion of internal iliac arteries in women with placenta accreta: literature review and analysis. Clin Radiol 2012;67(6):515-20.
15. Kim YJ, Yoon CJ, Seong NJ, et al. Failed pelvic arterial embolization for postpartum hemorrhage: clinical outcomes and predictive factors. J Vasc Interv Radiol. 2013;24:703-9.
16. Ballas J, Hull AD, Saenz C, et al. Preoperative intravascular balloon catheters and surgical outcomes in pregnancies complicated by placenta accreta: a management paradox. Am J Obstet Gynecol. 2012;207(3):e1-5.
17. Doumouchtsis SK, Nikolopoulos K, Talaulikar V, et al. Menstrual and fertility outcomes following the surgical management of postpartum haemorrhage: a systematic review. BJOG. 2014;121:382-8.
18. Sentilhes L, Gromez A, Clavier E, et al. Fertility and pregnancy following pelvic arterial embolization for postpartum haemorrhage. BJOG. 2010;117:84-93.
19. Andrews RT, Brown PH. Uterine arterial embolization: factors influencing patient radiation exposure. Radiology. 2000;217:713-22.
20. Tse G, Spies JB. Radiation exposure and uterine artery embolization: current risks and risk reduction. Tech Vasc Interv Radiol. 2010;13:148-53.

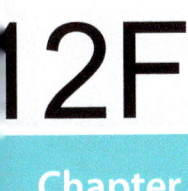

Chapter 12F: Newer Approaches in Management of Postpartum Hemorrhage

Savvas Argyridis, Sabaratnam Arulkumaran

INTRODUCTION

Globally, 300,000 women die each year of maternity related causes. This translates to 830 women dying each day and one every 2 minutes. Most of these deaths are in Sub-Saharan Africa and South East Asia—India contributing substantial numbers due to the absolute large number of births, i.e. 27 million births each year. Postpartum hemorrhage (PPH) is a major cause of maternal morbidity and mortality—30% of maternal deaths are due to PPH. Every 6-8 minutes, a woman dies of PPH. It is estimated that 15 million women suffer from PPH and 75,000 die. Most deaths can be prevented by prophylactic oxytocics and simple medical and surgical techniques. Paucity of health personal, nonavailability of effective medication and the delay in seeking care, delay in reaching a health facility, and delay in receiving treatment have been shown to be the main contributory factors. Despite these drawbacks, research has advanced effective treatment modalities to reduce the incidence and severity of PPH. This chapter deals with six newer approaches in management of PPH.

HEAT STABLE OXYTOCIN: OXYTOCIN AGONISTS

Carbetocin, a synthetic octapeptide analog to oxytocin, has agonist properties like natural oxytocin. It has a longer half-life than oxytocin (4-10 times) and can be administered as a single intramuscular (IM) or intravenous (IV) injection rather than a continuous infusion. The use of this drug as part of active management of the third stage of labor has been reported since early 1990s, with several trials assessing its efficacy and safety profile since then. The uterotonic properties of carbetocin are more sustained when administered as an IM rather than an IV bolus injection. IM injection of 10-70 µg, resulted in a tetanic contraction within 2 minutes that lasted up to 11 minutes and subsequent rhythmic contractions for 119 minutes.[1] The recommended dose for use is 100 µg IM or IV.

Compared to IM oxytocin and oral misoprostol administration, IM carbetocin has been a promising strategy regarding third stage blood loss prevention.[2] Four randomized trials have demonstrated significant reduction in need for additional uterotonics to prevent PPH following carbetocin administration for cesarean section compared to oxytocin.[3] Promising results have also been reported in high-risk vaginal deliveries, but more evidence was needed for use in low-risk cases and has now been accomplished by the CHAMPION (Carbetocin HAeMorrhage PreventION) trial conducted by the World Health Organization (WHO).[4] The WHO did not add carbetocin in the 2012 recommendations regarding PPH but was included in the 2018 revision.

Number of studies had concluded that compared to syntometrine, the carbetocin group required less additional uterotonics (13.5% vs 16.8%) following vaginal deliveries. Side-effects such as nausea and vomiting were more common in the syntometrine group than the carbetocin group.[5] Similar results were reported by another randomized controlled trial (RCT) that assessed carbetocin and syntometrine efficacy following vaginal deliveries. Carbetocin administration resulted in less blood loss (81.5 mL) and less hemoglobin reduction (0.3 g/dL).[6] A Cochrane review of 140 RCT, concluded that for prevention of blood loss of 500 mL or more following a vaginal delivery (VD), carbetocin is more effective than oxytocin alone.[7]

Quality audits have revealed that (a) about 74.2% of oxytocin injection samples failed the assay test[8] and (b) in 45.6% of oxytocin samples, the amount of active pharmacological ingredient was insufficient.[9] A heat-stable formulation of carbetocin has been developed and its stability has been assessed under ICH climate zone IV conditions (30°C, 75% humidity) for at least 3 years and at extreme temperatures up to 60°C for shorter periods of time. Results showed that 95% of drug purity was maintained for a minimum of 3 years at 30°C, 6 months at 40°C, 3 months at 50°C and 1 month at 60°C.[10] This formulation may be useful primarily in countries or areas where cold chain is unreliable or unavailable. A recent large, multicenter RCT by the WHO—the CHAMPION study has assessed 100 μg IM heat stable carbetocin injection compared to 10 IU IM oxytocin injection.[4] The results are summarized below:

- About 29,645 were randomized to receive 100 ug carbetocin or 10 IU oxytocin IM after VD
- Blood loss ≥500 mL or additional uterotonics; 14.5% in carbetocin and 14.4% in oxytocin group; relative risk (RR) 1.01 (CI 0.95–1.06)
- Blood loss ≥ 1000 mL 1.51% in carbetocin and 1.45% in oxytocin group; RR 1.04 (CI 0.87–1.25)
- Additional uterotonics, intervention to stop bleeding and adverse effects did not differ in the two groups.

Heat stable carbetocin is therefore non-inferior to oxytocin for blood loss prevention of up to 500 mL.[4]

Carbetocin is a third-line uterotonic when second-line options are unavailable or fail to control bleeding. According to International Federation of Gynaecology and Obstetrics (FIGO), 100 μg administered IM or IV over 1 minute is the recommended dose.

NETWORK META-ANALYSIS ON THE USE OF OXYTOCICS FOR PREVENTION OF PPH

Various drugs are available for prevention of PPH but there is little direct comparison of multiple drugs in the same study. But direct comparison between two drugs is available. Recent method of "network meta-analysis" by Cochrane collaboration permits indirect comparison to assess relative merits of the different drugs alone or in combination and to rank them based on their efficiency and side-effects profile.[7] The results of network meta-analysis comparing different drugs alone and in combination for effectiveness have been studied. However, they did not consider the dose of the drugs or route of administration. The summary of the network meta-analysis of 140 RCTs, consisting of 88,947 women who delivered beyond 37 weeks in hospital settings is given below.[7] In majority of trials, there was poor reporting of risks and hence there was uncertainty of risk of bias:

- Three most effective drugs identified for prevention of PPH > 500 mL compared with oxytocin were (1) ergometrine and oxytocin; (2) carbetocin; (3) misoprostol + oxytocin. Overall for the incidence of PPH:
  - Ergometrine and oxytocin; RR 0.69 (CI 0.57–0.83) moderate evidence

- Carbetocin; RR 0.72 (CI 0.52–1.0)—low quality evidence
- Misoprostol and oxytocin—RR 0.73 (CI 0.60–0.90) moderate quality.

The incidence of PPH > 500 mL was 10.5% with oxytocin; 7.2% with oxytocin and ergometrine; 7.6% with carbetocin and 7.7% with misoprostol and oxytocin.

The incidence of PPH > 1000 mL compared with oxytocin:
- Oxytocin and ergometrine—RR 0.77 (CI 0.61–0.95)
- Carbetocin—RR 0.70 (CI 0.38–1.28) * not enough numbers
- Misoprostol and oxytocin—RR 0.90 (CI 0.72–1.14).

There was no difference in maternal deaths or severe morbidity. The incidence is too low for analysis. The side-effect profile was as follows:
- Ergometrine and oxytocin—vomiting RR 3.10 (CI 2.11–4.56); hypertension RR 1.77 (CI 0.55–5.66)
- Misoprostol and oxytocin—higher risk of fever RR 3.18 (CI 2.22–4.55); 11.4% versus 3.6% cf oxytocin
- Carbetocin—similar risk of side effects like oxytocin* but low risk for hypertension.

Based on the above network meta-analysis one of the above three regimes are better than oxytocin. However, the side effects are more with oxytocin-ergometrine combination or oxytocin given along with misoprostol. Carbetocin has similar efficacy like the above combined regimes and less side effects but is more expensive than the other two regimes.

ANTIFIBRINOLYTIC AGENT—TRANEXAMIC ACID

Tranexamic acid (TXA) is an inexpensive, heat stable, and generic drug that reduces bleeding by inhibiting the breakdown of fibrinogen and fibrin. TXA used in surgery shows that it reduces bleeding by about one-third and when given soon after traumatic injury, it reduces deaths due to bleeding by a third [Clinical Randomisation of an Antifibrinolytic in Significant Hemorrhage 2 (CRASH-2 trial)].

As trauma and childbirth, have the same effect on plasmin activation, the use of TXA for reduction of PPH-related deaths and morbidity was considered. The WHO has included TXA in its recommendations since 2012 and suggested an IV dose of 1 g.[11] A 2015 systematic review of 12 RCT that randomized women in TXA administration and placebo, concluded that in women with PPH, risk of additional bleeding was reduced when TXA was administered (RR 0.52, 95% CI 0.42–0.63).[12]

The "WOMAN (World Maternal Antifibrinolytic) trial" was an extension of this hypothesis to see reduction of maternal deaths due to PPH with TXA. 20,060 women were randomized to get placebo or TXA 1 g IV when excessive bleeding was noticed.[13] This was in addition to the standard medications (prophylactic and therapeutic oxytocin/prostaglandins) given during such episode and needed surgical intervention (balloon tamponade/compression sutures). If bleeding continued for >30 minutes or stopped and restarted bleeding within 24 hours, another 1 g dose was given. It was an international, multicenter trial that studied the effect of TXA on death, hysterectomy, thromboembolic events, and other interventions for PPH.[13]

Death due to bleeding was significantly reduced in women who had TXA (155 of 10,036 women or 1.5%) compared with those who had placebo (191 of 9,985 women or 1.9%). The RR was 0.81 (95% CI 0.65–1.0). If the treatment was given within 3 hours of giving birth, the RR was 0.69 with a 95% CI of 0.52–0.91 (p = 0.008), i.e. a 30% reduction of maternal deaths due to bleeding and the maximal benefit was seen in those cases with bleeding due to uterine atony. There were other causes of smaller number of maternal deaths but they were not different between the placebo versus TXA group. The hysterectomy rates were not different between the two groups. One reason could be the ready recourse to hysterectomies for fear of inability to get adequate quantities of blood for transfusion. The need for repeat surgery for bleeding was reduced by 35% in the TXA group. Thromboembolic episodes on the arterial and venous side of the circulation were seen in small numbers but were equal in the placebo and TXA arms of the trial. Based on this trial, a 30% reduction of maternal death can be achieved by implementing a policy of early use of TXA in all cases of PPH.

Following the significant reduction in maternal deaths in the WOMAN trial, the WHO[14] came up with some recommendations and cautions about the use of TXA and are given below:
- Use TXA in all cases of PPH, regardless of whether the bleeding is due to genital tract trauma or other causes
- Use TXA within 3 hours and as early as possible after onset of PPH
- Do not initiate TXA more than 3 hr after birth unless being used for bleeding that restarts within 24 hours of completing the first dose
- Fixed dose of 1 g in 10 mL (100 mg/mL) IV at 1 mL/min—administered over 10 minutes
- Second dose of 1 g IV if bleeding continues after 30 minutes or if bleeding restarts within 24 hr of completing the first dose
- Bolus rapid injection has the potential risk of transient lowering of BP
- Tranexamic acid can be mixed with most IV solutions—electrolytes, carbohydrate, amino acid and dextran, and uterotonics
- Tranexamic acid should not be mixed with blood/products, penicillin, and mannitol
- Tranexamic acid should not be used if there is contraindication for use of antifibrinolytic agents including TXA (e.g. known thromboembolism during pregnancy, history of coagulopathy, active IV clotting, and known hypersensitivity to TXA).

INTERNAL UTERINE TAMPONADE

The principles of intrauterine tamponade include increasing intrauterine pressure that is higher than systemic arterial pressure and direct application of pressure on a bleeding site. A systematic review of the case series, retrospective studies regarding all available balloon types found an overall effectiveness of 91.5% in PPH management.[15] The tamponade maneuver is used as a prognostic test in cases where medical treatment was not effective to control bleeding. The original test used a Sengstaken-Blakemore esophageal catheter that was inserted and inflated in the intrauterine cavity. If no or minimal bleeding was observed, the test was positive and surgical intervention was avoided (87% of cases), while if significant bleeding continued, surgical intervention was needed.[16]

A systematic review that assessed all conservative methods following medically uncontrolled PPH, found that no method was significantly superior than the others, therefore uterine balloon tamponade should be the first step as it is the least invasive.[17] However, the technology has brought new players to the market in the form of double balloon tamponade and suction catheter negative pressure tamponade.

Double-balloon Catheter: Ebb Balloon

A dual-balloon polyurethane catheter (uterine and vaginal balloons) has been assessed in unresponsive PPH cases to medication following uterine atony or placenta previa. The results are comparable to other similar devices hence its popularity would be less because of its cost. A surveillance study of 51 patients found that in 98% of PPH cases, bleeding decreased or stopped following the dual-balloon catheter placement.[7]

Suction Tamponade Device

This device has an occlusion balloon, built into the device shaft which can be inflated at the level of the external cervical os to create a uterine seal. The distal end of the device is attached to a standard suction tubing to a regulated suction source with a one-liter collection canister, and set at 70 mm Hg vacuum. The suction created an immediate seal at the cervical os, with continuing suction 50–250 mL of residual blood could be evacuated from the uterine cavity into the vacuum canister. The uterus collapses and regains its tone within minutes. The hemorrhaging stopped in all cases in a study done in Indonesia and the other in India where there was no cervical occlusion balloon and higher pressures of 600 mm Hg were used.[18,19] The device should remain in place while vaginal and perineal lacerations are repaired. The device should be left in place for a minimum of 1 hour, and in the published studies they were kept in for up to 6.5 hours.

Suction collapse of the uterus to arrest PPH is a good concept and the initial trials are promising. More prospective descriptive studies on cases that warrant such intervention should provide us the information on the ideal suction pressure. The ongoing randomized control studies on balloon tamponade versus vacuum tamponade cross over trials should give us more information of its effectiveness (Fig. 1).

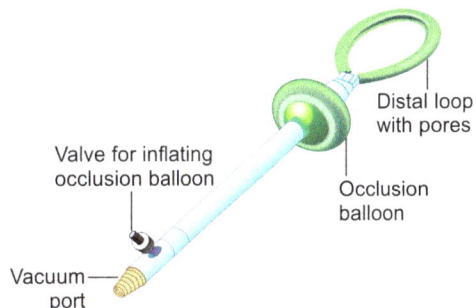

Fig. 1: In press suction device for tamponade.

TRIPLE P PROCEDURE FOR CONSERVING THE UTERUS IN CASES WITH PLACENTA ACCRETA

Morbidly adherent placenta is a major cause of maternal morbidity and mortality, with increasing incidence probably due to the rising number of cesarean sections which is a major risk factor. Conservative uterine-sparing techniques for future fertility include hemostatic sutures, balloon tamponade, leaving placenta in situ, pelvic devascularization, and uterine artery embolization. Further research is required about effectiveness of conservative treatment options (Doumouchtsis and Arulkumaran 2010).[20]

The triple P procedure was introduced by Chandraharan et al. in 2012, as a uterine conserving surgical technique in cases of morbidly adherent placenta.[21] It consists of perioperative placental localization and delivery of the fetus via a transverse incision above the upper border of the placenta, pelvic devascularization by radiologically-guided internal iliac artery balloon placement (before onset of surgery) and myometrial excision above and below the placenta and uterine wall reconstruction.[21] A subsequent study compared the triple P procedure to other conservative methods for placenta accreta and concluded that PPH and hysterectomy incidence is significantly reduced in the triple P group of patients.[22]

PELVIC PRESSURE PACK

It is used in the immediate postsurgical period to control bleeding from large surfaces and venous plexuses that other hemostatic measures have failed to do so. The most common type of this pack that is simple to make with cheap materials include a sterile bag filled with gauze rolls tied end-to-end that is placed intra-abdominally and the neck is delivered transvaginally through the open vaginal cuff. Suspension by a 1-liter bag of fluid is attached to neck of the bag to achieve optimal pressure. Most cases that have implemented this, have good bleeding control.[23] The Ebb balloon has also been proposed as an alternative for the gauze pack, but further research is required prior to recommending it.

CONCLUSION

We have reviewed the literature and decided to give two examples of newer approaches in medication (heat stable carbetocin and TXA); two examples of simple surgical techniques (double balloon tamponade and suction tamponade device) and two examples in advanced surgical techniques (triple P procedure and pelvic pressure pack). The textbook contains several chapters that cover a variety of conditions and methods to manage them—hence our brevity so as not to duplicate the contents in other chapters. We believe better knowledge of newer approaches may contribute to reduction in the incidence and severity of PPH thus reducing morbidity and mortality.

REFERENCES

1. Hunter DJ, Schulz P, Wassenaar W. Effect of carbetocin, a long-acting oxytocin analog on the postpartum uterus. Clin Pharmacol Ther. 1992;52(1):60-7.
2. Chong YS, Su LL, Arulkumaran S. Current strategies for the prevention of postpartum haemorrhage in the third stage of labour. Curr Opin Obstet Gynecol. 2004;16(2):143-50.
3. Su LL, Chong YS, Samuel M. Carbetocin for preventing postpartum haemorrhage. Cochrane Database Syst Rev. 2012;(4):CD005457.
4. Widmer M, Piaggio G, Najuyen TM, et al. Heat-stable carbetocin versus oxytocin to prevent haemorrhage after vaginal birth. N Engl J Med. 2018;379(8):743-52.
5. Su LL, Rauff M, Chan YH, et al. Carbetocin versus syntometrine for the third stage of labour following vaginal delivery-a double-blind randomized controlled trial. BJOG. 2009;116(11):1461-6.
6. Askar AA, Ismail MT, El-Ezz AA, et al. Carbetocin versus syntometrine in the management of third stage of labor following vaginal delivery. Arch Gynecol Obstet. 2011;284(6):1359-65.
7. Gallos ID, Williams HM, Price MJ, et al. Uterotonic agents for preventing postpartum haemorrhage: a network meta-analysis. Cochrane Database Syst Rev. 2018;4:CD011689.
8. Anyakora C, Oni Y, Ezedinachi U, et al. Quality medicines in maternal health: results of oxytocin, misoprostol, magnesium sulfate and calcium gluconate quality audits. BMC Pregnancy Childbirth. 2018;18(1):44.
9. Torloni MR, Gomes Freitas C, Kartoglu UH, et al. Quality of oxytocin available in low and middle-income countries: a systematic review of the literature. BJOG. 2016;123(113):2076-86.
10. Malm M, Madsen I, Kjellstrom J. Development and stability of a heat-stable formulation of carbetocin for the prevention of postpartum haemorrhage for use in low and middle-income countries. J Pept Sci. 2018;24(6):e3082.
11. WHO. WHO recommendations for the prevention and treatment of postpartum haemorrhage. Geneva: World Health Organization; 2012.
12. Novikova N, Hofmeyr GJ, Cluver C. Tranexamic acid for preventing postpartum haemorrhage. Cochrane Database Syst Rev. 2015;(6):CD007872.
13. Woman Trial Collaborators. Effect of early tranexamic acid administration on mortality,

hysterectomy and other morbidities in women with postpartum haemorrhage (WOMAN): an international randomized, double-blind, placebo-controlled trial. Lancet. 2017;389: 2105-16.
14. WHO. (2007). WHO recommendation on Tranexamic acid for treatment of Postpartum Haemorrhage. [online] Available from: https://www.who.int/reproductivehealth/publications/tranexamic-acid-pph-treatment/en/ [Last accessed July, 2019].
15. Georgiou C. Balloon tamponade in the management of postpartum haemorrhage: a review. BJOG. 2009;116(6):748-57.
16. Condous GS, Arulkumaran S, Symonds I, et al. The 'tamponade test' in the management of massive postpartum hemorrhage. Obstet Gynecol. 2003;101:767-72.
17. Dildy GA, Belfort MA, Adair CD, et al. Initial experience with a dual-balloon catheter for the management of postpartum hemorrhage. Am J Obstet Gynecol. 2014;210:136.e1-6.
18. Purwosunu Y, Sarkoen W, Arulkumaran S, et al. Control of postpartum haemorrhage using vacuum induced uterine tamponade. Obstet Gynecol. 2016;128(1):33-6.
19. Ram S, Ram S, Ram S, et al. Vacuum retraction of uterus for management of atonic postpartum haemorrhage. IOSR J Dental Med Sci. 2014; 13(11):15-9.
20. Doumouchtsis SK, Arulkumaran S. The morbidly adherent placenta: an overview of management options. Acta Obstet Gynecol Scand. 2010;89(9):1126-33.
21. Chandraharan E, Rao S, Belli AM, et al. The triple-P procedure as a conservative surgical alternative to peripartum hysterectomy for placenta percreta. Int J Gynaecol Obstet. 2012; 117(2):191-4.
22. Teixider Vinas M, Belli AM, Arulkumaran S, et al. Prevention of postpartum hemorrhage and hysterectomy in patients with morbidly adherent placenta: a cohort study comparing outcomes before and after introduction of the Triple-P procedure. Ultrasound Obstet Gynecol. 2015;46(3):350-5.
23. Dildy GA 3rd. Postpartum hemorrhage: new management options. Clin Obstet Gynecol. 2002;45:330-44.

Section 5

Critical Situations

- **Disorders of Hemostasis in Pregnancy**
  Sitalakshmi Subramanian
- **Peripartum Hysterectomy**
  Ashis Kumar Mukhopadhyay
- **Disseminated Intravascular Coagulation in Obstetric Hemorrhage**
  Anahita Chauhan, Madhva Prasad
- **Massive Transfusion Protocol: Role of Component Therapy**
  Shivaram Chandrashekar

Disorders of Hemostasis in Pregnancy

Sitalakshmi Subramanian

HEMOSTATIC CHANGES IN NORMAL PREGNANCY

Pregnancy is a physiological condition associated with hypercoagulable tendency which is likely a natural protective mechanism to ensure that the risk of bleeding during and immediately after delivery is reduced.

There are significant alterations in the components of hemostasis associated with normal pregnancy. The concentrations of most clotting factors are increased except factor XI. *Protein S which is one of the natural anticoagulants is decreased. The fibrinolytic activity is also decreased.* These changes together with a reduction in the activation of platelets result in a hypercoagulable condition leading to an increased tendency to develop thromboembolic complication during pregnancy and in the postpartum period. During pregnancy, the fibrinolytic activity is decreased due to the production of plasminogen activator inhibitor type 2 (PAI-2) by the placenta and this is restored to normalcy after delivery. D-dimer levels increase in pregnancy. However, it is not a marker of intravascular coagulation as fibrinolysis is depressed.[1,2] These D-dimers may be produced by the placenta. Normal pregnancy is associated with mild reduction in platelet count and the reduction is maximum in the last trimester due to hemodilution and excessive platelet destruction in the circulation. Most of these changes become normalized 4-6 weeks after delivery.

However, during the antepartum, intrapartum and in the immediate postpartum period, the chances of increased tendency to bleed or develop thrombosis are high. Disseminated intravascular coagulation (DIC) which can result in multiorgan failure can be secondary to eclampsia, HELLP (hemolysis, elevated liver enzymes, and low platelet count) syndrome, placental abruption and amniotic fluid embolism. Therefore, it is important to detect the abnormalities in hemostasis as early as possible to prevent complications.

Besides the systemic hemostatic changes, there are several changes occurring locally. The placental trophoblast expression of tissue factor is increased with reduction in production of tissue factor pathway inhibitor. The endothelial cells, platelets, placental trophoblasts produce microparticles which result in procoagulant effect. The local anticoagulant mechanisms contribute mainly in balancing the procoagulant effect. In patients with antiphospholipid antibodies (APLAs), autoantibodies to annexin V cause disruption of the anticoagulant mechanisms resulting in thrombotic complications in pregnancy.

Bleeding disorders among women are often unrecognized or misdiagnosed in obstetric cases. Certain pathological conditions unique to pregnancy result in bleeding tendencies. These are very rare causes of postpartum hemorrhage (PPH). However, in the absence of more common causes, these conditions should be considered. These include coagulopathy due to DIC associated with eclampsia, abruptio placentae and amniotic fluid embolism. *Sepsis and intrauterine death of the fetus are often associated with DIC.*

INHERITED BLEEDING DISORDERS IN PREGNANCY

Pregnant women who have been previously diagnosed to have a bleeding disorder or those who present with history of bleeding manifestation, e.g. bleeding gums, epistaxis or any other form of skin and mucous membrane bleeding or menorrhagia are at an increased risk of bleeding complications during pregnancy and delivery and hence require thorough investigation in order not to miss a pre-existing coagulation disorder. *Von Willebrand's disease (vWD), hemophilia A and hemophilia B due to factor VIII and factor IX deficiency respectively are the predominant causes in 95% of the cases.* Rare bleeding disorders (RBDs) which include inherited deficiencies of fibrinogen, factors II, V, V and VIII, VII, X, XI and XIII account for the remaining 3–5% of the cases.[3]

Von Willebrand's Disease

Von Willebrand's disease is the most common inherited bleeding disorder. The inheritance is autosomal dominant. Types 1, 2 and 3 are the three types of vWD. Type 1 and type 3 are characterized by deficiency of von Willebrand's factor (vWF) and type 2 is a defect in the structure of vWF. vWF is required to prevent the proteolysis of circulating factor VIII and for adhesion of platelets to the site of tissue damage. Type 2 has subtypes (2A, 2B, 2M, 2N). Type 1 vWD is the most common and has an incidence of 75%. It is the mildest form of vWD and is characterized by a mild deficiency of vWF. Type 2 is a structural defect of vWF and its subtypes are due to defective binding of vWF to glycoproteins and factor VIII. Type 3 vWD is very severe resulting from total deficiency of vWF. Type 2B is associated with thrombocytopenia. It is not always diagnosed because of the complexity of the disorder, varied clinical presentations, severity, and lack of diagnostic facilities in most laboratories. The predominant presenting manifestation of type 1 vWD in women is menorrhagia. Other mucocutaneous bleeding manifestations can occur like epistaxis, and excessive bleeding after tooth extractions or surgical procedures. vWF increases up to 200–375% in normal pregnancy. Patients with type 1 vWD disease can have normal factor concentrations as pregnancy progresses. The risk of developing a bleeding manifestation after the first trimester is minimal. In those with type 2 disease also, increase in vWF level is noted as pregnancy progresses. The defect in type 2 vWD is functional and hence these patients are at an increased risk of bleeding. Patients with vWD type 2B experience a further drop in platelet count as pregnancy progresses. Type 3 vWD cases are at increased risk of PPH as vWF level does not increase during pregnancy because of complete absence of vWF in their circulation. Laboratory diagnosis involves assay of vWF antigen, quantification of ristocetin cofactor (RiCof) activity and factor VIII levels. The outcomes of pregnancy in women with vWD are good.[4] This may be due to the protective effect of increases in fibrinogen, factor VII, factor VIII, factor X and vWF during pregnancy. It is essential to measure the amount of vWF antigen, RiCof activity and level of factor VIII in first trimester of pregnancy and in the last trimester to assess that levels are sufficient for normal delivery. Desmopressin (DDAVP) is considered safe for pregnant women with type 1 vWD. In type 2B vWD, the platelet count may reduce during pregnancy or be aggravated by pregnancy due to abnormal intermediate vWF multimers which are produced in excess and bind to platelets to cause spontaneous platelet aggregation.

Hemophilia A (Severe Factor VIII) and Hemophilia B (Severe Factor IX Deficiency)

It is a well-known fact that hemophilia is very uncommon in women; however, carrier state of hemophilia is not uncommon. It is reported that 35% of carriers have factor concentrations below the normal levels although a majority of them are asymptomatic. The presence of a carrier state may be detected in about less than 5% of women who complain of menorrhagia. The factor VIII or IX levels should be measured at conception and repeated at the third trimester of pregnancy in patients who are detected to have carrier status of hemophilia A or B. The factor VIII levels reach a peak in the last trimester of pregnancy, and in majority of patients who are hemophilia A carriers, the factor VIII levels will increase to the normal range.

Unlike factor VIII levels which usually increase by term to near normal levels, factor IX levels remain unaltered during pregnancy. Therefore, pregnant women with decreased factor IX levels or those with history of bleeding manifestation will require factor IX concentrates as replacement therapy before delivery. Specific factor concentrates as replacement therapy is the preferred treatment modality. However, DDAVP can be administered for bleeding prophylaxis in patients who are carriers of hemophilia A with borderline factor VIII levels in their circulation.

Recombinant activated factor VII acts as a powerful procoagulant used to activate the extrinsic pathway of coagulation, bind platelets, and help in the generation of a dose-dependent release of thrombin in patients with factor VIII or IX deficiency for restoration of normal hemostasis.

Factor eight inhibitor bypass activity (FEIBA) is one of the approaches for the management of patients who develop inhibitor to factor VIII.

Acquired Hemophilia

One of the rare, acquired complications that can occur during pregnancy or more commonly in the postpartum period is acquired hemophilia which is due to the development of an inhibitor which is acquired, an immunoglobulin G (IgG) antibody specifically directed against factor VIII. The bleeding manifestations are severe and bleeding occurs at different sites. In our experience, we encountered a case of a young lady in her third decade of life who had severe postpartum bleeding.[5] Laboratory testing typically showed activated partial thromboplastin time (aPTT) which is markedly prolonged and did not get corrected to normal on the addition of normal plasma. Factor VIII: C assay was less than 1%. Testing for factor VIII: C inhibitor by Bethesda assay showed high-titer inhibitor to factor VIII. She responded well to immunosuppressant therapy. The mortality is high due to severe bleeding. Most cases have a complete remission within 4–6 months. Timely recognition of the presence of inhibitor is crucial for effective management. If the inhibitor disappears completely, subsequent pregnancies will have a good prognosis.

Rarer forms of bleeding disorders: These include inherited deficiencies of clotting factors like fibrinogen, factors II, V, VII, X, XI and XIII, combined factor V and factor VIII deficiencies, and congenital deficiency of factor II, VII, IX and X which are the vitamin K-dependent factors.

Severe Factor XIII Deficiency

Factor XIII deficiency can present with recurrent pregnancy loss. Anuradha et al. reported a case of factor XIII deficiency with nine pregnancy losses who was treated effectively with regular cryoprecipitate transfusions once in 14 days from preconception till delivery in order to have a successful outcome of full term normal delivery.[6] If available, prophylaxis using high-dose factor XIII plasma concentrate or recombinant factor XIII is the preferred treatment modality. The frequency of dose should be increased from once in 4 weeks to once in 2-3 weeks to ensure that the plasma factor XIII concentration is more than 0.2 IU/mL. A dose of 10-40 IU/kg factor XIII concentrate is necessary during labor or before cesarean section.

Severe Fibrinogen Deficiency

Severe fibrinogen deficiency is also one of the causes of excessive bleeding in the intrapartum or postpartum period. Functional defect of fibrinogen predisposes the individual to thrombotic risk and pregnancy loss. When the level of active fibrinogen is reduced to values lower than 0.5 g/L, the pregnant woman will require prophylactic dose of fibrinogen concentrate 50-100 mg/kg twice a week initially. The trough fibrinogen activity should be adjusted to more than 1 g/L. It is recommended that the fibrinogen concentrate dose is increased as the pregnancy progresses to maintain fibrinogen activity. In order to control bleeding for patients in labor, it is desirable to maintain fibrinogen activity more than 1.5 g/L for 3 continuous days. Tranexamic acid is useful to treat minor bleeding manifestations.

The clinical phenotype of hypofibrinogenemia and dysfibrinogenemia is variable. Family history of similar manifestations will support the decision to plan aggressive therapy. Close monitoring is recommended for pregnant women for bleeding manifestations.

The risk of thrombosis is very high with fibrinogen replacement therapy and therefore requires careful monitoring. Thromboprophylaxis with low molecular weight heparin (LMWH) is considered for pregnant women with a qualitative defect in fibrinogen or other risk factors for thrombophilia, and with a minimal risk of bleeding.

Factor V Deficiency

Inherited factor X deficiency is extremely rare. The bleeding manifestation can be severe and mortality high if unrecognized. For women with factor V activity less than 0.2 IU/mL, 15-25 mL/kg fresh frozen plasma (FFP) is recommended when the patient is in labor or before cesarean section to achieve factor V activity 0.2-0.4 IU/mL. Additional dose of FFP 10 mL/kg at 12-hour intervals is given to ensure that the level of factor V is maintained at a level of 0.2 IU/mL for a minimum of 72 hours.

Severe Factor VII Deficiency

Recombinant factor VIIa 15-30 µg/kg every 4-6 hours plays an important role in the management of patients with severe deficiency of factor VII in the last trimester especially for those patients who have experienced bleeding manifestations in the past. Tranexamic acid (15-20 mg/kg or 1 g four times daily) has a role in the management of patients with mild bleeding manifestations. The use of recombinant factor VIIa 15-30 µg/kg every 4-6 hours is the recommended mode of treatment if clinically indicated, usually for a minimum of three doses for the management of severe bleeding.

Severe Factor X Deficiency

A case report by Shilpa, et al. in their case report have emphasized the management approach to a patient with severe factor X deficiency, who had a successful pregnancy with the rationale use of FFP.[7] Prothrombin complex concentrate 20-40 IU/kg (or factor X concentrate if available) may be used to achieve factor X activity more than 0.4 IU/mL in the management of pregnant women with factor X activity less than 0.3 IU/mL in the last trimester who have a history of bleeding manifestations and all those who require cesarean section. It is recommended that a dose of 10-20 IU/kg prothrombin complex concentrate be given once daily to maintain factor X activity more than 0.3 IU/mL for at least 3 days. For prophylaxis in the antenatal period in women with a history of recurrent bleeding manifestations or poor pregnancy outcome, a dose of prothrombin complex concentrate 20-30 IU/kg two or three times a week to maintain trough factor X more than 0.01 IU/mL is recommended.

Factor V and VIII Deficiency

Fresh frozen plasma is the preferred treatment of bleeding in women with combined deficiency of factor V and factor VIII. If factor V activity less than 0.2 IU/mL in the third trimester, once in established labor or before cesarean section, the recommended dose of FFP is 15-25 mL/kg to achieve factor V activity 0.2-0.4 IU/mL followed by further FFP 10 mL/kg once every 12 hours to maintain factor V activity more than 0.2 IU/mL for at least 3 days. Additional recombinant factor VIII if the factor VIII activity is less than 0.5 IU/mL in the third trimester is recommended.

Prothrombin (Factor II) Deficiency

Prothrombin (factor II) deficiency is extremely rare. Prothrombin complex concentrate 20-40 IU/kg is indicated if factor II activity is less than 0.2 IU/mL and there is significant bleeding, and for established labor or prior to cesarean section, to achieve factor II activity 0.2-0.4 IU/mL. Further prothrombin complex concentrate 10-20 IU/kg at 48-hour intervals is recommended to maintain factor II activity more than 0.2 IU/mL for at least 3 days. For women already receiving prophylactic prothrombin complex concentrate, the same can be continued throughout pregnancy.

In general, patients who present with bleeding disorders should be treated by a multidisciplinary team consisting of an obstetrician and hematologist

Abnormalities of Platelets

It can be qualitative or quantitative and are the most common hematological disorders during pregnancy.

Inherited Disorders of Platelet Function

These are a distinct group of disorders and may also pose a *challenge as the risk of bleeding during pregnancy is high.* These disorders are more common in South India where consanguinity rate is high.

Glanzmann Thrombasthenia

Deficiency of glycoprotein (GP) IIb/IIIa, the receptor responsible for platelet aggregation results in the disorder of platelet function referred to as Glanzmann thrombasthenia (GT) which is a severe, autosomal recessive bleeding disorder. Platelet aggregation tests or flow cytometry studies are the diagnostic tools available. Absence of aggregation response to adenosine 5'-diphosphate (ADP) agonists, collagen, adrenaline and arachidonic acid is the hallmark finding on platelet aggregometry. The absence of platelet aggregates in a finger prick smear (without anticoagulant) will provide a simple clue to the diagnosis. The risk of intrapartum and PPH is high. The management would include human leukocyte antigen (HLA)-matched platelet transfusions during labor and in the immediate postpartum period. Recombinant factor VIIa may be considered as a prophylactic treatment at delivery for patients with a history of bleeding. Depending on the severity of bleeding manifestation, repeat doses may be required. Tranexamic acid is recommended during labor and continued through the postpartum period. Maternal alloimmunization to fetal platelet antigens (GPIIb/IIIa) derived from the father may cause fetal thrombocytopenia and risk of bleeding in the fetus.[8]

Bernard-Soulier Syndrome

Deficiency of the platelet GP1b/IX/V receptor, which is required for adhesion of platelet to the vascular endothelium results in this disorder referred to as Bernard-Soulier syndrome (BSS) which is inherited as an autosomal recessive disorder. It is associated with moderate thrombocytopenia and giant platelets. Platelet aggregation tests and flow cytometry studies help in confirming the diagnosis. Platelet aggregometry shows normal aggregation response to ADP agonists, collagen, adrenaline and arachidonic acid, but absence of aggregation with the addition of ristocetin. *Patients with BSS often bleed excessively.* Where this is high consanguinity, the father may be tested for GPIb surface density using platelet flow cytometry. The chances of developing severe PPH and wound hematoma are high in these patients. The role of a multidisciplinary team in the effective management of delivery cannot be overemphasized. Prophylactic platelet transfusion at delivery or before cesarean section, in combination with tranexamic acid is recommended in patients with history of bleeding manifestations. To reduce the risk of development of alloantibodies and platelet refractoriness, platelets should be HLA-matched where possible.[9] Tranexamic acid should be given at the onset of labor and continued regularly through the postpartum period.

Secretory Disorders

These disorders result from deficiencies of alpha and/or dense granules. *They exhibit decreased aggregation with ADP, adrenaline and collagen.* Decreased dense granules are demonstrated by electron microscopy. Gray platelet syndrome is an autosomal dominant disorder which occurs due to decreased alpha granules resulting in gray appearance of platelets on the Romanowsky stained peripheral blood smear characterized by mild bleeding manifestations.

ACQUIRED PLATELET DISORDERS IN PREGNANCY

Gestational thrombocytopenia, idiopathic thrombocytopenic purpura (ITP) and hypertensive disorders like pre-eclampsia contribute to 99% of the cases of thrombocytopenia in pregnancy. Gestational thrombocytopenia (incidental) is the most common cause accounting for 75% of the cases. The onset of thrombocytopenia is usually after the first trimester. This is not of much clinical significance and the platelet count becomes normal 1–6 weeks after delivery. The diagnosis is of exclusion and at times may be difficult to differentiate it from immune thrombocytopenia. The platelet count is usually remains steady in gestational thrombocytopenia or ITP, whereas in pre-eclampsia, the platelet count can rapidly change and it is important to obtain serial platelet counts. It is important to note that platelet function is typically normal in gestational thrombocytopenia and ITP and may be abnormal in severe pre-eclampsia.

Immune Thrombocytopenia

Immune thrombocytopenic purpura is associated with thrombocytopenia due to the production of autoantibodies against glycoproteins on the platelet surface membrane, especially Ib/IX and IIb/IIIa. The antibody is IgG in nature. It crosses the placenta, especially in the third trimester of pregnancy and causes neonatal thrombocytopenia. The antibody may be secondary to drugs, human immunodeficiency virus (HIV) infection, or connective tissue disorders. It is idiopathic in most of the cases.

Destructive Thrombocytopenia Associated with Pre-eclampsia

Thrombocytopenia develops in 50% of the women with pre-eclampsia. In eclampsia or HELLP, the thrombocytopenia can be severe. In these cases, platelet activation, aggregation, and consumption occur due to endothelial injury results in the systemic microangiopathic vasculature leading to formation of multiple thrombi. Some of the patients with features of pre-eclampsia may develop HELLP. They can also present with severe liver dysfunction and overt coagulopathy.

The platelets are functionally abnormal and are decreased in number. Platelet counts >30 × 10^9/L are rarely associated with excess maternal bleeding. It is recommended to maintain a platelet counts >50 × 10^9/L toward term and for a normal vaginal delivery. For epidural analgesia and cesarean section, the recommended platelet counts are >80 × 10^9/L.

Platelet transfusion will be required to control the bleeding manifestations during childbirth and in the immediate postpartum period in most women with severe disorders of platelet function.

Thrombotic Microangiopathies

Pre-eclampsia, eclampsia, HELLP syndrome, thrombotic thrombocytopenic purpura (TTP), hemolytic-uremic syndrome (HUS) and DIC are a group of disorders associated with microvascular thrombi formation, consumption of coagulation factors and thrombocytes resulting in bleeding manifestations.[10]

HELLP (Hemolysis, Elevated Liver Enzymes, Low Platelets) Syndrome

HELLP syndrome is characterized by elevated bilirubin and liver enzymes, high lactate dehydrogenase with the presence of fragmented red cells in the peripheral blood smear and low platelet count below 100 × 10^9/L.

Pregnant women with severe pre-eclampsia are complicated by HELLP in 10% of the cases. It is also to be noted that severe thrombocytopenia and hepatic derangement can occur without hypertension and proteinuria. The features can aggravate in the immediate postpartum period. The risk of recurrence is up to 20% in subsequent pregnancies. The common complications are DIC and abruptio placentae in 16–20% of the cases and neonatal mortality in 10–15% cases.

Thrombotic Thrombocytopenic Purpura

Thrombotic thrombocytopenic purpura is a clinical syndrome. The features (pentad) that characterize TTP are: thrombocytopenia, microangiopathic hemolytic anemia (MAHA), renal failure, neurological disturbances and fever. It occurs rarely in pregnancy. Half the cases present in the first two trimesters. Deficiency of ADAMTS 13, vWF-cleaving protease leads to activation and consumption of platelets. The prognosis is bad if unrecognized early. Plasmapheresis is the treatment of choice. Platelet transfusions will worsen the condition and are therefore contraindicated. Fetal monitoring is required since placental infarcts can lead to fetal complications such as intrauterine growth restriction or death.

Hemolytic-uremic Syndrome

Hemolytic-uremic syndrome is a condition which is closely related to TTP characterized predominantly by renal dysfunction and is associated with prodromal diarrhea (due to verotoxin production by *Escherichia coli* O157:H7) in 90% of the cases. Unlike TTP, vWF-cleaving protease is normally present.

Disseminated Intravascular Coagulation

Disseminated intravascular coagulation is an uncontrolled widespread activation of the coagulation system leading to microvascular coagulation, excessive fibrinolysis and multiorgan failure. 0.1% of all pregnancies are complicated by DIC. Severe abruptions and PPH are associated with DIC in 35–40% of the cases. Damage to the vascular endothelium, release of tissue factor which promotes thrombosis, and production of procoagulant phospholipids contribute to the development of DIC. It occurs in conditions such as pre-eclampsia, HELLP, septicemia, hypovolemic shock, placental abruption, amniotic fluid embolism, and prolonged intrauterine fetal death.[11] Clinically the patient presents with bleeding. The coagulation screen reflects depletion of clotting factors with prolongation of the screening tests of coagulation like aPTT and prothrombin time (PT) with reduced levels of fibrinogen and evidence of fibrinolysis with increased D-dimers. Treatment of the underlying cause and providing adequate and timely hemostatic support with blood component therapy is necessary for recovery.

A DIAGNOSTIC APPROACH TO BLEEDING DISORDER IN PREGNANCY

The approach to the evaluation of a bleeding patient should begin with a complete blood count to evaluate for thrombocytopenia. A peripheral smear should be examined to evaluate platelet morphology and look for evidences of hemolysis.

Screening tests of coagulation like PT, aPTT and thrombin time should be performed as baseline. The need for additional testing will be decided based on patient history, family history, and laboratory results. In mild vWD and in some cases with type 2 vWD, the level of factor VIII will be sufficient enough to result in normal aPTT. Thus, a normal aPTT does not always rule out vWD. In patients with symptoms of mucosal bleeding and its vWF assay and vWF:RiCof activity are normal, platelet function studies should be performed to rule out a functional platelet disorder. In cases which show a high PT and/or aPTT, mixing tests and factor assays should be performed as appropriate to identify the factor deficiency or detect the presence of inhibitors to clotting factors.

Hemostatic status can be assessed by laboratory analyses and/or by point-of-care devices. Laboratory analyses are the most common assessment method; it is necessary to keep in mind that unlike point-of-care devices, laboratory analysis requires time for sample transport, testing and reporting the results. Hemostasis assessment by point-of-care devices is especially suitable in perioperative settings (cardiac surgery, liver surgery and obstetrics) and in intensive care units. The time is required for transportation of samples is avoided and the devices used for point-of-care testing provide faster results. Nevertheless, the staffs require training to use the point-of-care devices, perform the analyses and interpret results. The manufacturer's instructions should be followed to ensure proper functioning of the equipment.

Platelet count, aPTT, PT [international normalized ratio (INR)], fibrinogen assay, D-dimer and antithrombin levels are frequently used to assess the hemostatic function.

Platelet count: Reference range is 150–400 × 10^9/L. Increased risk of bleeding is rare at platelet count above 50 × 10^9/L and becomes more common particularly below 20 × 10^9/L, and especially below 10 × 10^9/L.

Activated partial thromboplastin time: Reference range is 30–40 seconds. It measures the overall activity of intrinsic and common pathway of coagulation (fibrinogen and factors II, V, VIII, IX, XI and XII). aPTT is prolonged when the activity (<25–30%) of any of these coagulation factors is significantly reduced.

Prothrombin time: Reference range is 13–15 seconds. It measures the overall activity of factors II, VII and X (vitamin K-dependent factors). Although factor IX is vitamin K-dependent, PT (INR) does not measure factor IX activity.

Fibrinogen: Reference range is 1.8–4.5 g/L. aPTT can be normal or near the upper reference range despite fibrinogen <1 g/L. Since fibrinogen is an acute phase protein, levels >5 g/L are common after surgery and during infection, as well as in pregnancy, especially in cases of pre-eclampsia.

D-dimer: Reference range is 0–0.5 mg/L. D-dimer represents degraded products of fibrin. Although D-dimer is a result of fibrinolytic activity, it is nonetheless a primary marker of increased coagulation as cross-linked fibrin is necessary to develop D-dimers. D-dimer is increased during pregnancy.

Thromboelastogram: The method follows the viscoelastic alterations that occur when clot is formed, providing data about clot formation, physical strength, stability, and fibrinolysis. The parameters obtained are:

- *R:* Reaction time, time from the start of a sample run until the first significant level of detectable clot formation (2 mm amplitude)
- *K:* K-time, time from R until a fixed level of clot firmness (20 mm amplitude)
- *Alpha (α) angle:* Measures kinetics of clot formation
- *MA:* Maximum amplitude, represents the strength of fibrin clot
- *LY30:* Lysis at 30 minutes after MA, represents clot lysis.

Management of bleeding disorders in pregnancy is challenging and requires a coordinated approach between obstetrician, hematologist and neonatologist.

Pregnant women are likely to be in a state of hypercoagulability during pregnancy primarily due to increased resistance to the effects of activated protein C, reduction in protein S activity and total/free protein C antigenicity, increases in serum fibrinogen, factors II, VII, VIII and X, and increased fibrinolytic inhibitors, especially PAI-1 and PAI-2. In addition, there is increased pressure on the pelvic veins and decreased flow in the lower extremities secondary to a gravid uterus contributes to the thrombophilic state. Thrombophilia in pregnancy will be discussed separately.

KEY POINTS

- Hemostatic changes are common in pregnancy. Although pregnant women are known to be in a hypercoagulable state, bleeding is a common complication of pregnancy.
- Gestational thrombocytopenia, ITP and hypertensive disorders like pre-eclampsia contribute to 99% of the cases of thrombocytopenia in pregnancy. *Gestational thrombocytopenia (incidental) is the leading cause accounting for 75% of the cases.*
- Inherited clotting factor deficiency is not uncommon in pregnancy. vWD, fibrinogen deficiency, factor XIII deficiency, factor V deficiency and rarely factor X deficiency and combined factor V and VIII deficiency have been described.
- Correct diagnosis by relevant laboratory tests is the key to effective management. Diagnostic approach includes baseline screening tests and confirmatory tests to identify the factor deficiency. Thromboelastography used as an adjunct diagnostic modality is of added value.
- Disseminated intravascular coagulation occurs in conditions such as pre-eclampsia, HELLP, septicemia, placental abruption, amniotic fluid embolism, and prolonged intrauterine fetal death.
- *Management of bleeding disorders in pregnancy is challenging and requires a coordinated approach between obstetrician, hematologist and neonatologist.*

REFERENCES

1. Ebrahim SH, Kulkarni R, Parker C, et al. Blood disorders among women implications for preconception care. Am J Prev Med. 2010;38 (4 Suppl):S459-67.
2. Prisco D, Ciuti G, Falciani M, et al. Hemostatic changes in normal pregnancy. Haematol Rep. 2005;1(10):1-5.
3. Thornton P, Douglas J. Coagulation in pregnancy. Best Pract Res Clin Obstet Gynaecol. 2010;24(3):339-52.
4. Gringeri A. Congenital bleeding disorders and pregnancy. Haematol Rep. 2005;1(10):43-6.
5. Shanthala Devi AM, Anuradha S, Sitalakshmi S, et al. Clinicohaematological profile of two cases of inhibitors to factor VIII. Indian J Pathol Microbiol. 2001;44(3):365-6.
6. Anuradha S, Sitalakshmi S, Shanthala Devi AM, et al. Good, bad and ugly facts of factor XIII deficiency. Indian J Hematol Blood Transfus. 2003;XX1(Suppl 1).
7. Venkatesh S, Ross C, Ramkumar V. Severe factor X deficiency in pregnancy: an obstetric challenge. Int J Pregnancy Child Birth. 2017; 2(1):14-5.
8. Diz-Kucukkaya R. Inherited platelet disorders including Glanzmann thrombasthenia and Bernard-Soulier syndrome. Hematology Am Soc Hematol Educ Program. 2013;2013:268-75.
9. Alamelu J, Liesner R. Modern management of severe platelet function disorders. Br J Haematol. 2010;149:813-23.
10. Gernsheimer TB. Congenital and acquired bleeding disorders in pregnancy. Hematology Am Soc Hematol Educ Program. 2016;2016(1):232-5.
11. Thachil J, Toh CH. Disseminated intravascular coagulation in obstetric disorders and its acute haematological management. Blood Rev. 2009;23:167-76.

Chapter 13B

Peripartum Hysterectomy

Ashis Kumar Mukhopadhyay

INTRODUCTION

Peripartum hysterectomy, described as an explicit marker of severe acute maternal morbidity (SAMM), is defined as removal of uterus after delivery or at cesarian section (CS) or performed within 24 hours of a delivery.[1] It is also called obstetric hysterectomy.

If uterus has to be removed due to complications during cesarean like severe postpartum hemorrhage (PPH) not managed conservatively, it is termed as cesarean hysterectomy, similarly if a woman needs hysterectomy post vaginal delivery, due to various complications, it is termed as peripartum hysterectomy. It is a last resort and lifesaving procedure for a woman though it can be quite challenging.

INCIDENCE

Incidence varies from 0.2 to 5.4 in 1,000 deliveries worldwide. And number of peripartum hysterectomies performed in an institute reflects the health care status of that area. The range of prevalence is wide (0.2–5.4/1,000), and mostly in developing countries. Furthermore, most of these reports were hospital-based and high-risk referral patterns were likely to influence this figure.[1] On the other hand, if we consider three population-based studies, they showed prevalence at the lower end of the scale: 0.3/1,000 in the Netherlands,[2] 0.5/1,000 in Israel,[3] and 0.5/1,000 in one Canadian province.[4] Overall, peripartum hysterectomy rate doubled in a decade in Canada.[5] In Denmark, incidence of emergency peripartum hysterectomy (EPH) is 0.24/1,000,[6] in turkey 0.41/1,000,[7] and 0.36/1,000 in UK.[8] And overall incidence is 0.4/1,000.[9,10] It is less than North America (0.77–1.4/1,000), this is due to increased vaginal birth after cesarean (VBAC) and low primary cesarean rate in Europe.[11-14]

In an excellent review of prevalence of EPH and the relationship with other comorbid associates, Flood et al. from Ireland, over 40 years studied 872,379 women, with 358 EPH, rate of 0.4/1,000 and concluded that risk of EPH has decreased over last 4 decades though there is an increased cesarean rate and incidence of placenta accreta.[15]

Farah Lone et al. reported an incidence of 0.6/1,000 over a period of 20 years, who did not agree to the reduction in the rate of EPH and concluded that "Despite the introduction of pharmacologic agents and new surgical techniques to control PPH, there was no reduction in the prevalence of EPH. Previous cesarean delivery with associated placenta previa or placenta accreta was a major contributor toward EPH".[16] Most of the studies in developing world have shown higher figures of EPH. Indian studies: A 2-year study from Bengaluru showed a high EPH rate of 10.1/1,000 deliveries, the highest contributor being atonic PPH.[17] A one-year study from Vishakhapatnam, Andhra Pradesh has shown a prevalence rate of EPH of 3.53/1,000 deliveries.[18] Our experience at CSS College of Obstetrics, Gynecology and Child Health, Kolkata: The prevalence rate of EPH as the ultimate resort to saving lives of mothers used to be around 5.77/1,000 deliveries, happening 10 years ago. In the last 5 years, the rate of EPH has come down to 2.77/1,000 deliveries, but at the same time, the incidence rate of placenta accreta and low-lying placenta has increased significantly. A 5-year study from Lahore, Pakistan, involving 10,030 deliveries showed 22 cases of EPH, giving an incidence rate of 2.1/1,000 deliveries, but the striking difference was that 3/4th of all cases had scarred uterus.[19] Basnet et al. from BPKIHS, Dharan, Nepal, reported 29 cases of EPH out of 19,539 births, giving a prevalence rate of 1.48/1,000 births, and rupture uterus was the most common indication.[20] Sepsis on the other hand played a major role in a South African study being an indication of EPH in more than 60% of cases, and the total prevalence rate of EPH was 2.77/1,000 deliveries.[21]

The incidence of EPH is on rise in various countries due to higher cesarean delivery rates and concomitant increases in placenta previa and/or accreta in subsequent pregnancies. We can assume that obstetric hysterectomy rates will continue to rise as we are facing increasing cesarean delivery rate.[1] Multiple pregnancy rates are also rising due to assisted reproductive treatments, and the need for critical care and hysterectomy is higher in these women.[22,23]

Francois et al. found that women with multiple pregnancies were six times more prone to EPH compared to singleton pregnancies and an almost 24-fold increase in higher order multiple pregnancies.[22] Other changing maternal demographic factors such as increasing age and obesity also contribute to rising cesarean delivery rates.

On the other hand, it is also true that due to improved conservative management techniques like active management of the third stage of labor (AMTSL), balloon tamponade, compression sutures and stepwise devascularization, incidence of EPH has reduced. But still it is a lifesaving procedure in those who do not respond to any conservative management. It is associated with excessive blood loss, maternal death consecutive to hemodynamic instability, disseminated intravascular coagulation (DIC), intraoperative complications, significant postoperative morbidity and adverse perinatal outcome.

A BIT OF HISTORY OF PERIPARTUM HYSTERECTOMY

In 1869 in the United States, Horatio Storer performed the first hysterectomy during cesarean. The patient died in 68 hours after surgery even though uterus was removed successfully.

In 1876, first cesarean hysterectomy was described by Eduardo Porro Head of Midwifery School in Milan in which both mother and baby survived.

Primiparous dwarf 144 cm height, Julia Cavallani after cesarean section had to undergo hysterectomy. Cintrat's constrictor was used as tourniquet to compress uterine arteries. Once uterus was removed, stump was brought through abdominal wound and closed externally with silver wire. Modifications were done by Lawson and Godson is 1890 and 1884, respectively.

INDICATIONS

Common indications are intractable hemorrhage due to conditions like:
- Atonic PPH
- Placenta previa with/without accreta
- Concealed abruptio placentae
- Uterine rupture
- Sepsis.

EPH: AT CROSSROADS—DO OR NOT TO DO

It is well-known that at times PPH can be refractory to medical management. We are dealing with a huge number of deliveries annually, hence this is quite expected. One finds himself at obstetric crossroad when the lifesaving decision of opening up for EPH or conservative management has to be taken within a very short period of time. Expertise and experience play a key role here, because every moment is vital.

SURGICAL PRINCIPLES OF EMERGENCY PERIPARTUM HYSTERECTOMY

Decision making is of utmost importance in situations of crisis requiring EPH. Ultimately, one has to decide with alternative conservative methods with less morbidity, but which may be futile in few conditions leading to excessive bleeding, delay in definitive treatment resulting in even DIC, or to move on lifesaving procedure like peripartum hysterectomy with increased morbidity and mortality. This should depend on judgment of experienced obstetrician.

Though the technique of obstetric hysterectomy has a similar principle to that of total abdominal hysterectomy in gynecological conditions, there are surgical difficulties due anatomic and physiological changes in pregnancy.

- *Abdominal entry*: It is very crucial to adopt a "Quick in quick out" policy, because patient may be in an exsanguinated condition; although entry can be made by any incision, it should preferably be done by midline/paramedian vertical incision because it provides better exposure.

Technique involves exteriorizing uterus from abdominal walls, straight clamp to be applied involving round ligament, fallopian tube and utero-ovarian ligament thus compressing the collateral blood flow to uterus from ovarian vessels which are markedly enlarged and distended, one should be careful as the pelvic tissues are edematous and quite friable. Tourniquet by rubber catheter to be applied to compress the uterine arteries at the level of lower uterine segment (LUS) incision to prevent excessive blood loss.

- Clamp, cut and drop technique (Mickel and Plauche) is preferable as it saves time and secures early hemostasis.
- All pedicles ligated as close to uterus and cervix as possible (sliding off technique), adequate size of the stump must be kept in order to prevent slipping off.
- Round ligament should be separately ligated due to the invariable presence of Sampson's artery which bleeds if not ligated separately.
- Double clamps to be applied at cornual and vascular areas as they will be thick and edematous, free tie to be applied after removing proximal clamp and transfixing suture used to displace distal clamp. This ensures that there is no hematoma formation at pedicle.
- Clamps on vascular pedicles should be manipulated as little as possible to avoid traction and trauma causing loose stumps which bleed.
- It is always wise to remain in midline while dissecting bladder. Laterally dilated venous plexuses of Santorini may bleed. Adhesions of bladder with LUS require sharp dissection.
- Bladder wall is edematous. In order to protect the edematous bladder, a mop should be kept between bladder and Doyen's retractor.
- Lower limit of cervix in most of the cases can be defined by making an incision in the lower segment or through lower segment cesarean section (LSCS) incision.
- Uterosacrals should always be excised and sutured as separate pedicles.
- When tying last cardinal ligament take angle of friable and edematous vagina in it to prevent angle bleeding.
- Before closing the abdomen, inspect pedicles carefully.
- Do not do reperitonization.

- Keep two drains (14 no.), one in pelvis and one superficial.
- Do not forget to count mops and instruments.
- Perioperative antibiotic prophylaxis (broad spectrum) for 24–48 hours.
- If necessary thromboprophylaxis to be given with low molecular weight heparin (LMWH) if one is sure about hemostasis.
- Detailed record of events should be documented including the indication, intraoperative findings and amount of blood loss.

Choice of Hysterectomy (Total/Subtotal)

In those cases where LUS is not involved as in atonic PPH, rupture of uterus, subtotal hysterectomy will be sufficient to secure hemostasis, which is our primary objective. It is easier and safer to perform with less bowel and bladder injuries. However, in cases where LUS is involved as in placenta previa, total hysterectomy is required for hemostasis. Main concern with subtotal hysterectomy is vaginal discharge, bleeding and rare instances of stump carcinoma and the need for regular cytology.

COMPLICATIONS

- Excessive blood loss is a most frequent complication of peripartum hysterectomy and may need transfusion of blood and blood products. Blood loss is mainly due to delay in decision-making. Tissue edema and adhesions due to previous surgery, pre-existing cause and inherent risk of coagulation can also cause bleeding.
- The bladder is particularly vulnerable and it is not uncommon to injure bladder in cases of previous cesarean while dissecting the bladder. Hence, bladder should be examined intraoperative to check for integrity. One can try to examine bladder wall to see if Foley's bulb is visible or retrograde filling of bladder can be done with methylene blue to check for any leak. Tears of bladder should be repaired with 3-0 Vicryl. For other tissues, Vicryl 1-0 can be used.
- While clamps over uterine arteries chances of injuring ureters by applying clamps or ligating ureters are high, there are <1% reported incidences of ureteric injuries. Integrity of the ureters after bladder repair can be checked by cystoscopy by observing flow of urine at ureteric orifices or by use of indigo carmine dye. It is best to diagnose and manage urological injuries intraoperatively to prevent increased morbidity, need for extensive investigations and second surgery and to prevent the chances of litigation.
- Other complications are gaping of wounds, sepsis, prolonged hospital stay, paralytic ileus, urinary tract infections, etc.

ELECTIVE EMERGENCY PERIPARTUM HYSTERECTOMY

If the risk factors for placenta previa/accreta are identified from beforehand by high-resolution ultrasonography (USG) or magnetic resonance imaging (MRI), one may need elective or semielective EPH. Due to increased primary cesarean rate, the incidence of adherent placenta is on the rise, the need of the hour is to be proficient in doing peripartum hysterectomy, hence residents in obstetrics should learn to perform this lifesaving procedure.

CONCLUSION

Peripartum hysterectomy is the "near miss event" in both developed and developing countries. It contributes significantly to morbidity and mortality of a woman as it is riskiest operation. It has to be prevented. High-risk cases to be identified, refer at the earliest, cesarean section to be timed properly, careful monitoring and resort to conservative procedures can reduce the near miss event. Though peripartum hysterectomy is a lifesaving procedure in emergency obstetric conditions, it represents a painful dilemma for the obstetrician. The decision to perform this operation, especially in a primigravida or in patients with no living children remains a difficult one. So, it should be performed judiciously weighing the need to sacrifice the obstetric future of the patient in favor of patient's life. Special provision of blood transfusion facilities, dialysis facilities, and good ventilatory support is necessary round the clock. Availability of multidisciplinary team involving an experienced obstetrician, anesthetist, neonatologist, urologist, interventional radiologist and a physician round the clock is necessary. Availability of communication and transport facilities for these emergency patients are required. Provision of emergency ambulance facility provided by the government has played a huge role in quicker access for health care facilities. Further, such measures will help in reducing maternal and perinatal morbidity in EPH. Training of obstetricians in EPH and various conservative procedures is very much necessary to reduce the morbidity and mortality associated with this procedure. The role of simulation exercises in training birth attendants and paramedical staff in basics of prevention and management of EPH like slow delivery of the infant, AMTSL can help a long way in reducing the need for hysterectomy. As cesarean section is one of the major contributors to this morbidity, the rate of primary cesarean section should be kept under check and also a trial of labor after cesarean (TOLAC) should be encouraged. Women requesting for cesarean section should be educated about the immediate and long-term complications of cesarean section like increased risk of placenta accreta/percreta need for EPH. Interventional radiology has emerged as a ray of hope in minimizing morbidity related to adherent placenta previa. More research and inventions in this specialty, availability of equipment and specialists can further improve the quality of life of women at risk of EPH.

KEY POINTS

- Peripartum hysterectomy is a marker of SAMM.
- Incidence varies worldwide, as facilities of improved maternal service not available everywhere. It has got a wide range from 0.3 to 5.6/1,000 deliveries.
- Incidence has decreased over the years as obstetric service has improved, especially the conservative management of PPH.
- But the chief concern seems to be an increase in the rate of cesarean section worldwide leading to an increased incidence of adherent placenta.
- Incidence of multiple pregnancies and in vitro fertilization (IVF) pregnancies has led to an increased incidence of placenta previa which has led to more intrapartum hemorrhage and more placental problems.
- There is a changing pattern in the causation also—atonic PPH as indication for EPH has decreased over the years; it has been outnumbered by the adherent placenta, not only in developed nations, but also in developing countries.
- Decision making on conservative versus EPH management is crucial and has to be taken by a senior and experienced obstetrician.
- In laparotomy, a "Quick in quick out technique" is followed, and proper hemostasis must be achieved before closure.
- Bladder or ureteric injuries are not uncommon. Extreme care must be taken to prevent them.

- Subtotal EPH is enough in most of the cases of EPH; it is lifesaving, quick and effective; however, in cases of placenta previa where bleeding continues from LUS, or adherent placenta in LUS, total hysterectomy is indicated.

REFERENCES

1. Baskett TF. Epidemiology of obstetric critical care. Best Pract Res Clin Obstet Gynaecol. 2008;22:763-74.
2. Kwee A, Bots ML, Visser GH, et al. Emergency peripartum hysterectomy: a prospective study in the Netherlands. Eur J Obstet Gynecol Reprod Biol. 2006;124:187-92.
3. Sheiner E, Levy A, Katz M, et al. Identifying risk factors for peripartum cesarean hysterectomy. A population-based study. J Reprod Med. 2003;48:622-6.
4. Baskett TF. Emergency obstetric hysterectomy. J Obstet Gynaecol. 2003;23:353-5.
5. Wen SW, Huang L, Liston RM, et al. Severe maternal mortality in Canada, 1991–2001. Can Med Assoc J. 2005;173:759-63.
6. Sakse A, Weber T, Nickelsen C, et al. Peripartum hysterectomy in Denmark 1995-2004. Acta Obstet Gynecol Scand. 2007;86:1472-5.
7. Kayabasoglu F, Guzin K, Aydogdu S, et al. Emergency peripartum hysterectomy in a tertiary Istanbul hospital. Arch Gynecol Obstet. 2008;278:251-6.
8. Knight M, Kurinczuk JJ, Spark P, Brocklehurst P, for the UKOSS. Cesarean delivery and peripartum hysterectomy. Obstet Gynecol. 2008;111:97-105.
9. Eniola OA, Bewley S, Waterstone M, et al. Obstetric hysterectomy in a population of South East England. J Obstet Gynaecol. 2006;26:104-9.
10. N Smith J, Mousa HA. Peripartum hysterectomy for primary postpartum haemorrhage: incidence and maternal morbidity. J Obstet Gynaecol. 2007;27:44-7.
11. Kastner ES, Figueroa R, Garry D, et al. Emergency peripartum hysterectomy: experience at a community teaching hospital. Obstet Gynecol. 2002;99:971-5.
12. Forna F, Miles AM, Jamieson DJ. Emergency peripartum hysterectomy: a comparison of cesarean and postpartum hysterectomy. Am J Obstet Gynecol. 2004;190:1440-4.
13. Whiteman MK, Kuklina E, Hillis SD, et al. Incidence and determinants of peripartum hysterectomy. Obstet Gynecol. 2006;108: 1486-92.
14. Glaze S, Ekwalanga P, Roberts G, et al. Peripartum hysterectomy 1999 to 2006. Obstet Gynecol. 2008;111:732-8.
15. Flood KM, Said S, Geary M, et al. Changing trends in peripartum hysterectomy over the last 4 decades. Am J Obstet Gynecol. 2009;200:632. e1-632.e6.
16. Lone F, Sultan AH, Thakar R, et al. Risk factors and management patterns for emergency obstetric hysterectomy over 2 decades. Int J Gynaecol & Obstet. 2010;109(Issue 1):12-5.
17. Amudha S, Sarojini. Clinical study of emergency peripartum hysterectomy for postpartum hemorrhage. Int J Reprod Contracept Obstet Gynecol. 2016;5(4):1171-3.
18. Mokkana S, Pratha AR, Isukapalli V. Critical analysis of peripartum hysterectomies at a tertiary level hospital in 1 year; International Archives of Integrated Medicine. 2016;3(8): 179-84.
19. Rasul S, Tahir S, Riaz L, et al. Clinical analysis of emergency peripartum hysterectomy. Journal of Rawalpindi Medical College (JRMC). 2016; 20(2):132-5.
20. Basnet P1, Thakur A1, Agrawal A1, et al. Peripartum hysterectomy and analysis of risk factors. NJOG. 2017;23(1):46-9.
21. South African Society of Obstetrics and Gynaecology 2016 Congress (1-4th May 2016), Sepsis, 2016.
22. Francois K, Ortiz J, Harris C, et al. Is peripartum hysterectomy more common in multiple gestations? Obstet Gynecol. 2005;105:1369-72.
23. Baskett TF, O'Connell CM. Maternal critical care in obstetrics. J Obstet Gynaecol Can. 2009;31:48-53.
24. Gilmour DT, Baskett TF. Disability and litigation from urinary tract injuries at benign gynaecological surgery in Canada. Obstet Gynecol. 2005;105:109-14.

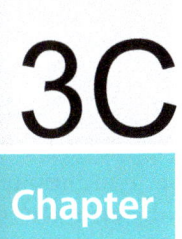

Chapter 3C

Disseminated Intravascular Coagulation in Obstetric Hemorrhage

Anahita Chauhan, Madhva Prasad

INTRODUCTION

All mechanisms in the body are built on the principles of *homeostasis*—a tendency toward a relatively stable equilibrium between interdependent elements. The physiological process of hemostasis attempts the same, i.e. to remain in equilibrium even when pushed to the limit. The net effect of a disturbance of equilibrium in the hemostatic process is "disseminated intravascular coagulation (DIC)". Recent commentators opine that "disseminated intravascular microthrombosis" is a better terminology.[1]

Dupuy (1834) and Trousseau (1865) first described what is now called DIC. Lasch, McKay, Ratnoff and others in the 1960s described obstetric cases with DIC, especially fetal death/amniotic fluid embolism (AFE).[2] Understanding why DIC occurs is essential for obstetricians to aid them to make independent decisions, especially when help from physicians/intensivists may not be immediately available.

The coagulation cascade as we commonly understand it, consists of the intrinsic and extrinsic pathways culminating in coagulation. It also involves the complement pathway and many inflammatory mediators. In the context of obstetric hemorrhage, there is a phase of raised hepatic synthesis of clotting factors, which is like an acute phase response. However, this hypercoagulability which occurs is overcome by the actual blood loss which is characterized by a complete consumption of clotting factors, which leads to a tendency of bleeding.

ETIOLOGICAL FACTORS OF DISSEMINATED INTRAVASCULAR COAGULATION

There is a wide range of conditions which can cause DIC: sepsis, massive trauma, vascular disorders, cancer, immunological disorders, drugs, fulminant liver failure, shock, and massive transfusion. Immaterial of the cause, there is a final common pathway which gives rise to the typical presentation of DIC.[3]

PATHOGENESIS[2,3]

The various mechanisms which result in DIC are endothelial injury, cytokine and tissue factor release, elevation in level and activity of thrombin and platelets, upregulation of inflammatory proteins (interleukins) and proinflammatory role of fibrinogen and fibrin. These above mechanisms enhance the coagulant pathways. Dysregulation of natural anticoagulant pathways involving protein C, protein S, antithrombin, dysregulation of fibrinolysis and dysregulated release of vasoactive molecules such as nitric oxide leads to consumption of hemostatic factors. Depending on which factor is depleted or enhanced, either bleeding, thrombosis, or both can occur.

CONDITIONS IN OBSTETRICS WHICH CAUSE DISSEMINATED INTRAVASCULAR COAGULATION

Rattray et al. reported the obstetrical causes associated with DIC, which are placental abruption (37%), postpartum hemorrhage (PPH) or hypovolemia (29%), pre-eclampsia/HELLP (14%), acute fatty liver (8%), sepsis (6%), and AFE (6%).[4] A study from Thailand estimated the occurrence of DIC to be 1 in 1,355 deliveries, and the associated conditions were somewhat similar [abruptio placentae 24%, hypertension/HELLP syndrome 32%, AFE 16%, acute fatty liver of pregnancy (AFLP) 16%].[5] A brief overview of the obstetrical conditions that can result in DIC is offered here.

Abruptio Placentae

DeLee is believed to have described the first few cases of severe abruptio placentae with DIC. There is a sudden release of massive amounts of tissue factor from the damaged placenta and uterus, resulting due to the sudden rupture of uterine spiral arteries. The degree of placental separation correlates with the DIC severity. Elderly multiparous parturients are at highest risk of DIC after abruption.

Amniotic Fluid Embolism

Life-threatening coagulopathy appears to occur in around 12% of cases with AFE. While almost 40% of cases with AFE have a maternal mortality, in the surviving, DIC is rapid in onset, approximately in 4 hours in almost half of the cases. Procoagulant substances in the amniotic fluid lead to cytokine and complement action resulting in consumptive coagulopathy. Fibrinolysis occurs secondary to activation of the coagulation cascade and due to urokinase-like plasminogen activators in the amniotic fluid.[6]

Pre-eclampsia/HELLP Syndrome

The pre-eclampsia/eclampsia continuum contributes significantly to obstetric DIC. The main overlapping feature is the HELLP syndrome, where thrombocytopenia is a major component. DIC in these cases is due to endothelial dysfunction leading to widespread deposition of fibrin along injured blood vessels, exposure of general circulation to placental tissue factor, and raised thrombin generation in various amounts. Endothelial dysfunction appears to be the triggering factor. Subcapsular hematomas are a common feature.[7]

Sepsis

There is diffuse activation of the coagulation system with inflammation, causing consumption of coagulation factors. Disturbed endothelial cells, activated mononuclear cells cause increase in proinflammatory cytokines and promote coagulation. The microorganisms associated can be gram-negative bacteria, streptococci (Group A), and clostridial group. The occurrence of fulminant DIC is frequent. Endovascular entry of the pathogens can occur during failure of asepsis during abortion, amnionitis following rupture of membranes, endometritis during labor or urinary tract infection. When compared with other causes of DIC, the occurrence of end organ damage is more common with sepsis, as is maternal mortality; currently a global awareness campaign regarding this is in progress.[8]

Dead Fetus Syndrome

Recent trend involving prompt termination of pregnancy has decreased the occurrence of DIC in fetal demise.

Acute Fatty Liver of Pregnancy

The occurrence of DIC in AFLP is around 80%. While fibrin degradation products (FDPs) are cleared rapidly, and fibrinogen levels improve rapidly after treatment of abruption, time to achieve normalcy is much longer in AFLP. Prolonged reticulocytosis, nucleated blood cells, prolonged hyperbilirubinemia, persistent hemolysis and a much longer lasting coagulopathy are characteristics of AFLP.[9]

Placenta Previa Spectrum

While excessive hemorrhage due to a low-lying placenta can cause consumption of coagulation factors and DIC, the more important emerging cause of DIC is the morbidly adherent placenta. This is strongly associated with DIC and can lead to obstetric hysterectomy also. In one series from our institution, DIC occurred in 3 out of 25 patients requiring obstetric hysterectomy due to various causes.[10] In another series of 50 cases of obstetric hysterectomy, the main causes of mortality were the occurrence of DIC.[11]

■ PATHOPHYSIOLOGY OF DISSEMINATED INTRAVASCULAR COAGULATION IN OBSTETRIC HEMORRHAGE

In obstetric hemorrhage, multiple factors are in play.

- *Dilutional coagulopathy*: In antepartum and PPH, there is brisk loss of blood. The first step is usually active attempts to replenish blood volume with crystalloid and colloid infusions to counteract blood loss. However, this increased blood volume leads to dilution of concentration of coagulation factors and platelets.
- *Consumptive coagulopathy*: As an oversimplification, all available coagulation factors rush to the uterine bed and attempt to cause coagulation, leaving the rest of the body deprived of coagulation factors. In abruptio placentae, this is an important mechanism.
- Fibrin deposition and fibrinolysis occur to a variable extent contributing to the DIC. In HELLP syndrome and abruptio placentae, this is a common feature.

■ CLINICAL FEATURES

A commonly used classification of DIC was previously based only on severity, i.e. overt and nonovert. In overt DIC, there is a host of clinical manifestations with varying severity (Table 1). There are no specific pathognomonic features of DIC.

Organ	Manifestation
Skin	Bleeding from injury sites, purpura, hemorrhagic vesicles, focal necrosis and acral gangrene
Cardiovascular	Acidosis, shock, cerebrovascular events, myocardial infarction and thromboembolic phenomena
Renal	Acute tubular necrosis, hematuria, oliguria and renal cortical necrosis
Liver	Jaundice, fulminant hepatic failure
Lungs	Hypoxemia, pulmonary edema, hemorrhage and acute respiratory distress syndrome (ARDS)
Gastrointestinal	Mucosal necrosis, intestinal ulceration and ischemia
Central nervous system	Coma, convulsions and focal lesions

TABLE 1: Systemic manifestations of disseminated intravascular coagulation.

Clinicopathological Correlation

There appears to be a pathoclinical correlation between the underlying pathological process and the clinical presentation. Table 2 shows the possibilities based on the amount of fibrinolytic activity and coagulation activation. Abruptio placentae is prototypical of the enhanced fibrinolytic type, while a septic abortion may lead to DIC with reduced fibrinolysis.[12]

The syndrome of DIC can progress in any direction; a simplification is depicted in Figure 1. When the severity of fibrinolysis or coagulation is minimal, there is an *asymptomatic type*. When fibrinolysis predominates, there is a *bleeding type*. When coagulation predominates, there is the *organ failure type*. When there is coexisting persistent coagulation and fibrinolytic abnormalities, there is a *massive bleeding type*.[13] In nonovert DIC, there are no discernible clinical features. Most of the available classification systems concentrate on the identification of overt DIC. Due to the rapidly progressive nature of the condition, laboratory diagnosis forms a very important aspect in the management of the condition.

DIAGNOSIS AND MONITORING

Identification of the coagulation abnormality is important and the options available are:
- Clinical observation
- Laboratory testing
- Point-of-care testing.

Clinical Observation Tests

After cleansing with sterile saline, a puncture is made on the index finger pulp using a lancet. The finger is held taking care not to squeeze it. Every 20 seconds, a nonalcoholic cotton swab is used to gently wipe off the trickled blood. The time taken for the bleeding to stop is noted (which corresponds to platelet plug formation); the normal range is 1–9 minutes. A drop of blood is taken on a clean transparent slide and a needle is used to hold a microdrop of the blood and moved gently away from the blood drop. This is performed every 30 seconds. When "clotting" has taken place, a fine fibrin strand will be noted. The usual clotting time ranges from 4 minutes to 10 minutes. The "clot retraction test" and "clot lysis test" are tests for fibrinolysis. Trainee

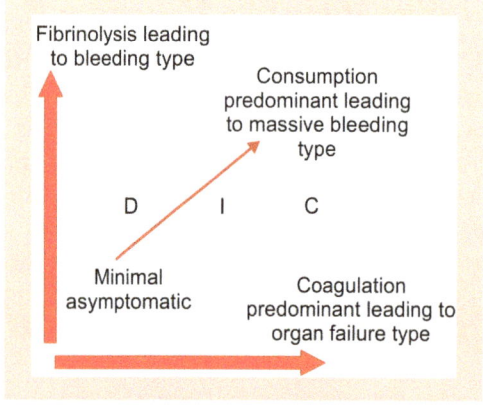

Fig. 1: Progression of disseminated intravascular coagulation.

TABLE 2: Pathophysiological correlates in disseminated intravascular coagulation.

Coagulation activation	Fibrinolysis	D-dimer elevation	Typical diseases	Organ symptoms	Bleeding symptoms
++++++	++	+	Sepsis	+++	+
++++	++++	++++	Cancer	++	++
++	++++++	++++++	Abruptio placentae	+	+++

resident doctors may be taught these skills which may be needed in primary care settings. However, in the context of an active ongoing hemorrhage, the clinical utility of these bedside tests is limited.

Laboratory Tests

The disadvantage of the laboratory tests is that they consume time and actually represent a "situation in the past". By the time results are available, the bleeding may have evolved and the current situation may be very different. It is important to note that coagulation abnormalities may worsen rapidly; a trend in values is more important to understand the evolution of the problem rather than any one particular reading.

- *Prothrombin time (PT)*: Tests the extrinsic pathway. In DIC, PT increases. An elevation of more than 1.5 times the normal is considered abnormal.
- *Activated partial thromboplastin time (aPTT)*: Tests the intrinsic pathway. In DIC, aPTT increases. An elevation of more than 1.5 times the normal is considered abnormal.
- *Fibrinogen*: Fibrinogen should always be included in the initial analysis because among other coagulant molecules, there is an early decrease in its level, even before there is a significant clinical worsening. Compared to PT/aPTT raise, fibrinogen fall occurs first.
- *Platelet count*: Platelet count is an important investigation. A count of more than 100,000/mm^3 is considered adequate for coagulation.
- *Fibrin degradation products*: They are markers of the extent of fibrinolysis. When the fibrinolytic pathway gets activated, the circulating FDPs increase. This is a nonspecific test, and no consensus is available regarding a particular cutoff point at which this value should be taken as diagnostic of DIC.
- *D-dimer*: D-dimer is the dimer of the degraded fibrin molecule when there is extensive clot formation. The diagnostic value of this molecule is mainly in algorithms of pulmonary thromboembolism, and is less reliable in DIC.

The use of FDPs and D-dimer investigations is only adjunctive, and if cost is prohibitive, it may be omitted. Since no single test can make a conclusive diagnosis of DIC, multiple scoring systems have been studied.

The International Society on Thrombosis and Hemostasis (ISTH) has described scoring systems for DIC. One such validated score is presented in Table 3.

A score greater than 5 is suggestive of overt DIC, and less than 5, of nonovert DIC. It is recommended that patients with score more

TABLE 3: ISTH scoring system for disseminated intravascular coagulation (DIC) (not specific to pregnancy).

Parameter	3	2	1	0
Underlying disorder associated with DIC	–	Present	–	Absent
Platelet count	–	<50,000/mm^3	50,000–100,000/mm^3	>100,000/mm^3
Fibrin degradation products (FDP)	Strong increase	–	Moderate increase	No increase
Fibrinogen level	–	–	<100 mg/dL	>100 mg/dL
Prothrombin time	–	>6 seconds	3–6 seconds	<3 seconds

TABLE 4: Pregnancy-specific disseminated intravascular coagulation scoring system.

Parameter	Value	Score assigned
PT difference	<0.5	0
	0.5–1	5
	1–1.5	12
	>1.5	25
Platelet concentration	<0.5	1
	0.5–1	2
	1–1.85	1
	>1.85	0
Fibrinogen concentration	<3 gm/L	25
	3–4	6
	4–4.5	1
	>4.5	0

than 5 should have the scoring repeated on a daily basis, while those with score less than 5 can be monitored on alternate days. However, this is not specific for obstetric patients. Due to the drawbacks of each of the available criteria, there is considerable debate and many different validations are in progress.

The reason why the scoring systems of DIC are not directly applicable to pregnancy is because of the physiological changes in the levels of fibrinogen, platelet concentration and the various coagulation parameters. After detailed analysis of the relative contribution of each biochemical parameter in the severity of DIC, and after accounting for the physiological changes associated with gestation, a pregnancy-specific scoring system has been developed by Erez et al. A modification of this scoring system is shown in Table 4.[14]

The question that arises is: faced with a clinical situation where there is brisk ongoing obstetric hemorrhage, can these scoring systems be used?

Goksever Celik et al. have tested this scoring system and in their study, the median score was 37. A discriminatory score of 26 points appeared to be ideal to suggest overt DIC. A large number of patients who would have otherwise been transfused with blood products, in the absence of a scoring system, were identified. It was concluded that use of an objective scoring system to determine which patient needed transfusion, reduced the rate of unnecessary transfusion and related risks and complications.[15]

It is suggested that these scoring systems be incorporated into our clinical practice, with refinements based on local data and studies.

Point-of-Care Testing

Thromboelastography and thromboelastometry studies: Since results of conventional coagulation studies can take some time, reliable tests for bedside assessment of coagulation abnormalities have led to interest in thromboelastometry. The strength and speed of clot formation and the speed of fibrin lysis are assessed, which leads to specific patterns which can be translated into electrical signals and graphs. Unique graphical patterns have been observed for specific coagulation disorders. Thromboelastogram (TEG), rotational thromboelastometry (ROTEM), intrinsic elastometry (INTEM), extrinsic elastometry (EXTEM) and fibrinogen thromboelastometry (FIBTEM) have been recently validated in pregnancy. In each of these, particular values of these graphical patterns correspond to well-established biochemical values.[16] A few of the recent guidelines have started relying heavily on the viscoelastic parameter values. Studies have also suggested a significant advantage of using these testing methods.[17] Thromboelastography in India is in its early stages, and there is still a long way to go before these can be used in the management of PPH.[18]

TREATMENT

The principles of management of DIC involve:
- Removal of the trigger which caused the DIC (in obstetric hemorrhage, it is the arrest of the cause of the bleeding which is the most important step)
- Restoration of blood volume
- Restoration of coagulation hemostasis.

The goal is to ensure adequate tissue perfusion and prevent or arrest any end organ damage.

Removal of the Trigger

In obstetric hemorrhage causing DIC, removal of specific trigger constitutes treatment of the underlying obstetric condition. Treatment of pre-eclampsia/abruptio placentae involves prompt delivery of the fetus and control of blood pressure using appropriate agents. Treatment of AFLP includes prompt delivery and liver failure management measures. Treatment of AFE involves prompt identification, prevention of uterine contraction, prompt delivery and cardiorespiratory support. Treatment of sepsis-related DIC consists of antibiotics, support of vital organ functions and surgical intervention to consider removal of any focus of infection. In case of severe sepsis, hysterectomy may be resorted to.

Restoration of Blood Volume

The replacement of blood is dictated by the amount of blood loss that has occurred and the hemodynamic status of the patient. A variety of protocols suggest various methods of replacement of blood volume. It is suggested that each institute develops its own protocol based on consensus between obstetricians, hematologists and intensivists.

Cross-matched blood should be transfused. If cross-matched blood is not available, O negative blood group should be considered for transfusion. Western literature is replete with well-set "protocols" in place, which are activated by the clinicians upon identification of massive obstetric hemorrhage. This leads to the immediate issuing of blood and blood products in various combinations:

- *Example 1*: A set of 4 units of packed red cells, 4 units of fresh frozen plasmas (FFPs) and 4 units of platelets. This is sometimes referred to as "shock pack". Some studies suggest such a 1:1:1 ratio of blood product replacement can sometimes lead to overtransfusion of platelets.[19]
- *Example 2*: 6–10 units of red cell units (O negative), 4 units of AB plasma and an apheresis platelet unit.[20,21] Many such combinations exist, but considering resource constrained situations in India, such protocols do not appear to be in place, and blood and products are issued "as per demand". This results in a large heterogeneity in the pattern of blood product usage in India.

Restoration of Coagulation Status

Fresh Frozen Plasma

- Fresh frozen plasma should be transfused if PT/aPTT is more than 1.5 times the normal. The dosage is 12–15 mL/kg (supported by RCOG guideline)[22]
- Recent German guideline recommends more than 20 mL/kg (up to 30 mL/kg)
- Empirical FFP administration along with massive red blood cell (RBC) transfusion in 1:1 (supported by ACOG guideline), 3:2 or 6:4 protocol.[23]

Use of FFPs has shown to reduce the requirement of further blood and blood product transfusion. Tanaka et al. have reviewed the various studies which commented on the ratio of FFP/RBC units in obstetric hemorrhage. The consensus was to maintain a ratio of more than 1:1, that is, for every unit of RBC transfused one unit of FFP should be transfused.[24,25] The drawback of these studies that have arrived at conclusions regarding hemostatic resuscitation is that they are retrospective in nature. Moreover, the heterogenic nature of the study (few utilizing 100 mg/L and others 150–200 mg/L as the target for fibrinogen value) also creates a need for further clarification in this matter. However, some commentators argue against early use of FFPs due to association with circulatory overload and acute lung injury.

Cryoprecipitate

Cryoprecipitate is given if fibrinogen is <1 g/L. However, if there is continuous ongoing resistant hemorrhage, some authorities consider that 2 g/L can be considered as a cutoff.[17] The aim is to maintain fibrinogen above 1–1.5 g/L, especially in cases where administration of FFP proves insufficient. A unit of cryoprecipitate has the ability to increase plasma fibrinogen by 0.5 g/L. However, it depends on how much the consumptive environment is and the intended dose that is targeted. Heterogeneity exists regarding target of fibrinogen chosen in various studies. Cryoprecipitate also contains good concentration of factor VIII, von Willebrand's factor (vWF) and factor XIII.

Fibrinogen Concentrate

Fibrinogen concentrates are available in Western countries, but is not popular in India. The dosage is about 60 mg/kg for an increase of 100 mg/L. It is currently not recommended.

Platelet Transfusion

As has been described with FFPs, platelets are to be transfused when a value of 75,000/µL is reached. While 50,000/µL is suggested as adequate for hemostasis, the rationale is that when a 75,000/µL value is observed in ongoing hemorrhage, by the time of receipt of platelets for transfusion, the actual value *in vivo* may have reached closer to 50,000. Recent German guideline suggests much higher target of 100,000/µL. The options are random or single donor platelets. Single donor platelets typically take time to prepare and test, and are not suitable during acute massive hemorrhage. Random donor platelets are the mainstay, and as such do not require grouping and typing. One unit raises the platelet count by around 5,000/µL.

Fibrinolytic Agents

The use of tranexamic acid for the control of PPH is now well-established. This agent should always be considered in prevention of DIC and if not yet used by the time DIC has set in, addition should be considered. The easy availability of this agent and its effectiveness makes this a strong recommendation.[26]

The availability of testing and the availability of blood products are presented in Flowcharts 1 and 2.

Recombinant Factor VIIa[27]

Though few trials have some proven efficacy, no specific recommendations exist regarding the usage of recombinant factor VIIa (available as Novoseven). While there are sporadic case reports from India, the use of its agents cannot be recommended at present. Consideration for this agent arises when PPH is ongoing, but there are no detectable laboratory abnormalities. It is one of the resources in the Jehovah's witness patients. The optimal dosage is around 60–90 µg/kg body weight, up to a maximum of two doses.

Vasopressin

Few authorities have also suggested the use of desmopressin at 0.3 µg/kg body weight with monitoring of electrolytes.[25]

CHAPTER 13C: Disseminated Intravascular Coagulation in Obstetric Hemorrhage

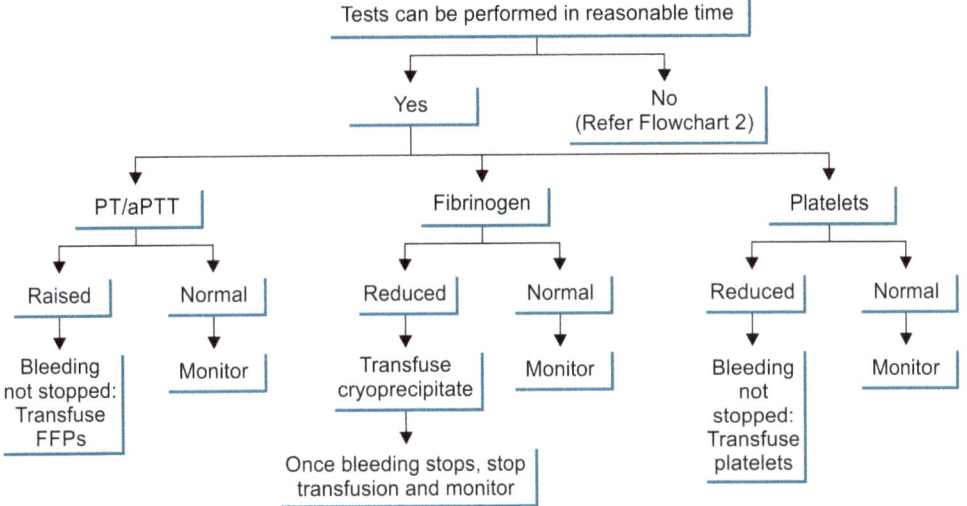

Flowchart 1: Management algorithm—tests can be performed in reasonable time.

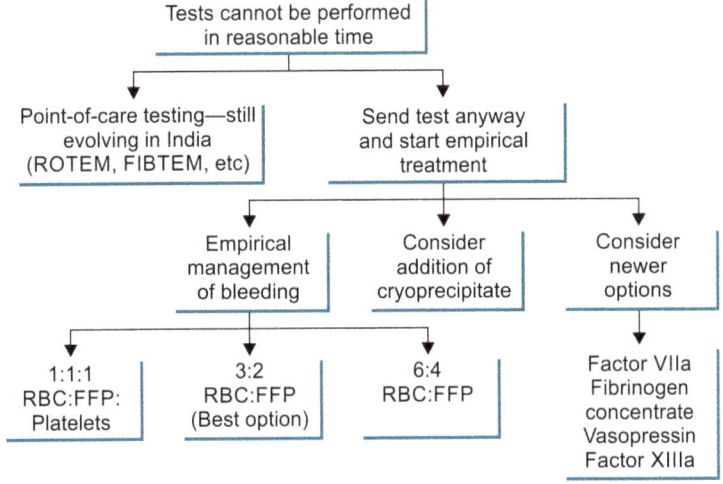

Flowchart 2: Management algorithm—tests cannot be performed in reasonable time.

Prothrombin Complex Concentrates

Prothrombin complex concentrates at initially 1,000–2,500 IU (25 IU/kg body weight) is suggested by one guideline, but the risk of thrombotic events has to be kept in mind. It is not well proven by randomized controlled trials (RCTs).

Factor XIII Concentrate

One to two bags of factor XIII 1,250 IU (15–20 IU/kg body weight) are suggested. The availability of these in the Indian scenario is doubtful.

Once hemostasis has been achieved and 24 hours have passed, a short duration

TABLE 5: Abnormalities in disseminated intravascular coagulation: quick recall.

Test	When to act?	Treatment options
Fibrinogen	<100 mg/dL	Cryoprecipitate
Platelet count	<75,000	Platelets
Prothrombin time	>1.5 times normal	Fresh frozen plasma
Activated partial thromboplastin time	>1.5 times normal	Fresh frozen plasma
Fibrin degradation products, D-dimer	No specific threshold has been found in PPH. They are only a marker of severity of the coagulopathy	

of thromboprophylaxis such as heparin should be considered for a short duration ranging between 1 week and 6 weeks. There is a possibility of recurrence of PPH, and DIC in subsequent pregnancies. Hence, appropriate measures should be taken. Simplified management algorithms are presented in Flowcharts 1 and 2.

SUMMARY

- Consider the possibility of DIC while managing patients who have obstetric diagnoses with high propensity of DIC.
- The mechanisms which give rise to DIC in various obstetric conditions are varied.
- Overt DIC can be bleeding type, coagulation type or massive bleeding type. The pathoclinical correlates in each are different.
- Diagnosis of DIC can be based on bedside clinical tests, laboratory investigations and point-of-care testing.
- Bedside tests mainly serve as screening test, but all practitioners should be familiar with it. Laboratory testing includes fibrinogen, PT, activated PT and platelet count.
- Scoring systems for DIC should be considered for incorporation into local protocols.
- Thromboelastography and its congeners are of growing interest.
- The main principles of management of DIC include resolution of the trigger, maintenance of blood volume and restoration of coagulation status.
- Resolution of the trigger involves treatment of the obstetric problem.
- Maintenance of blood volume may involve massive transfusion protocols.
- Consider the following values when correcting coagulation abnormalities (Table 5). Do not transfuse if bleeding has already stopped.

REFERENCES

1. Chang JC. Disseminated intravascular coagulation: is it fact or fancy? Blood Coagul Fibrinolysis. 2018;29(3):330-7.
2. Levi M, Selingsohn U. Disseminated intravascular coagulation. In: Kaushansky K, Beutler E, Seligsohn U, Lichtman MA, Kipps TJ, Prchal JT (Eds). Williams Hematology, 8th edition. New York: McGraw-Hill; 2010.
3. High KA, Valder A. Disorders of coagulation. In: Longo DL, Kasper DL, Jameson JL, Fauci AS, Hauser SL, Loscalzo J (Eds). Harrison's Principles of Internal Medicine, 18th edition. New York: McGraw-Hill; 2012. p. 1432.
4. Rattray DD, O'Connell CM, Baskett TF. Acute disseminated intravascular coagulation in obstetrics: a tertiary centre population review

(1980 to 2009). J Obstet Gynaecol Canada. 2012;34(4):341-7.
5. Kor-anantakul O, Lekhakula A. Overt disseminated intravascular coagulation in obstetric patients. J Med Assoc Thai. 2007; 90(5):857-64.
6. Rath WH, Hoferr S, Sinicina I. Amniotic fluid embolism: an interdisciplinary challenge: epidemiology, diagnosis and treatment. Dtsch Arztebl Int. 2014;111(8):126-32.
7. Hypertenisve disorders. In: Cunningham FG, Leveno KJ, Bloom SL, Spong CY, Dashe JS, Hoffman BS (Eds). Williams Obstetrics, 24th edition. New York: McGraw-Hill; 2014. p. 748.
8. Bonet M, Souza JP, Abalos E, et al. The global maternal sepsis study and awareness campaign (GLOSS): study protocol. Reprod Health. 2018; 15(1):16.
9. Nelson DB, Yost NP, Cunningham FG. Hemostatic dysfunction with acute fatty liver of pregnancy. Obstet Gynecol. 2014;124(1):40-6.
10. Satia MN, More V. Obstetric hysterectomy: an emergency lifesaving procedure. Int J Reprod Contracept Obstet Gynecol. 2016;5:2338-42.
11. Mayadeo NM, Swaminathan G. Obstetric hysterectomy: analysis of 50 cases at a tertiary care hospital. Int J Reprod Contracept Obstet Gynecol. 2018;7:2882-7.
12. Asakura H. Classifying types of disseminated intravascular coagulation: clinical and animal models. J Intensive Care. 2014;2(1):20.
13. Wada H, Matsumoto T, Yamashita Y. Diagnosis and treatment of disseminated intravascular coagulation (DIC) according to four DIC guidelines. J Intensive Care. 2014;2(1):15.
14. Erez O. Disseminated intravascular coagulation in pregnancy: clinical phenotypes and diagnostic scores. Thromb Res. 2017;151:S56-60.
15. Goksever Celik H, Celik E, Ozdemir I, et al. Is blood transfusion necessary in all patients with disseminated intravascular coagulation associated postpartum hemorrhage? J Matern Fetal Neonatal Med. 2019;32(6):1004-8.
16. Katz D, Beilin Y. Disorders of coagulation in pregnancy. Br J Anaesth. 2015;115:75-88.
17. Snegovskikh D, Souza D, Walton Z, et al. Point-of-care viscoelastic testing improves the outcome of pregnancies complicated by severe postpartum hemorrhage. J Clin Anesth. 2018;44:50-6.
18. Ahmad A, Kohli M, Malik A, et al. Role of thromboelastography versus coagulation screen as a safety predictor in pre-eclampsia/ eclampsia patients undergoing lower-segment caesarean section in regional anaesthesia. J Obstet Gynaecol India. 2016;66(Suppl 1):340-6.
19. Collis RE, Collins PW. Haemostatic management of obstetric haemorrhage. Anaesthesia. 2015;70 Suppl 1:78-86, e27-8.
20. Guasch E, Gilsanz F. Massive obstetric hemorrhage: current approach to management. Med Intensiva. 2016;40(5):298-310.
21. Butwick AJ, Goodnough LT. Transfusion and coagulation management in major obstetric hemorrhage. Curr Opin Anaesthesiol. 2015;28(3):275-84.
22. Royal College of Obstetricians and Gynaecologists. (2019). Postpartum hemorrhage, prevention and management (Green-top guideline no. 52). [Online] Available from https://www.rcog.org.uk/en/guidelines-research-services/guidelines/gtg52/ [Last accessed July, 2019].
23. Committee on Practice Bulletins-Obstetrics. Practice bulletin no. 183: postpartum hemorrhage. Obstet Gynecol. 2017;130: e168-86.
24. Tanaka H, Matsunaga S, Yamashita T, et al. A systematic review of massive transfusion protocol in obstetrics. Taiwan J Obstet Gynecol. 2017;56(6):715-8.
25. Lier H, von Heymann C, Korte W, et al. Peripartum haemorrhage: haemostatic aspects of the new German PPH guideline. Transfus Med Hemother. 2018;45(2):127-35.
26. Brenner A, Shakur-Still H, Chaudhri R, et al. The impact of early outcome events on the effect of tranexamic acid in post-partum haemorrhage: an exploratory subgroup analysis of the WOMAN trial. BMC Pregnancy Childbirth. 2018;18(1):215.
27. Welsh A, McLintock C, Gatt S, et al. Guidelines for the use of recombinant activated factor VII in massive obstetric hemorrhage. Aust N Z J Obstet Gynaecol. 2008;48(1):12-6.

13D Chapter

Massive Transfusion Protocol: Role of Component Therapy

Shivaram Chandrashekar

■ MAJOR OBSTETRICAL BLEEDING

Globally obstetrical bleeding, in particular postpartum hemorrhage (PPH), is often a life-threatening emergency and is the leading cause of maternal mortality requiring prompt action. PPH accounts for over one-third of all maternal deaths worldwide. Risk of maternal mortality due to hemorrhage is 1 in 1,000 deliveries or 100/100,000 live births. Majority of deaths occur in the low- and middle-income countries[1] mostly due to delays in obstetric care, home deliveries, or substandard care due to paucity of doctors or sufficient trained personnel. Management of hypovolemic shock can be a real challenge in resource-constrained regions lacking good transfusion support.

Postpartum Hemorrhage

Postpartum hemorrhage is defined as blood loss of 500 mL after vaginal delivery[2] or 1,000 mL after cesarean section. Another simpler definition would be loss of sufficient blood that causes hemodynamic instability in the mother. PPH is called primary, if bleeding occurs within 24 hours of delivery and secondary if it occurs more than 24 hours after delivery. While death is the worst outcome of PPH, other serious effects are the result of lack of blood, wrong choice of components or complications of transfusion of blood in large quantities. Shock resulting from hypovolemia, transfusion-related acute lung injury (TRALI) mimicking acute respiratory distress syndrome, transfusion-associated cardiac overload (TACO) due to excessive fluids/blood transfusion coagulopathy resulting from dilution of platelets and clotting factors and loss of fertility when hysterectomy is undertaken as a lifesaving measure are some of the outcomes.[3]

Factors Associated with Major Obstetrical Hemorrhage

Obstetrical bleeding may be caused by a variety of causes (Box 1). However, uterine atony[4] is the most common cause of PPH. Although PPH is more common in developing countries, uterine atony does not differentiate between developed and developing countries. The incidence of PPH in developed countries is also on the rise and is mostly attributed to uterine atony.[5]

Other factors causing major obstetrical bleeds include placental abruption, placenta previa, multiple pregnancy and obesity but not high parity. Estimates of its incidence in the literature vary widely from 3% to 15% of deliveries.[6]

> **Box 1:** Causes of massive blood loss/obstetric hemorrhage.
>
> - Early pregnancy, e.g. ectopic pregnancy, cervical pregnancy
> - Antenatal and intrapartum conditions—placental abruption, placenta previa, coagulopathy secondary to amniotic fluid embolism
> - Postpartum, e.g. uterine atony, retained products of conception, genital tract laceration

Factors known to put a woman at higher risk[7] for acute PPH include a history of PPH, prolonged, augmented or rapid labor, pre-eclampsia, operative delivery, chorio-amnionitis, and overdistended uterus due to macrosomia, twins, or hydramnios.

What is Massive Blood Loss?

Massive blood loss is arbitrarily defined as the loss of one blood volume within a 24-hour period (Mollison et al.). However, recognizing the fact that not all patients with acute blood loss may survive for 24 hours, alternative definitions (Box 2) have been proposed. These include a 50% blood volume loss in 3 hours or loss of blood at a rate faster than 150 mL/minute (Fakhry and Sheldon, 1994). The latter, acute definitions are more dynamic and may be more helpful in routine practice.[8]

PATHOPHYSIOLOGY OF TRAUMATIC SHOCK IN MASSIVE BLOOD LOSS

What is Traumatic Shock?

Shock is a condition characterized by tissue hypoxia caused by a variety of mechanisms. Following trauma and major blood loss shock is caused initially by the decrease in circulating blood volume due to hemorrhage and is called hemorrhagic (hypovolemic) shock. Next, comes the phase of anemic shock caused by the dilution of blood by fluids infused to resuscitate the patient and maintain circulating volumes. During the initial stages, tissue perfusion is maintained by increasing the heart rate in the conscious patient or the stroke volume in an anesthetized patient. When the heart is no longer able to do this circulatory failure results from diminished pumping by the heart and the same is called cardiogenic shock. Cardiogenic shock may also occur initially as a result of direct injury (neurogenic) or when it occurs later, it is secondary to hypoperfusion or reperfusion injuries. In presence of cardiac disease,[9] the response to fluid resuscitation may be blunted and decompensation may set in much earlier. Finally myogenic shock is caused by loss of vascular tone. All mechanisms act together in traumatic shock.[10] Various mechanisms act at various stages (Box 3).

Box 2: Definitions of massive blood loss.
- Replacement of one blood volume over 24 hours
- Replacement of half of total blood volume (TBV) within 3 hours
- Transfusion of >4 units of packed red blood cells (PRBCs) in 1 hour in the presence of continued bleeding
- Blood loss faster than 150 mL/minute

Box 3: Types of shock.
- Hemorrhagic (hypovolemic)
- Anemic
- Cardiogenic shock
- Myogenic

Stages of Shock

Initially the heart compensates for traumatic shock by increasing the heart rate, or by increasing the stroke volume. This coupled with vasoconstriction of nonvital blood vessels helps to maintain our body in a state of compensated shock. Decompensated traumatic shock is a stage where in the increase in heart rate or stroke volume is unable to maintain perfusion due to the failing heart. This is more likely to set in early in the aged or those with cardiopulmonary disease. Hypoperfusion resulting from a failing myocardium leads to build up of toxic metabolites and these can cause injury later on when perfusion is restored. Yet these, two stages are reversible with prompt intervention. In the absence of proper obstetrical care or in the presence of risk factors, the patient may progress to the subacute or acute phases of

TABLE 1: Stages of shock.

1.	Compensated shock	Tissue oxygenation is maintained by increasing heart rate or stroke volume
2.	Decompensated shock	Heart begins to fail; metabolic wastes accumulate
3.	Subacute shock	Multiorgan failure caused by toxic effects of hypoxia and build-up of toxic metabolites which cause reperfusion injury
4.	Acute shock	Marked by ongoing bleeding, hypothermia, acidosis and dilutional coagulopathy

TABLE 2: Response to shock.

Cell level	Cellular ischemia/cell edema/inflammation
CNS level	Neuroendocrine response aimed at maintaining the functions of vital organs heart, brain and kidneys
Heart	Maintenance of blood volume by increasing heart rate or stroke volume Susceptible to reperfusion injury
Kidneys	Maintains glomerular filtration rate but is unable to concentrate urine
Lungs	Pile up of inflammatory mediators. Responsible for multiorgan failure
Liver	Synthetic function of liver stops. Affected by reperfusion injury

shock. In the subacute phase, the patient develops multiorgan failure secondary to build up of toxic effects of ischemia and metabolites. Finally ongoing bleeding coupled with hypothermia, acidosis, and dilutional coagulopathy often produces acute irreversible shock (Table 1).

ORGAN RESPONSE TO SHOCK

Cellular ischemia coupled with cell edema and inflammation induced by trauma can lead to multiorgan failure and death. In response to a traumatic event, the central nervous system (CNS) acts through the neuroendocrine system (Table 2). The goal of resuscitative measures is to preserve the functions of the vital organs the CNS, heart and the kidneys. Blood flow to the heart is well maintained by fluid resuscitation till the later stages of shock, but eventually decompensation sets in. The kidney is able to maintain glomerular filtration rate (GFR) by vasoconstriction but loses its ability to concentrate urine. Action of inflammatory mediators is predominantly seen in the lungs.

The lungs are at the center for multiple organ system failure (MOSF) in traumatic shock patients.[11,12] The gastrointestinal tract (GIT) also exhibits vasoconstriction early in the traumatic process. The liver like the heart can be affected by reperfusion injury and death is imminent if any of the critical organs like the heart, kidney or liver does not recover. The liver is more likely to be affected by reperfusion injury.[13]

MASSIVE BLOOD LOSS: MANAGEMENT

Infusion of large quantities of crystalloids or colloids is often the first line of treatment aimed at maintaining perfusion of vital organs. This no doubt helps compensate for the traumatic shock transiently, but if this is not quickly corrected with appropriate blood components hemodilution and hypothermia set in leading to dilutional thrombocytopenia, dilutional coagulopathy leadings to multiorgan failure and death. Originally it was believed that such patients should be transfused with whole blood or red cells and then followed up with platelet concentrates and/or fresh frozen plasma (FFP) depending on clinical scenario and the results of bleeding/coagulation tests. Today it is believed that starting transfusions with red cells early and adding on FFP and platelets early can prevent irreversible complication of traumatic shock.

Indicators of Massive Blood Loss

Blood pressure (BP)—systolic and diastolic along with heart rate have prognostic value in the setting of massive blood loss as that seen with PPH. Additionally mean arterial pressure and pulse pressure are also useful.

Some studies[14] recommend shock index (SI) [heart rate/systolic BP (SBP)] as a guide to the outcome of PPH. SI has been shown to compare favorably with conventional vital signs in predicting intensive care unit (ICU) admission and other outcomes in PPH. SI <0.9 indicates relative safety whereas a SI ≥1.7 indicates a need for urgent intervention. SI has been used more often in the nonobstetrical setting but it is believed that it is of value in obstetrics too (Table 3).

Activation of Massive Transfusion Protocol

There are no national guidelines for activating the massive transfusion protocol (MTP). However, the Australian Red Cross has given the following guidelines with a view to standardize the transfusion trigger for MTP. The criteria are varied and include:

TABLE 3: Shock index (SI).

Shock Index	Heart rate/Systolic BP
SI <0.9	Good prognosis
SI ≥1.7	Urgent action needed to save life

- Need for 4 units of red cells in 4 hours—actual or expected
- Acute blood loss of 50% of blood volume in 3 hours—actual or ongoing
- Clinical or laboratory evidence of coagulopathy, e.g. disseminated intravascular coagulation (DIC)
- The Transfusion service can activate the MTP on its own when a request for 4 or more emergency O negative red cells is made by the treating team.

ABC Score for Identification of Patients Needing Massive Transfusion

According to one study[15] identification of patient needing activation of MTP may be done using the following criteria. Assign a value of 0 or 1 to the following:
- Penetrating injury
- Systolic BP on arrival <90 mm Hg
- Tachycardia >120 beats/minute
- Presence of free fluid in the peritoneum detected by ultrasound.

A score of 2 or more is considered positive.

When to Initiate Massive Transfusion Protocol

Initiation can be based on one or more of the following criteria:[16]
- ABC score of 2 or more
- Hemodynamic instability—uncorrected and persistent
- Ongoing bleeding requiring surgery or embolization
- Blood transfusion in the emergency room (ER).

Once the protocol is activated, the blood center should have a mechanism for quick and fast dispatch and delivery of blood components to facilitate resuscitation. Dependence on hematology and coagulation laboratory must be reduced during the acute resuscitation phase. Development of a massive transfusion card or an emergency transfusion card could play an important role in ensuring correct communication with the blood center.

Teamwork is the key to handling massive blood losses. The team comprises of the obstetric surgeons, anesthetists, hematologists and blood bank staff working together to secure hemostasis, restore circulating volume, and effectively managing blood component therapy.[17]

Recommendation for Management of Massive Blood Loss [Based on British Committee for Standards in Haematology (BCSH) Guidelines[18]]

Restoration of Circulating Volume

First all patients with a massive blood loss have diminished circulating volume and therefore it is important to restore circulating volumes using crystalloids and colloids using a 14-gauge peripheral or central cannula. Some prefer two cannulae for faster transfusion of blood or intravenous (IV) fluids. However, it is important to note that no other medication other than normal saline may be transfused with blood. It is equally important to assess the clinical situation, the need for transfusion, the need for activating MTPs before activating the MTP team.

Surgical Intervention

Early obstetrical intervention with or without interventional radiology may be needed to arrest the bleeding. Interventional radiological procedures like uterine artery embolization procedures play an important role when supportive measure are unable to stop the bleeding and help in management of emergent obstetrical bleeding.

Laboratory Tests

Order a battery of predetermined tests which may include complete blood count (CBC), prothrombin time (PT), activated partial thromboplastin time (aPTT), thrombin time, arterial blood gas, biochemistry profile and pulse oximetry.

Blood Bank

Send blood samples to blood bank for ABO and Rh grouping, antibody screening and compatibility testing.

Blood Transfusion

Pending the availability of tests it is often wise to transfuse blood components as follows:

Cell salvage: Cell salvage is a technique where the patients cells shed during trauma or surgery are passed through filters and returned to the patient thereby reducing the need for allogenic transfusions. Such equipment, called cell savers are able to salvage the red cells from shed blood in a closed system, filter the same and reinfuse the blood. Cell salvage techniques are particularly helpful in case of patients with a rare group (Bombay Oh negative) or when there is unexpected blood loss with little time for arranging for donors. Cell savers are commonly used by cardiac surgeons and orthopedicians in the operation theaters to minimize allogenic transfusions but may be employed in obstetrics as well. Manual methods of filtering red cells using gauze are fraught with risks and are not advisable in this age and time.

Red cell concentrates: Start red cell transfusions with O negative blood or O positive blood in the absence of O negative blood if the hemoglobin (Hb) = <6 g/dL and when there is a blood loss of over 30%. Group-specific-matched blood may be used once the same becomes available. Uncrossmatched blood is acceptable in the setting of massive blood loss.

Box 4: Goals of treatment in massive blood loss.
- Maintain circulating blood volume with crystalloids and colloids
- Maintain Hb above 6 g/dL or HCT of at least 20% by red cell transfusions in the presence of bleeding
- Transfuse platelets to maintain a platelet count over 50,000/µL
- Transfuse FFP to keep PT/aPTT below 1.5 and fibrinogen >1 g/L
- Correct metabolic disturbances like hypothermia, hypocalcemia, hyperkalemia and acid-base balance Temperature >35°C; pH >7.2; Ca^{++} >1.3 mmol/L and lactate <4 mmol/L
- Temperature >35°C (infuse only warm fluids and blood warmers for transfusion)
- Maintain plasma oncotic pressure using albumin or FFP

Fresh frozen plasma: If the estimated blood loss is over 1-1.5 times, the blood volume anticipate dilutional coagulopathy and treat with FFP at the rate of 12-15 mL/kg. This means 4 units of FFPs are needed for a patient weighing 50 kg, 5 units for a patient with 60 kg and 6 units for a patient with 70 kg.

Increase in PT/aPTT above 1.5 could be due to underlying microvascular bleeding and indicates need for FFP transfusions. Infusion of concomitant calcium is necessary to arrest microvascular bleeding. Target an ionized Ca^{++} of over 1.13 mmol/L.

Cryoprecipitate: Transfusion with cryoprecipitate is indicated only when the bleeding cannot be controlled by FFP or when the fibrinogen levels are <1 g/L. Two units of pooled cryoprecipitate or 10 units of cryoprecipitate are the standard adult dose for correction of hypofibrinogenemia. Pooled cryoprecipitate is not a licensed product in India. Major obstetrical bleeds often present with low fibrinogen levels (<1 g/L) and early fibrinogen supplementation using lyophilized fibrinogen or cryoprecipitate with hemostatic resuscitation can stabilize a catastrophic situation.[19]

Platelet transfusions: When the platelet count is less than 50,000/uL, it can be assumed that the patient has lost the equivalent of two blood volumes and platelet transfusions are indicated immediately. Target a platelet count of 75,000/uL. Transfuse 6 random donor platelets (RDP—whole blood derived) or 1 single donor platelets (apheresis—SDP) at once. Both are equally efficacious and one needs to be guided by availability more than anything else in the emergency situation.

The goals of treatment[20] in massive blood loss are as given in Box 4.

ROLE OF MASSIVE TRANSFUSION PROTOCOLS

What is Massive Transfusion Protocol?

We now understand the pathophysiology of hemorrhagic shock and its resuscitation better. Instead of starting volume replacement and transfusing blood components later, we now follow a more proactive approach of straight away using blood components in a fixed ratio. This method of treating massive blood loss using blood components in a predefined ratio is what is called as a MTP. Each institute should design its own MTP protocol after an understanding of its importance, benefits and adverse effects. Appropriately designed MTPs help to mitigate the complications arising from acidosis, hypothermia and coagulopathy that are common accompaniments of massive blood loss and fluid resuscitation.

Rationale for Massive Transfusion Protocol

Physicians involved in treating war injuries noticed that early administration of FFP during massive transfusion decreased coagulopathy and improved morbidity and mortality. Recent studies have also shown that increasing the ratio of FFP to red blood cell (RBC) transfusion has a beneficial effect compared to the traditional approach of adding FFP after knowing the results of laboratory studies only.[21-23]

When whole blood is being lost, transfusing fresh whole blood would seem ideal. However, in this era of nucleic acid testing (NAT), the only way for a blood center to provide fresh whole blood would be to give blood tested by the least sensitive rapid immunochromatographic tests which endanger patients' lives. Further use of components helps to adjust dosages better and blood components are hence widely accepted as the only rational way of treating bleeding and conserving the precious resource. When whole blood is stored for even a few days, the platelets are rendered nonviable and there is significant loss of labile coagulation factors. Therefore, administering RBCs to correct hypoxia, adding FFP and platelets to correct the clotting factor and platelet depletion gives the closest resemblance to fresh whole blood and is a good alternative.

Although it is a good practice to be guided by laboratory tests in all clinical settings, massive blood loss does not always give enough time for accurate laboratory estimations. It is well established that while plasma substitutes—crystalloids and colloids help in the initial restoration of circulating volume, fluids given in excess of 1.5 times the blood volume are very likely to precipitate dilutional anemia, dilutional coagulopathy, and dilutional thrombocytopenia. It is also estimated that loss of more than two blood volumes will reduce the platelet counts below 50,000/µL. This being the case it is felt by many that starting treatment with massive transfusions using red cell concentrates, FFP and platelet concentrates, right in the beginning could prevent the complications of massive fluid therapy and herald early recovery.

Newer Insights into Massive Transfusion: Advantages of Increased RBC:FFP:Platelet Ratios

Transfusion of packed RBCs (PRBCs), plasma, and platelets in a proportion similar to that of fresh whole blood may help mitigate the effects of dilutional coagulopathy and hypovolemia.

Some studies have shown that increasing the ratio of FFP to RBC to (1:1 or 1:2) confers a survival advantage to recipients by reducing mortality in massive transfusion after trauma. Other studies have shown that an increased platelet:red cell transfusion ratio is also beneficial.[24,25] This is the rational for using red cells:FFP:Platelets in a 1:1:1 ratio by many centers.

Early trauma-induced coagulopathy (ETIC) is one of the prime factors associated with mortality. Predefined MTPs having an increased ratio of RBCs, FFP/cryoprecipitate and platelets units in each pack (e.g. 1:1:1) may prove beneficial in such patients.[26,27]

When everything fails, recombinant factor VIIa may be used an adjunct to treat consumptive coagulopathy together with standardized MTPs. Although the authors of recent studies have advocated a 1:1:1 ratio of PRBCs to FFP to platelet transfusions in patients requiring massive transfusion, each institution needs to weigh this against the risks of plasma transfusion such as TRALI and devise their own MTP protocol (1:1:1 or 2:1:1).

In addition to a MTP, all efforts must be directed toward damage control resuscitation. This includes control of surgical bleeding and correction of the complications of coagulopathy described above.

Point-of-care testing: Arterial blood gas helps to detect hypoxia and acidosis early. Thromboelastography (TEG) helps to guide transfusion therapy particularly in the choice of blood components and also guides cessation of transfusion. Electrolyte and lactate levels can be estimated bedside quickly. Most tests will need to be repeated hourly and after blood transfusions to direct further management in this rapidly changing dynamic scenario of massive blood loss or massive transfusions.

Benefits of Massive Transfusion Protocol

- A trauma call (messaging system) eliminates the need for unnecessary phone calls by treating clinician and ensures attendance of all specialists needed for therapy
- Facilitates quick response upon initiating the MTP by the blood center
- Massive transfusion card which forms a part of the MTP ensures correct communication regarding the urgent need for blood and ensures prompt action by the blood center.

Drawbacks of Massive Transfusion Protocols

- There are no internationally accepted guidelines for initiating the MTP
- There is no optimum ratio of RBC:FFP:Platelets. Whether to use 1:1:1 or 2:1:1 or not to use any MTP at all is a matter of institutional choice
- Triggering MTP for mild-moderate blood losses may lead to issue of large quantities of blood leading to wastage
- Fresh frozen plasma thawed and kept must be used preferably within 6 hours and maximally within 24 hours otherwise the same is wasted
- Easy availability of blood in response to call may lead to unnecessary transfusions leading to late complications.

Blood Groups Switch in Massive Transfusion

It is obvious that large quantities of blood components are needed in handling massive blood loss and the desired group may not be available. Further paucity of time to provide the first few units of blood necessitates abbreviated pretransfusion testing and hence wherever possible high-risk blood transfusion consent must be obtained from the patient. Blood centers that do not have adequate stock of blood necessarily try to store a few units of O negative and O positive red cells units to meet emergency situations like an unexplained PPH. AB group plasma does not have any antibody and hence may be used as universal plasma. While group-specific platelets are desirable the same are not essential. The Rh(D) antigen is not present on platelets. Hence platelets are also commonly used across Rh barriers except when the platelets are contaminated with red cells and appear pink in color. The goal during management of massive blood losses is to provide blood as quickly as possible, not necessarily the most compatible blood group. It is useful to have a chart showing the various blood group switches possible in apron pockets or the same may be displayed in the wards ER, ICUs for ready reference (Figs. 1A and B, Blood groups switches chart).

Other Hemostatic/Blood Replacement Strategies

A number of other adjunctive treatments have been proposed in unresponsive patients.[28]

Recombinant factor VIIa (rFVIIa)—the role of rFVIIa is not clear. However, it must be

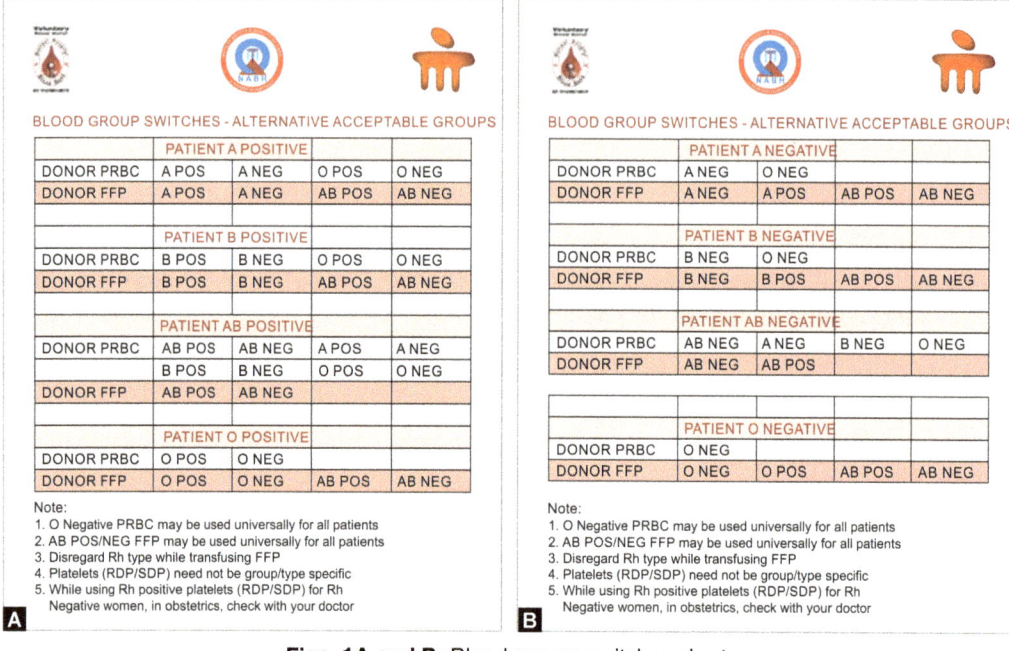

Figs. 1A and B: Blood groups switches chart.
Source: Manipal Hospitals.

considered in all patients who fail to respond to conventional hemostatic therapy or in the presence of life-threatening hemorrhage with no time for conventional therapy to take effect. Treatment can be initiated with a dose of 200 µg/kg followed by a repeat dose at 100 µg at 1 hour and 3 hours if needed.

Antifibrinolytic drugs like tranexamic acid may also be useful in bleeding associated with fibrin degradation. Administration of tranexamic acid in bleeding trauma patients helps to significantly reduce mortality.

Termination of Massive Transfusion Protocol

The MTP is called off when the following conditions are satisfied:
- Anatomic control of bleeding
- Normalization of hemodynamic status
- Normalization of hematological parameters.

Late Complications of Massive Blood Loss/Massive Transfusions

Late complication of massive blood loss followed by massive fluid or blood replacement therapy can lead to TACO. Massive transfusions may also lead to TRALI, sepsis and thrombosis. Citrate toxicity causing hypocalcemia and also hypomagnesemia due to the large amounts of citrate being infused with blood may also occur. Hyperkalemia is related to the age of the red cells. Every unit of PRBCs adds an acid load of approximately 6 mEq. Acidosis directly reduces activity of both extrinsic and intrinsic coagulation pathways.

■ SUMMARY

The ABCDE of massive transfusions[29] comprises of:
- Assessing the need for massive transfusion and its Activation

- Blood components for correction of dilutional coagulopathy
- Correction of Complications by drugs like rFVIIa, tranexamic acid, etc
- Damage control resuscitation measures—e.g. correction of hypothermia and acidosis
- Employing MTPs help effective management of massive obstetrical bleeding.

Current studies have shown the benefit of early aggressive MTPs using red cell concentrates to FFP to platelet concentrates in a ratio of 1:1:1 to be beneficial in avoiding dilutional and consumptive coagulopathy and thrombocytopenia, together with reduction in morbidity. Every institution needs to evolve its own MTP and also methods of activating and terminating the same together with constitution of MTP team for effective management of massive blood loss.

REFERENCES

1. World Health Organization. Postpartum haemorrhage. [Online] Available from http://www.who.int/medicines/areas/priority_medicines/Ch6_16PPH.pdf [Last accessed July, 2019].
2. World Health Organization. Managing complications in pregnancy and childbirth. Geneva: World Health Organization; 2000.
3. Newsome J, Martin JG, Bercu Z, et al. Postpartum hemorrhage. Tech Vasc Interv Radiol. 2017;20(4):266-73.
4. Makin J, Suarez-Rebling DI, Varma Shivkumar P, et al. Innovative uses of condom uterine balloon tamponade for postpartum hemorrhage in India and Tanzania. Case Rep Obstet Gynecol. 2018;2018:4952048.
5. Butwick AJ, Goodnough LT. Transfusion and coagulation management in major obstetric hemorrhage. Curr Opin Anaesthesiol. 2015;28(3):275-84.
6. Sentilhes L, Daniel V, Darsonval A, et al. Study protocol. TRAAP—tranexamic acid for preventing postpartum hemorrhage after vaginal delivery: a multicenter randomized, double-blind, placebo-controlled trial. BMC Pregnancy Childbirth. 2015;15:135.
7. American College of Obstetricians and Gynecologists. ACOG Practice Bulletin: Clinical Management Guidelines for Obstetrician-Gynecologists Number 76, October 2006: postpartum hemorrhage. Obstet Gynecol. 2006;108:1039-47.
8. Patil V, Shetmahajan M. Massive transfusion and massive transfusion protocol. Indian J Anaesth. 2014;58(5):590-5.
9. Dark PM, Delooz HH, Hillier V, et al. Monitoring the circulatory responses of shocked patients during fluid resuscitation in the emergency department. Intensive Care Med. 2000;26:173-9.
10. Dutton RP. Pathophysiology of traumatic shock. Semin Anesthesia Perioperative Med Pain. 2001;20(1):7-10.
11. Demling R, LaLonde C, Saldinger P, et al. Multiple-organ dysfunction in the surgical patient: pathophysiology, prevention, and treatment. Curr Probl Surg. 1993;30:345-414.
12. Horovitz JH, Carrico CJ, Shires GT. Pulmonary response to major injury. Arch Surg. 1974;108:349-55.
13. Chun K, Zhang J, Biewer J, et al. Microcirculatory failure determines lethal hepatocyte injury in ischemic/reperfused rat livers. Shock. 1994;1:3-9.
14. Nathan HL, El Ayadi A, Hezelgrave NL, et al. Shock index: an effective predictor of outcome in postpartum haemorrhage? BJOG. 2015;122(2):268-75.
15. Cotton BA, Dossett LA, Haut ER, et al. Multicenter validation of a simplified score to predict massive transfusion in trauma. J Trauma. 2010;69 Suppl 1:S33-9.
16. ACS TQIP. Massive transfusion in trauma guidelines. [Online] Available from https://www.facs.org/~/media/files/quality%20programs/trauma/tqip/massive%20transfusion%20in%20trauma%20guildelines.ashx [Last accessed July, 2019].
17. Stainsby D, MacLennan S, Hamilton PJ. Management of massive blood loss: a template guideline. Br J Anaesth. 2000;85(3):487-91.
18. British Committee for Standards in Haematology, Stainsby D, MacLennan S, et al. Guidelines on the management of massive blood loss. Br J Haematol. 2006;135(5):634-41.
19. Matsunaga S, Takai Y, Seki H. Fibrinogen for the management of critical obstetric hemorrhage. J Obstet Gynaecol Res. 2019;45(1):13-21.

20. Hewitt E, Machin J. ABC of transfusion. Massive blood transfusion. BMJ. 1990;300:107-9.
21. Kashuk JL, Moore EE, Johnson JL, et al. Postinjury life-threatening coagulopathy: is 1:1 fresh frozen plasma:packed red blood cells the answer? J Trauma. 2008;65:261-70; discussion 270-1.
22. Riskin DJ, Tsai TC, Riskin L, et al. Massive transfusion protocols: the role of aggressive resuscitation versus product ratio in mortality reduction. J Am Coll Surg. 2009;209:198-205.
23. Snyder CW, Weinberg JA, McGwin G Jr, et al. The relationship of blood product ratio to mortality: survival benefit or survival bias? J Trauma. 2009;66:358-62.
24. Phan HH, Wisner DH. Should we increase the ratio of plasma/platelets to red blood cells in massive transfusion: what is the evidence? Vox Sang. 2010;98(3 Pt 2):395-402.
25. Pham HP, Shaz BH. Update on massive transfusion. Br J Anaesth. 2013;111 Suppl 1:i71-82.
26. Nunez TC, Young PP, Holcomb JB, et al. Creation, implementation, and maturation of a massive transfusion protocol for the exsanguinating trauma patient. J Trauma. 2010;68:1498-505.
27. O'Keeffe T, Refaai M, Tchorz K, et al. A massive transfusion protocol to decrease blood component use and costs. Arch Surg. 2008;143:686-90.
28. Meng ZH, Wolberg AS, Monroe DM 3rd, et al. The effect of temperature and pH on the activity of factor VIIa: implications for the efficacy of high-dose factor VIIa in hypothermic and acidotic patients. J Trauma. 2003;55:886-91.
29. Jackson DL, DeLoughery TG. Postpartum hemorrhage: management of massive transfusion. Obstet Gynecol Surv. 2018;73(7):418-22.

Index

Page numbers followed by *b* refer to box, *f* refer to figure, *fc* refer to flowchart, and *t* refer to table.

A

ABC score 279
Abdominal pregnancy, laparoscopic view of
 secondary 95*f*
Abortion 42, 131
 classification of 97*fc*
 common cause of 131
 complications of unsafe 203
 incomplete 43, 97
 medical methods of 134
 spontaneous 138
 varieties of 97*fc*
Abruptio placenta 33, 40, 44, 65, 143, 162, 169, 260, 266, 268
Absorbable gelatin matrix 220
Absorbent delivery mats 4
Accredited Social Health Activists 5
Actinomycin-D 120
Activated partial thromboplastin time 166, 200, 251, 257, 269, 274, 280
Acute hemolytic transfusion reaction 70
Acute lung injury, transfusion-related 68, 276
Acute respiratory distress syndrome 39, 40, 68
 development of 168
Adenosine 5-diphosphate agonists 253
Adequate fluid resuscitation, signs of 57
Adherent placenta 28
Adjuvant medical therapy 113
Airway mucosa 78
Alcohol 163
 consumption 162
Alopecia 109
Amenorrhea 42
 history of 94
American College of Obstetrics and Gynecology 208, 210
Amniocentesis 163
Amniotic fluid 64
 embolism 65, 249, 265, 266

Anemia 39, 165, 193
 correction of 67
 risk of 9
 severe 40
Anesthesia 37, 156, 187
 general 194
Antepartum arterial balloon occlusion 235
Antepartum hemorrhage 33, 42, 43, 141, 143, 162, 204
Antepartum period 173
Antepartum uterine rupture 174
Antibiotics 104, 228
Anticipation 31
Anti-D prophylaxis 68
Antifibrinolytic
 agent 241
 clinical randomisation of 241
Antimicrobial therapy 104
Aorta clamp 187*f*
Aortic compression 7, 210
Arterial balloon occlusion 235
Arterial blood gas 56, 280
Arterial embolization 159
Artery, internal 214*f*
Aspirin 194
Assisted reproductive technology 90, 114, 143
Atonic postpartum hemorrhage 6*t*, 12, 197, 203, 260
 management of 50
Atonic uterus, management of 135*b*
Atony 99
Audit
 cycle 12
 process, types of 12
Automated external defibrillator 32
Auxiliary nurse midwife 5

B

Backache 165
Bacteroides fragilis 102
Bakri balloon 25, 209*f*

Balloon
    condom catheter 50, 51f
    tamponade 7, 157, 210
Bernard-Soulier syndrome 254
Beta human chorionic gonadotropin 87, 112, 127
Bimanual compression 7, 210
    suture 82f
Bimanual palpation 124
Biochemistry profile 280
Birth
    trauma 65
    weight, low 166
Bladder fistula, formation of 110
Bleeding 219
    anatomic control of 284
    causes of 4
    control of 119
    disorders 133, 138, 194, 225, 226, 249, 251, 256
        inherited 250
        management of 258
    first trimester 163
    history of 143
    intraperitoneal 121, 235f
    life-threatening 121
    posthysterectomy 136
    reduce
        intraoperative 187
        risk of 154
    symptoms 268
    third stage 31
    uncontrolled 90
    warning bout of 182
Blood 3, 64, 200
    bag 69
    bank 280
    collected, measuring 61
    collection vacutainer and tubes 48f
    color of 144
    components 66, 71
        therapy 53f, 67, 200t
        types of 66
    count
        complete 166, 280
        full 6, 65
    culture 227
    grouping 166
    groups switches chart 283, 284f
    loss 45, 54, 60, 61, 98, 201b
        acute 66
        assessment of 60, 63f, 64, 198t
        estimation of 4, 64, 77, 204, 237
        excessive 262
        measurement of 46, 63
        monitoring 4
        objectifying 61
        quantification of 64
        quantify 60
        volume 63
    pressure 6, 18, 76, 165, 197, 201, 203, 230, 279
        raised 165
        systolic 39, 54, 61, 198, 279
    product 52, 69
        transfusions 131
        use of 215
    replacement 271
        strategies 283
    sample bottles 5
    set 5
    transfusion 4, 6, 57, 68, 71, 201, 279, 280
        in management, role of 65, 66
        indications of 66
        purpose of 66
        role of 52
    urea nitrogen 167
    use of 215
    volume 76
        loss 204
        restoration of 271
    warming 69
B-lynch sutures 211f
Body
    mass index 163, 204
    surface area 88
Brass V drape 45f, 62f
British Committee for Standards in Haematology guidelines 280
Broad-spectrum antibiotic coverage 137
Bronchospasm 49
Bucket-handle tears 222

C

Cancer 268
Cannula
    large intravenous 65
    test 99
Carbapenem 104
Carbetocin 48, 239, 241
Carboprost 49
Cardiac disease 40

Cardiac overload, transfusion-associated 276
Cardiology 37
Cardiotocography 163, 165, 169
Cardiovascular system 76
Catheter 5
Cell salvage 215, 280
Cellular hypoxia 75
Central nervous system 267, 278
Central venous
    catheters 47*f*
    pressure 65
Cephalic version, external 162
Cervical
    ectopic pregnancy 90, 108, 123, 125*t*, 128
        classification 125
        diagnosis 124
        differential diagnosis 125
        etiopathogenesis 123
        incidence 123
        management 126
        medical management 126
        risk factors 123
        treatment for 126*fc*
    erosions 153
    injuries 99, 133, 136
    laceration 99, 132, 197
    lesions 225
    polyp 143, 151
    pregnancy 87
        incidence of 123
        management of 90
    preparation 101
    priming 137
    ripening 101
    stenosis 134
    tear 222
        minor 222
    tumor 125
Cervicoisthmic apposition sutures 213*f*
Cervix 123
Cesarean
    delivery 63, 209
        planned repeat 171
    hysterectomy 159
        steps for 159
    scar ectopic pregnancy 95*f*
    scar pregnancy 91, 107, 108, 109*t*
        diagnosis of 108
        number of 91
        treatment modalities for 109*t*
        types of 108
        ultrasound of 108*b*
    section 18, 21, 226, 259
        number of previous 143
        previous lower segment 172
Chemotherapy 121
Childbirth 21
Cho's square sutures 212, 212*f*
Chorioamnionitis 162, 163
Choriocarcinoma 119, 121, 121*f*, 225, 226
    bleeding in 121
Chorionic vessels 151*f*
Circulatory failure, management of 56
Circulatory overload, transfusion-associated 70, 216
Clamp, cut and drop technique 261
Clindamycin 104
Clinical audit 12, 17
    process of 12
Clinical observation tests 268
Clostridium
    perfringens 228
    welchii 102
Clot lysis test 268
Clot retraction test 268
Clotting factor correction 67
Coagulation
    activation 268
    disorders 65, 197
    failure 31
    screen 6
    status, restoration of 271
    study 166
Coagulopathy 99, 200
    early trauma-induced 282
    in pregnancy, pathophysiology of 77
    management of 168
    risk of 6
Cocaine 163
    abuse 162
Colloid 47, 200, 210
Color Doppler 148, 155, 227
Community rehabilitation centers 38
Component therapy, role of 276
Comprehensive emergency obstetric care 205
Compression sutures 157, 209
    hemostatic 199
    use of 158
Computed tomography scan 227, 230
Connective tissue disorders 255

Constrict placental bed vessels 81
Consumptive coagulopathy 166, 267
Continuous electronic fetal heart monitoring 167
Conventional color Doppler 150*f*, 151*f*
Cord
    insertion, marginal 152*f*
    traction, controlled 194
Cornual pregnancy 91, 114
Cornual wedge resection 112
Cornuostomy 91, 112
Corticosteroids, antenatal 176
Cotton swabs 5
Couvelaire uterus 85*f*
Crash kit 46, 49, 50*f*
C-reactive protein 103, 227
Creatinine 167
Cryoprecipitate 58, 66, 200, 272, 281
Crystalloid 75, 200, 210
Cyclophosphamide 120
Cytomegalovirus 69

D

D-dimer 257, 269, 274
    elevation 268
Dead fetus syndrome 266
Decidua, deficiency of 86, 132
Delivery
    assisted 219
    mode of 155
    normal 121
    timing of 176
Demography, clinical governance and audit 1
Dengue hemorrhagic fever 235*f*
Devascularization
    site of 214*f*
    stepwise 212
Diabetes 37, 40
    mellitus 163
        gestational 39, 180
Digital subtraction angiography 230
Dilutional coagulopathy 267
Disseminated intravascular coagulation 7, 157, 208, 228, 230, 249, 256, 260, 265, 266, 268*t*, 269*t*, 274*t*, 279
    diagnosis of 68
    etiological factors of 265
    pathophysiology of 267
    progression of 268*f*
    risk of 105
    systemic manifestations of 267*t*

Disseminated intravascular microthrombosis 265
Dopamine 57
Double-balloon catheter 242
Drugs 22, 194

E

Early pregnancy 107
    bleeding in 42, 44, 119
Eclampsia 40
Ectopic gestation sac 89
Ectopic pregnancy 40, 65, 87, 88*t*, 94*f*, 123
    abdominal 91
    expectant management of 87
    history of 93
    management of 87
    medical management of 87
    nontubal 90
    preventing hemorrhage in 87
    ruptured 43
    surgery, type of 89
    surgical management of 89
    unruptured 43
Elastometry
    extrinsic 270
    intrinsic 270
Electric vacuum aspiration 134
Electronic fetal monitoring 169
Elevated liver enzyme 39, 40, 149, 249, 255, 266
Embolization coil 233*f*
Embryo transfer 107
Emergency
    codes and alerting systems 28*f*
    kits for safety 24
    obstetric care 10
    peripartum hysterectomy 259
        surgical principles of 261
    tray 46
Empty uterine cavity 125*f*
End organ damage 75
Endometrial cavity 227
    normal 227
Endomyometritis 102
Endotoxic shock management 101*b*
Endovascular management 231
Episiotomy 194, 197, 221
Ergometrine 6, 49, 199, 241
Erythrocyte sedimentation rate 227
Escherichia coli 102, 256
Ethylenediaminetetraacetic acid 55
Etoposide 120

F

Factor eight inhibitor bypass activity 251
Fallopian tube 87, 89
    arteriography of 83*f*, 84*f*
    interstitial part of 90
Fatty liver, acute 266
Febrile nonhemolytic transfusion reaction 70
Federation of Obstetric and Gynaecological Societies of India 12, 194
Fertility
    after treatment 128
    after uterine arterial embolization 237
    sparing treatment 90
Fetal
    death 265
        management of 102
    distress 165
    growth restriction 166
    heart rate 182
        abnormal 173
    macrosomia 194
    movements, loss of 165
    status monitoring 167
Fetus
    and placenta 75
    delivery of 175
    normal 44, 119
Fibrin
    degradation product 68, 266, 269, 274
    deposition 267
    sealants 220
Fibrinogen 200, 257, 269, 274
    concentrate 272
    correction of 67
    deficiency, severe 252
    level 269
    thromboelastometry 270
Fibrinolysis 267, 268
Fibrinolytic agents 272
Fibroid 163
    uterus 194
Filling bladder 159
First trimester complications 107
First-line drug 48
Fluids 3, 197
    therapy 47, 200*t*
    transfusion 6
Foley's bulb 262
Foley's catheter 7, 65

Folic acid
    deficiency 162
    supplementation 193
Fresh frozen plasma 6, 53, 58, 66, 167, 200, 252, 271, 274, 279, 281
    transfusion of 68
Fundal rupture, intraoperative findings of 174*f*

G

Gefitinib 90
Gelatin sponge 234
Genital tract 9, 31, 200, 233, 234
Genital tumor 143
Gentamicin 104
Gestational age 181
Gestational sac 87
    implantation of 91
Gestational trophoblastic
    disease 119
        bleeding in 119
        neoplasia 119
Glanzmann thrombasthenia 253
Glomerular filtration rate 278
Glycoprotein, deficiency of 253
Golden hour 193
    concept and first response 193
Grand multiparity 162, 194
Gravimetric method 62
Great arteries 4
Growth assessment protocol 25

H

Hayman's sutures 210, 211*f*
Heart
    disease 37, 39
    rate 279
        stabilizing 9
Heat stable oxytocin 239
Heavy bleeding, control 121*f*
HELLP syndrome 40, 65
Hematocrit 166
Hematological parameters, normalization of 284
Hematological system 76, 76*f*
Hematomas 218
    incidental 115
    infralevator 222
    intra-amniotic 166
    management of 222

marginal 166
size of 115
Hematometra 100
Hematuria 173
Hemodynamic status, normalization of 284
Hemoglobin 17, 31, 39, 105, 200, 203, 227, 235f
Hemogram, complete 55
Hemolysis 39, 40, 149, 249, 255, 266
Hemolytic uremic syndrome 255, 256
Hemoperitoneum 93f
laparoscopy in presence of 89
Hemophilia
A 226, 250, 251
acquired 251
B 226, 250, 251
Hemorrhage 19, 55, 99, 102, 131, 203
abortion-related 134
abortion, management of 99
acute 144
after abortion 100t
amount of 143
causes of 99
class 204
classification of 61t
early 144
estimation of 134
high risks of 108
in early pregnancy 73
intracranial 58
nature of 143
prophylaxis 92
resolving 144
risk group 100
risk of 90
sepsis, and pregnancy 35
specific issues of 98
uncontrolled 57, 91
Hemorrhagic emergencies 4
Hemostasis 128
disorders of 249
monitoring 52
Hemostat drugs, administration of 207t
Hemostatic status 256
Heparin 194
Hepatic function 88
Hepatitis
B 68
C 68
Heterogeneous signal intensity within placenta 148

Heterotopic pregnancy 87, 92, 111
treatment of 92
High dependency unit 18, 21, 37, 39-41, 206, 220
care 39t
management of 39
Homeostasis, principles of 265
Hospital emergency alerting systems 27
Hospital-acquired infection 26
Human chorionic gonadotropin 88, 126-128
production of 119
Human immunodeficiency virus 6, 68
infection 255
Hydatidiform mole, evacuation of 119
Hyperhomocysteinemia 162
Hypertension 19, 143, 266
chronic 162
gestational 163
pregnancy induced 65
severe 39
Hypertensive disorders 17, 40, 41, 203, 254
Hypoperfusion, acute 75
Hypotension 165
Hypothermia 159
Hypovolemia 159, 266, 276
Hypoxia 67
Hysterectomy 8, 109, 121f, 159, 175, 213, 216, 228
choice of 262
specimen of subtotal 120f
steps of 188
Hysteroscopic
excision 109
guidance 110
resection 90, 92, 95f
Hysterotomy, high vertical 172

I

Idiopathic thrombocytopenic purpura 254
Iliac artery
common 214f
external 214f
internal 81, 214f
right internal 84
Immune thrombocytopenia 255
In vitro fertilization 107, 263
program 123
Incision, site of 156
Infection
control systems 26
transfusion-related 70

Infusion syringe pump 48*f*
Initial fluid replacement 54
Intensive care unit 18, 31, 36, 37, 75, 186, 206, 279
International Federation of Obstetrics and Gynaecology 184
International normalized ratio 53, 166
International Society on Thrombosis and Hemostasis 269
Interstitial pregnancy 90, 111, 112, 113*t*
    management of 112*fc*
    treatment of 111
Interventional radiology 237
    advantages of 237
    selective arterial embolization 223
    techniques 157, 230
Intracervical canal 125*f*
Intraoperative cell salvage 70
Intrapartum period 173
Intrauterine
    balloon tamponade 158
        use of 158
    contraceptive device 123
    fetal death 169
    growth restriction 165
    insemination 93
    manipulator 90
    pregnancy 93
    tamponade 242
        principles of 242
Intravenous infusion 4
Invasive mole 120*f*
    bleeding in 120
    Doppler appearance of 120*f*
Iron 193

J

Janani Shishu Suraksha Karyakram 10
Janani Suraksha Yojana 10
Jehova's witness 215
Jugular vein distention 70

K

Kerala Federation of Obstetrics and Gynaecology 185
Kerr's incision 210
Kidney injury, acute 40
Klebsiella 102

L

Labor
    active management of third stage of 194, 260
    after cesarean delivery, trial of 171, 263
    and delivery complex 22*f*
    delivery and recovery 24
        number of 22
    management of third stage of 31
    obstructed 172
    preterm 165
    prolonged third stage of 194
    unsupervised 172
    ward 26, 195
        complex, reception for 23
        preparedness 195
        safety in 21
        trolley parking area 23
        working station for 23
Laparotomy 174, 175, 175*f*
Left internal iliac artery 83
Left ovarian ectopic pregnancy, laparoscopic view of 94*f*
Left uterine artery 83, 84
    angiography 234*f*
Lethal anomaly, without 44
Ligament artery, round 83
Liver 267
    disorders 40
    failure 235*f*
    function test 55
Living ligatures 80*f*
Local embryocidal agents 110
Low molecular weight heparin 262
Low platelet
    count 39, 40
    syndrome 149, 249, 255, 266
Lower genital tract
    hemorrhage 219
    trauma 223
Lower left vaginal artery 83, 84
Lower segment cesarean section incision 75, 261
Lower uterine segment 173, 261
Lung 267
    injury, transfusion-associated 216

M

Massive blood loss 67, 277, 277*b*, 281*b*
    causes of 276*b*
    indicators of 279

late complication of 284
management of 278, 280
Massive hemorrhage 90, 112, 182
management of 200
Massive transfusion 53, 58, 279, 282-284
therapy indication in 58*t*
Massive transfusion protocol 52, 207, 215, 276, 279, 281
activation of 279
benefits of 283
drawbacks of 283
rationale for 281
role of 281
termination of 284
Maternal anatomy 79
Maternal cardiovascular changes 77*f*
Maternal coagulopathy 162
Maternal complications 35, 91
Maternal death 17, 35, 36
causes of 33
surveillance and response 19
Maternal health 19
services 40
Maternal morbidity 60, 65, 175
severe acute 14, 18, 259
Maternal mortality 35, 65, 175
causes of 12, 87
rates 35
ratio 3, 12
Maternal near miss 18
Maternal pulse 165
Maternal respiratory changes 78*f*
Maternal resuscitation 34
Maternal safety pyramid 36*f*
Maternal vital signs stable 181
M-cross double ligation 159
Mean arterial pressure 61, 198
Medical abortion 98, 105
Medical management 4, 51
Medical Termination of Pregnancy 97, 131
Membrane, preterm premature rupture of 163, 180
Mental status 54
Metabolic acidosis 56
Metabolic alkalosis 56
Methergine 5
Methotrexate 87, 88, 88*t*, 112, 120, 126-128
administration 90, 92
doses of 109
therapy 127*t*

toxicity 89
treatment protocol 127*t*
Methylergometrine 5, 6, 49, 5, 207, 228
maleate 100
Metronidazole 104
Microangiopathic hemolytic anemia 255
Midwifery team safety principle 29
Minute ventilation 78
Miscarriage 42, 97
complete 43
inevitable 43
risk of spontaneous 115
threatened 43
Misoprostol 5, 49, 100, 135, 199, 207, 228, 241
prostaglandin 6
Mitochondrial deoxyribonucleic acid 164
Modified early obstetric warning 59*f*
score 46*t*, 59
system 219
Molar pregnancy 43
Monsel's solution 158
Morbidly adherent placenta 184, 189
Mortality compared 3
Moth-eaten hypoechoic areas 149
Mucositis, development of 88
Müllerian anomaly 114
Multidisciplinary teams 21
Multifetal gestation 143
Multiple gestation 163
Multiple organ system failure 278
Multiple placental infarctions 151*f*
Multiple pregnancy 194
Muscle cells 80
Myelosuppression, development of 88
Myometrial margin, loss of 149*f*
Myometrial nodules, highly vascular 120*f*
Myometrium 80

N

Nausea 109
Nausicaa compression suture 8
Near miss audit 18
Neonatal resuscitation bay 23
Nephrology 37
Nestor embolization coil 234*f*
Neurology 37
Nomenclature 184
Noninflatable antishock garment 51*f*

Noninvasive blood pressure 40
	monitoring 48*f*
Nonpneumatic antishock garment 7, 199, 210, 216, 216*f*, 220
Nonstress test 168
Nonvertex presentation 163
Nuchal translucency 180
Nucleic acid testing 282
Nulliparous 90

O

O'leary sutures 8
Obesity 40
Obstetric anal sphincter repair 28
Obstetric care
	complete 37
	complexities of 21
Obstetric complications 37, 39
Obstetric handover board 26
Obstetric hemorrhage 13, 39, 42, 75, 79, 132, 265, 267
	causes of 276*b*
	clinical audit in 13, 15*t*
	maintenance of 4
	major 58, 65
	management of 42, 65
	massive 65
	operating procedure for 31
	prevention 42
Obstetric
	high-dependency unit 35, 37, 38
	hysterectomy 40, 235*f*
	intensive care unit 37
	management 33, 168
	shock index 4
	surgery, role of 67
Obstetrical bleeding, major 276
Obstetrical hemorrhage 276
O-Leary stitch 158
Oligemic shock, management of 75
Operation theater 21
	shifting 208
Operative delivery 194
Operative trauma 65
Organ
	dysfunction 39
	response 278
Ovarian artery 81
	right 83

Ovarian ligament 159
Ovarian pregnancy 87, 91
Ovarian reconstruction 94
Ovary, arteriography of 83*f*, 84*f*
Oxygen saturation 6
Oxytocics 3
Oxytocin 5, 6, 48, 49, 98, 100, 199, 207, 228, 241
	administration of 157
	analog 48
	inadvertent use of 172

P

Pain 165
	abdominal 107, 173
	causes of 165
Palacios-Jaraquemada 81
Pallor 165
Partial thromboplastin time 68
Patient's urine 64
Pelvic
	artery embolization, selective 228
	hematomas 218
	pressure pack 244
	rest 116
	vasculature 75
Penetrating injury 279
Periclitoral lacerations 221
Perinatal morbidity 176
Perinatal mortality 176
Perineal lacerations 194
Perineal tear repair 220
Peripartum hysterectomy 259, 262
	bit of history of 260
	elective emergency 262
Peripheral blood smear, Romanowsky stained 254
Peripheral villous trees 152*f*
Peritrophoblastic blood flow 125*f*
Periurethral lacerations 221
Photometric technique 61
Photometry 61
Piperacillin 104
Placenta 32, 63, 116
	accreta 65, 85, 116, 147, 148, 155, 159, 185, 194, 243
	evaluation of 104
	rule out 181
	spectrum 184
	types of 85*f*

circumvallate 44, 163
increta 147, 235*f*
location of 154
low lying 147, 147*f*
percreta 147
position of 159
previa 33, 40, 44, 65, 79, 84, 85*f*, 116, 125, 143, 145, 146, 148*f*, 154, 156, 157, 182, 260
    asymptomatic 180, 181
    complete 146
    expectant management of 180
    magnetic resonance imaging for 148
    marginal 146
    partial 146
    spectrum 267
    symptomatic 181
    true 147, 147*f*
thickened heterogeneous 149*f*
Placental abnormality 234
Placental abruption 144, 162*t*, 249
    location of 144
    types of 145*f*
    ultrasound diagnosis of 144
Placental adherence 86
Placental cord insertion 152*f*
Placental infarction 150
Placental migration 147
Placental myometrial interface, normal 149*f*
Placental polyp 225
Placental site trophoblastic tumor 119
Placental tissue 197, 199
Placentation, abnormal 84, 107, 117, 132, 136
Plasma protein 66
    A, pregnancy associated 164
Plasminogen activator inhibitor type 2 249
Plaster to fix cannula 5
Plastic bag, ordinary 4
Platelet 58, 67, 71, 200, 274
    abnormalities of 253
    concentrate 66
    count 200, 257, 269, 274
    deficits 67
    disorders, acquired 254
    function, inherited disorders of 253
    rich concentrate 67
    rich plasma 67
    transfusion 272, 281
Pneumonia 109
Point-of-care testing 270, 283
Polyglycolic acid 157

Polyhydramnios 143, 194
    sudden decompression in 162
Polyvinyl alcohol 233
Poor health infrastructure 3
Postabortion
    hemorrhage 131
        causes of 132
        management for 134, 134*t*
    syndrome 133
    treatment of hemorrhage in 101*t*
    triad 133
Postnatal care 168
Postpartum hemorrhage 3, 12, 18, 24, 26*f*, 31, 40, 42, 50, 155, 157, 193-195, 201, 203, 210, 218, 231, 231*t*, 239, 259, 276
    antenatal risk factors for 204*t*
    anticipate 46
    audit of 14
    box 5*t*
    causes of 3
    diagnosis of 45
    drills 4
    endovascular management of 230
    identification of 218
    intrapartum risk factors for 205*t*
    management of 4, 24, 64, 156, 195, 196, 208, 239
    massive 6
    morbidity, prevent 46
    mortality, prevent 46
    pharmacological management of 199*t*
    prevention of 219
    previous 194
    risk factors for 194*t*
        secondary 226*t*
    risk of 3
    secondary 9, 52, 225, 235, 236*f*
    standards for 18*t*
    stepwise management of 195
    structured audit in 13
Postpartum intrauterine contraceptive device 24
Postpartum maternal complications 169
Postpartum period 174
Postvaginal delivery 206
Potassium chloride 110, 112, 126
    injection of 91
Practical skills 4
Preconceptional health and care 42
Pre-eclampsia 115, 163, 165, 194, 255, 266
Pregnancy 35, 37 38, 40, 75, 249
    abdominal 87, 91

angular 113, 113*t*, 114
complications, management of 79
hemostatic changes in normal 249
medical termination of 98
physiology in 75
preterm 44
second trimester termination of 101
specific disseminated intravascular coagulation scoring system 270*t*
Pregnant women 78
Premature ovarian aging 110
Primary hemostasis 81
Primigravida 44
Progesterone therapy 116
Prostaglandin 5, 98
    F2 alpha 228
Prothrombin complex 65
    concentrates 273
Prothrombin deficiency 253
Prothrombin time 166, 200, 207, 256, 257, 269, 274, 280
Pseudomonas 102
Pulmonary edema 216
Pulmonology 37
Pulse 61
    oximetry 280
    pressure 54
    rate 54, 197, 201
        monitoring 6

Q

Quick in quick out
   policy 261
   technique 263

R

Radiation exposure 237
Random donor platelets 281
Randomized controlled trial 240, 273
Red blood cell 17, 61, 66, 186, 271, 282
    packed 53
    radioactive tagging of 61
Red cell
    concentrates 280
    transfusions 67
Referral transportation 8
Regular hospital care 37
Renal curve 233

Renal failure 166
    acute 39
Renal function 88
    tests 167
Reproductive function 121
Respiratory
    acidosis 56
    alkalosis 56
    center 78
    physiology 78
    rate 54, 197, 201
Resuscitation 227
Resuscitative hysterotomy 79
Retained placenta 65, 194, 199
Retained placental tissue 225
    ultrasound examination for 227
Retained tissue 52, 99, 132, 137
Retroplacental collection 166
Rh-negative platelets 68
Ringer lactate 5
Robertson uterine artery 233
Rotational thromboelastometry 270
Royal College of Obstetricians and Gynaecologists 156, 203, 210, 221
Rubin's criteria 124
Rudimentary horn pregnancy, right 94
Rupture uterus 40
    diagnosis of 174

S

Safe labor ward 29
Safety
    maternity dashboard for 27
    signage for 26
    staffing for 25
    training for 25
Salpingectomy 89, 90
Salpingostomy 89
    incision 94*f*
Sampson's artery 261
Scar
    previous 99
    tenderness 173
Scarred uterus, rupture of 171
Scissors, pair of 5
Secretory disorders 254
Sepsis 40, 194, 260, 266, 268
    causes of 102
Septic abortion 97, 102

clinical features 102
complications 103
investigations 103
management 103
mode of infection 102
pathology 102
phases of 103f
prevention 103
Serum
　beta-human chorionic gonadotropin 227
　electrolytes 103
　fibrinogen 167
　vacutainers, plain sample for 55f
Shift handovers serve 26
Shock 165, 278, 278t
　acute 278
　clinical 201b
　compensated 278
　decompensated 278
　hemorrhagic 54, 54t, 75
　hypovolemic 54
　index 42, 279, 279t
　management of 55
　stages of 46t, 277, 278t
　subacute 278
　types of 277b
Short umbilical cord 163
Shoulder dystocia 28
Single donor platelets 281
Skilled birth attendant 38
Skin 267
Sliding off technique 261
Sliding sign 108
Special hemostatic measures 113
Specialized care units, types of 37
Speculums, large 5
Spontaneous circulation, return of 79
Staff lounge 23
Standard operating procedure 31, 32
Staphylococcus 102
　aureus 102
Sterile gloves 5
Sterile trays 22
Stomatitis 109
Subchorionic abruption, ultrasonic image of 144f
Subchorionic hematoma 115, 116, 166
Suburethral nodule 121, 121f
Suction apparatus, blood collected in 63f
Suction tamponade device 243
Sudden severe sharp pain 165

Supralevator hematoma 214, 223
Surgery, laparoscopic 111
Surgical challenges 154
Surgical compression suture 82f
Surgical intervention 280
Syntometrine 49
Systemic methotrexate 109

T

T2 dark intraplacental bands 148
Tachycardia 165, 279
Tamponade 208, 243f
Tazobactam 104
Tears, management of 220
Tenderness over uterus, mild 165
Testing, time of 56
Therapeutic management 114
Thrombin 3, 197
　time 280
Thrombocytopenia 255
　destructive 255
　gestational 254, 258
Thromboelastogram 257, 270
Thromboelastograph 52f
　signature waveform 52f
Thromboelastography 270, 283
Thromboelastometry studies 270
Thromboembolism 242
Thrombophilia 163
Thrombosis, factors affecting 78f
Thrombotic microangiopathies 255
Thrombotic thrombocytopenic purpura 255
Tissue 3, 75, 197
　hypoxia 159
　perfusion 61, 198
Tone 3
Tools, standardization of 14
Total blood volume 277
Total hysterectomy 215
Tranexamic acid 157, 207, 228, 241
　role of 6, 228
Transabdominal excision 92
Transabdominal ultrasonography 181
Transcatheter arterial embolization 237
Transfusion
　complications 70
　reactions
　　acute 70
　　chronic 70
　　common 70

Transvaginal route 110
Transvaginal sonography 147, 154, 181
Transvaginal ultrasound 126
Trauma 3, 143, 150, 162, 163, 197, 233
    history of 143
Traumatic cervical injuries 98
Traumatic postpartum hemorrhage 9, 218
    causes of 218
    management of 220
Traumatic shock 277
    pathophysiology of 277
Treponema pallidum 69
Trigger, removal of 271
Triple P procedure 243
Trisodium citrate 56
Trophoblastic hyperplasia 119
Tubal ectopic pregnancy 87, 111
    ruptured right 93*f*
    unruptured right 94*f*
Tubal rupture 87
    risk of 88
Tubes and ovary, blood supply of 83*f*
Twin
    pregnancy 119
    with hydatidiform mole 119
Tying uterine vessels 158
Typical diseases 268

U

Ultrasonography 143, 151, 166, 173
    high-resolution 262
Ultrasound imaging 180
Uninterrupted power supply 23
Unscarred uterus, rupture of 171, 172
Upper vaginal segment, arteriography of 83*f*, 84*f*
Urea 6
Urinary tract 175
Urine
    output 54
    pregnancy test 93, 94
    routine 167
Urobag 5
Uterine 83
    arterial embolization 230, 237
        technique of 233
    arteriovenous malformation 226, 235
    atony 65, 80, 132, 135, 233
    body 84
    bulging 148
    cavity 94, 120
    contour, abnormal 173
    contraction 81*f*
    curettage 226
    embolization procedure 84*f*
    evacuation 228
    infection 225
    injury 101
    lesions 225
    massage 7
    muscle, circular 80*f*
    packing 5, 7, 210
    pathology 225
    perforation 133, 137
    position 133
    rudimentary horn, right 94*f*
    scar rupture, repair of previous 175*f*
    segments 83*f*
    septum 163
    sound 137
    surgery 226
    tetany 165
Uterine artery 214*f*, 232
    angiogram 234*f*
    branches of 234*f*, 235*f*
    embolization 101, 105, 109, 110, 126, 136, 209, 210
    ligation, bilateral 8
    right 83, 84
Uterine myometrium 90
    defective 92
Uterine rupture 65, 171, 175, 177, 260
    clinical presentation of 173
    complete 171
    incomplete 171
    prediction of 172
    prevention of 176
    previous 172
Uterine tamponade 50, 228
    internal 242
Uterotonic drugs 4, 100, 228
    administration of 207*t*
    storage of 6
Uterotonics 4
Uterus 44
    anteroinferior wall of 236*f*
    arteriography of 83*f*, 84*f*
    blood supply of 83*f*
    complete rupture of 171*f*
    conserving 243

contraction of 165
hour glass appearance of 124f
inversion of 199
perforation of 120, 120f, 121
puerperal inversion of 225
rupture of 143, 171, 197
woody 165

V

Vacuum aspiration, manual 98, 134
Vagina 84
   blood supply of 83f
Vaginal artery
   middle
      left 83
      right 83
   upper left 84
Vaginal births 63
Vaginal bleeding 109, 173
   mild 165
   severe 235f
Vaginal delivery 31, 168, 240
Vaginal lacerations 197
Vaginal metastasis 121
Vaginal packing 221
Vaginal tear
   repair 221
   superficial 221
Vasa previa 143, 151, 152f

Vascular coagulation 110
Vascular ligation 8
Vasopressin 57, 272
Vasopressors 58
Velamentous cord 152f
Ventouse-related lacerations 222
Vincristine 120
Visual assessment 61, 64
Vital parameters monitored 138
Volume replacement 67
von Willebrand's disease 226, 250
von Willebrand's factor 250
Vulvovaginal infections 143

W

Wash area 23
Waste management 21
Wedge resection 91
Whole blood 66
   transfusion 52
Workflow design for labor, delivery and recovery 22f
World Health Organization 193, 210, 239
World Maternal Antifibrinolytic Trial 241

Y

Young-laplace equation 81f

Milton Keynes UK
Ingram Content Group UK Ltd.
UKHW050925020824
446396UK00003B/18